RECENT ADVANCES
IN PÆDIATRICS

Recent Advances in Pædiatrics

EDITED BY

DOUGLAS GAIRDNER

M.A. (Cantab.), D.M. (Oxon.), F.R.C.P.

*Pædiatrician to Addenbrooke's Hospital, Cambridge,
and the Cambridge Maternity Hospital; Associate
Lecturer in Pædiatrics, University of Cambridge*

THIRD EDITION

With 86 Illustrations

LITTLE, BROWN AND COMPANY

BOSTON

1965

First Edition .   .   . 1954
Translated into Spanish 1957
Second Edition   .   . 1958
Third Edition   .   . 1965

Printed in Great Britain at the Pitman Press, Bath

Published in London by J. & A. Churchill Ltd. 104 Gloucester Place, W.1

CONTRIBUTORS

A. G. BAIKIE, M.B., F.R.C.P.E., M.C.Path.

First Assistant, University of Melbourne Department of Medicine, St. Vincent's Hospital, Melbourne, Australia.

J. A. BLACK, M.D., M.R.C.P.

Pædiatrician, Children's Hospital, Sheffield; Late Senior Lecturer in Child Health, Institute of Child Health, The Hospital for Sick Children, London.

MARTIN BODIAN, M.D., M.R.C.P.

Pathologist, The Hospital for Sick Children, Great Ormond Street, London.

OLOV CELANDER, M.D.

Associate Professor of Pediatrics, University of Göteborg, Sweden.

G. S. DAWES, D.M., B.SC.

Director of the Nuffield Institute for Medical Research, University of Oxford.

R. F. A. DEAN, F.R.C.P.

Director of the Medical Research Council Infantile Malnutrition Unit, Mulago Hospital, Kampala, Uganda.

CECIL MARY DRILLIEN, M.D., D.C.H.

Lecturer, Department of Child Life and Health, University of Edinburgh.

JAMES W. FARQUHAR, M.D., F.R.C.P.E.

Reader in Child Life and Health, University of Edinburgh; Associate Consultant Pædiatrician, Royal Edinburgh Hospital for Sick Children and the Simpson Memorial Maternity Pavilion, Royal Infirmary of Edinburgh.

DOUGLAS GAIRDNER, D.M., F.R.C.P.

Pædiatrician, Addenbrooke's Hospital, Cambridge, and the Cambridge Maternity Hospital; Associate Lecturer in Pædiatrics, University of Cambridge.

DOUGLAS HUBBLE, M.D., F.R.C.P.

Professor of Pædiatrics and Child Health, University of Birmingham; Director of the Institute of Child Health; Pædiatrician, United Birmingham Hospitals.

PETTER KARLBERG, M.D.

Professor of Pediatrics, University of Göteborg, Sweden.

G. H. MACNAB, M.B., F.R.C.S.

Surgeon, Westminster Hospital and The Hospital for Sick Children, Great Ormond Street, London.

GERALD NELIGAN, D.M., M.R.C.P.

Senior Lecturer in Child Health, University of Newcastle upon Tyne.

A. P. NORMAN, M.D., F.R.C.P., D.C.H.

Deputy Director, Institute of Child Health, University of London; Physician, The Hospital for Sick Children, Great Ormond Street, London; Pædiatrician, Queen Charlotte's Maternity Hospital, London.

B. G. OCKENDEN, M.B.

Assistant Morbid Anatomist, The Hospital for Sick Children, Great Ormond Street, London.

R. H. R. WHITE, M.B., M.R.C.P., D.C.H.

Assistant to the Director, Department of Pædiatrics, Guy's Hospital, London.

O. H. WOLFF, M.D., F.R.C.P., D.C.H.

Reader in Pædiatrics and Child Health, University of Birmingham.

PREFACE

This third edition of *Recent Advances in Pædiatrics* follows much the same lines as its two predecessors. Two chapters, those on Hydrocephalus and Spina Bifida Cystica, bear the same titles as in the last edition, but their content, like that of all the remaining chapters, is fresh.

The subjects chosen are those which have developed interestingly in recent years and have reached a stage where to pause and take stock seems profitable. The scope of the different chapters varies widely, from, for instance, D. V. Hubble's analysis of the large subject of growth and its disorders, to J. W. Farquhar's monograph on the more circumscribed subject of diabetic pregnancy and its outcome. The two chapters on fœtal and neonatal physiology by G. S. Dawes and by P. Karlberg and O. Celander display the mutually stimulating effects that the experimental physiologist and the pædiatrician caring for the newborn baby continue to exert upon one another's ideas. Common to all the contributions is the fact that their authors have been actively engaged in the study of the subject they deal with; as a result much hitherto unpublished work will be found incorporated in the book, while two chapters, Aspects of Cancer by the late M. Bodian and Renal Biopsy by J. A. Black and R. H. R. White, are based entirely on their authors' original observations.

An important function of a book of this kind is to provide a guide to further reading, and over 1200 references are quoted.

My first debt of gratitude must be paid to the sixteen contributors on both sides of the North Sea and in the Antipodes, who (to repeat what I wrote in the last edition) have suffered with good-humoured resignation the cajolings, criticisms and textual excisions received at the hands of an editor, himself often sorely pressed by exigencies of time and space.

Almost equally responsible for the present volume are the contributors to its two predecessors—four of the present authors have thus earned a double measure of my thanks—because the standard already set by them made my task in assembling a new team a gratifyingly easy one.

My ability to undertake this book has again depended upon my continued good fortune in having in Dr Janet Roscoe a colleague always ready to shoulder more than her share of our joint responsibilities, while my family have maintained an attitude of kindly tolerance to my inevitable domestic deficiencies during the past year.

Lastly, Mr J. A. Rivers of J. & A. Churchill, Ltd. has once again smoothed my way unfailingly.

CAMBRIDGE   D. M. T. G.

CONTENTS

CHAPTER 1

THE CIRCULATION, RESPIRATION AND GENERAL METABOLISM OF THE NEWBORN

G. S. DAWES

ALTHOUGH the alterations which occur in the circulation at birth are now given a brief description in most textbooks of physiology, there is almost no other recognition of the fact that the fœtus and the newborn mammal have special physiological problems. A previous essay in the last edition of this book was written primarily to describe what was known of the cardiovascular changes at birth (Dawes 1958). The apparently mechanical nature of these changes had suggested that they were completed wholly and abruptly within a short period of time. We know now that this is not so, the transition from fœtal to extrauterine life is indeed abrupt but various adjustments continue to take place over a period which may last several weeks. Thus there is a condition of the circulation, transitional between that of the fœtus and that of the adult, which is only to be found in the immediate newborn period and whose characteristics deserve especial consideration.

The purpose of the present chapter is firstly to bring up to date the description of the circulatory changes at birth, and secondly to demonstrate that over a wide field of general physiology, comprising respiration and the response to asphyxia, temperature regulation and carbohydrate and fat metabolism, the physiological behaviour of the newborn differs in a variety of ways from that of the adult.

The Fœtal Circulation

The course of the fœtal circulation has been the subject of intermittent controversy for many centuries. The period of direct experiment started in 1927 when Huggett showed that it was possible to deliver a fœtal goat and maintain it in good physiological condition, while still attached to the mother by an intact umbilical cord. Within the next 15 years the main anatomical problems of the fœtal circulation were solved by the use of cinéangiography (Barclay, Franklin and Prichard 1943, Barcroft 1947) and subsequent measurements with other methods have confirmed the general conclusions arrived at. The next phase of the problem has been to try and understand the physiological mechanisms which regulate the circulation in the fœtus.

The umbilical circulation and placental development. In the fœtus the two sides of the heart work in parallel to pump blood from the great veins to the pulmonary trunk and the aorta, which are linked by the ductus arteriosus (Fig. 1). The P_{O_2} and P_{CO_2} of the arterial blood supplying the fœtal tissues must in part depend on the volume of fœtal blood flowing through the placenta relative to that flowing through the fœtal tissues, since both streams mix in the great veins and the heart. What, then, determines the volume of umbilical blood flow, through the fœtal side of the placenta?

Simultaneous measurements of the pressures at different points in the umbilical circulation of fœtal lambs have shown that more than two-thirds of the pressure drop occurs between the cotyledonary arteries and veins of the placenta (Dawes 1962a). Hence most of the resistance to blood flow through the whole umbilical circulation (from the end of the aorta to the entry of the hepatic veins into the inferior vena cava) occurs across the fœtal villi, *within the placenta itself*. During moderate hypoxæmia there is no change in the resistance offered to blood flow; during acute severe hypoxæmia there is a small increase. Hence this is a relatively passive part of the circulation. The changes in it during growth and development are

GREAT VEINS

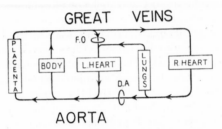

AORTA

Fig. 1. Simplified diagram of the fœtal circulation, to show that the right and left sides of the heart work in parallel to pump blood from the great veins to the aorta, by way of the foramen ovale (F.O.) and ductus arteriosus (D.A.).

nevertheless of considerable interest. In the sheep the fœtus increases in weight from about 500 g. at 90 days to 3–5 kg. at term (147 days). The placenta reaches its maximum weight at 90–100 days; the resistance to umbilical blood flow offered by the placenta *decreases* between 90 and 115 days gestation, *but not thereafter*. Consequently, in order to maintain an adequate umbilical blood flow commensurate with fœtal growth, the arterial pressure of the fœtus has to rise rapidly during the last few weeks of gestation. In fœtal lambs with exceptionally small placentas the blood pressure was unusually high. The larger fœtuses did not necessarily have larger placentas or ones with a lower resistance to blood flow, and hence the larger the fœtus the higher was its arterial pressure.

No similar measurements have been undertaken on other species, but if the same principles apply to man one would expect that in larger fœtuses or in ones with infarcted placentas, the arterial pressure would be greater. The idea that the infant has to adapt itself to the placenta with which it is endowed is an old one, and is supported by these quantitative measurements. It is an hypothesis which evidently bears further examination.

The O_2 environment of the fœtus. The partial pressure of O_2 in the arterial blood of the fœtus is only 20–25 mm. Hg, compared with about 90 mm. Hg in the adult. It has repeatedly been stated, or implied, that the lower the O_2-tension of umbilical arterial blood on delivery the worse is the condition of the baby and often it is suggested that it has been worse over a hypothetical period of time previously. If there is little or no O_2 in the umbilical arterial blood the infant is evidently in bad case, but what are we to think if the O_2-tension is 15 or 10 or 8 mm. Hg? Where is the dividing line between what is tolerable for fœtal survival and what is fatal? No simple answer can be given to this question because it depends, in part, on the volume of umbilical blood flow. With better methods for measuring umbilical flow it is evident that it is often much greater than was formerly thought. In some immature fœtal lambs it has exceeded 300 ml./kg.min. A reduction in umbilical blood flow below 100 ml./kg.min causes a fall in fœtal O_2-consumption, but in some mature fœtal lambs this fall in O_2-consumption is actually *accompanied by a rise* in umbilical arterial O_2-saturation (Dawes and Mott 1964). Moreover analysis of simultaneous blood samples have shown that there are often large differences between the O_2-contents of carotid and umbilical arterial blood, particularly when umbilical blood flow is reduced and conditions are unsteady, as they are likely to be on delivery.

The conclusion to be drawn from these observations is that the O_2-saturation or -tension of human umbilical arterial blood on delivery is likely to be an untrustworthy index of the physiological condition of the baby. The pH or P_{CO_2} gives a better quantitative measure of acute asphyxia at birth (see p. 17). There is as yet no adequate functional measure of "placental insufficiency."

Breathing

The onset of breathing. *In utero* the normal fœtus is believed to make respiratory movements from time to time (Windle 1940, Barcroft 1946) but during the last half of gestation these movements are uncommon even though the arterial P_{O_2} is low and the P_{CO_2} about 40 mm. Hg. A fœtal lamb can be delivered by cæsarean section from its mother under local or spinal anæsthesia and, if it is kept warm with the umbilical cord intact, can be handled extensively without inducing either arousal or respiratory movements. Only when the umbilical cord is tied does gasping start, and then only after an interval of half a minute or more during which the arterial P_{O_2} has fallen and the P_{CO_2} has risen considerably. There is little doubt that these changes stimulate the systemic arterial chemoreceptors and the brain and hence initiate the first respiratory efforts. What is puzzling is that half an hour later a newborn lamb or monkey is breathing gently and rhythmically, quite adequately to maintain an arterial P_{O_2} of up to 75 mm. Hg and a P_{CO_2} of 35–45 mm. Hg. It is evident that although asphyxia at birth can explain the expansion of the lungs by gasping, the changes in arterial and alveolar gas tensions alone cannot explain the maintenance of breathing. Something else must happen as well.

After birth the lungs are expanded, there are changes in the circulation and a rise in arterial P_{O_2}. There are also alterations in the external environment (such as cold) and a greater sense of weight on delivery from within the warm amniotic fluid. The fact that a fœtal lamb can be handled after delivery without starting breathing suggests that neither tactile nor gravitational stimuli are of the first importance. But if fœtal lambs (with an intact umbilical cord and a saline filled reservoir attached to a tracheal cannula) are cooled, even under general anæsthesia, so that their rectal temperature falls below 37°C, rhythmic respiratory movements usually begin (Dawes and

Mott, unpublished). Application of ice or ice-cold water to the face is often effective in starting these regular rhythmic efforts, which cause intrapleural pressure changes of only 10–20 mm. Hg, very different from the large pressure changes caused by gasping. When the cold stimulus is removed the lamb stops making respiratory movements, so the cold stimulus was necessary both for their initiation and their continuation. Further work is needed to establish what other factors may be involved. The explanations usually given for the onset of breathing at birth may be quite adequate, but almost no attention has been given to the question of why the baby goes on breathing. More work is clearly necessary.

Respiratory reflexes. The evidence that the systemic arterial chemoreceptors are functional at birth is good. Even in the rabbit, which is very immature at birth, injection of cyanide causes an increase in the rate and depth of breathing (Lim and Snyder 1945) which is abolished by denervation of the carotid bifurcations (Dawes and Mott 1959a). Further experiments on newborn rabbits also showed that it was possible to reproduce the phenomenon reported by Cross and Oppé (1952) in the human baby. Administration of 15% O_2 caused a temporary increase in the minute volume of breathing, which increase disappeared after a few minutes. Cross and Oppé concluded that the respiratory stimulation was due to excitation of the systemic arterial chemoreceptors, and that the failure to maintain the response was due to a depressant effect of O_2 lack upon the respiratory centres. The experiments on rabbits suggest an alternative explanation. In newborn rabbits at 35°C hypoxia (breathing 10% O_2) caused a well-maintained and large hyperpnœa, with no change in O_2-consumption (Dawes and Mott 1959a, Adamsons 1959). The fact that hyperpnœa was well-maintained showed that the respiratory centre was not depressed by the consequent hypoxæmia in rabbits. Exposure to a cooler environment caused an increase in O_2-consumption and a moderate hyperpnœa; hypoxia then caused a decrease in O_2-consumption and only a small transient change in breathing. The failure of hypoxia to cause maintained hyperpnœa in a cool environment could be due to a fall in arterial P_{CO_2} consequent on the fall in O_2-consumption and hence in CO_2-production. Hence it is possible that Cross and Oppé's observations on human babies might have been carried out at a temperature which, for them, was relatively cool. Exposure of newborn babies to 15% O_2 also caused a fall in O_2-consumption (Cross, Tizard and Trythall 1958). Of course an extreme reduction in arterial P_{O_2} will cause respiratory depression, but it seems most unlikely that this would happen in a *normal* child while breathing 15% O_2.

Apart from the chemoreceptors, the Hering-Breuer reflexes are also functional at birth (Dawes and Mott 1959a) and injection of lobeline or nicotine into newborn rabbits induces rapid, shallow breathing, abolished by vagotomy and attributed to an action on other pulmonary receptors. The cough reflex is also present. In a stimulating paper Cross, Klaus, Tooley and Weisser (1960) showed that when the lungs are rapidly inflated in newborn babies a further inspiratory effort is often observed. They suggest that this may be due to Head's paradoxical reflex, and propose that it may serve a useful purpose when respiration is first being established. The reaction was only seen in very young infants. A similar phenomenon has been observed while resuscitating asphyxiated newly delivered monkeys. At a certain stage of recovery positive pressure inflation of the lungs initiates a further active inspiration. More work is still required to establish the mechanisms with certainty.

It is evident that the principal reflexes are functional at birth. It would indeed be surprising if this were not so in a physiological system which demands such precise control and variation with the rate of metabolism, and which is essential to survival. There may be quantitative differences in the details and the precision of control in the newborn as compared with the adult, and no quantitative analysis of the interaction of stimuli on breathing has been undertaken in the newborn. Until this is done we shall not have the information needed to say whether the threshold or sensitivity of the sensory centres, central and peripheral, are different in the newborn from the adult. The fact that the arterial and alveolar P_{O_2} and P_{CO_2} are very similar in the newborn and adult suggest that they may not be very different, but we still have to explain why the fœtus does not continuously make respiratory efforts.

The Pulmonary Circulation

In the fœtus pulmonary arterial pressure is greater than aortic pressure, and a large part of the output of the right heart flows through the ductus arteriosus. After birth, when normal breathing has been established, pulmonary arterial pressure falls, the ductus arteriosus closes, and the whole of the right cardiac output passes through the lungs. It is reasonable to infer, and direct measurement has confirmed, that there is a fall in pulmonary vascular resistance after birth, which results from gaseous inflation of the lungs. What is the mechanism of this change in the pulmonary circulation at birth? and what are the physiological factors which regulate the pulmonary circulation in the fœtus and the newborn? We may start by considering what is known in the adult.

The pulmonary circulation in the adult. In adults the pulmonary blood vessels have, until recent years, been regarded as comparatively inert, accepting passively the output of the right heart. Although the investigations of I. de Burgh Daly and his colleagues demonstrated that they were under nervous control, the changes produced reflexly or by sympathetic stimulation were comparatively small. However, in 1946 von Euler and Liljestrand found that hypoxia (breathing 10% or less O_2 in N_2) caused a large rise in pulmonary arterial pressure in adult cats, attributed to pulmonary vasoconstriction.

The conclusion that the vascular resistance of the adult lung can be altered very considerably receives support from three other lines of evidence. Firstly, using cardiac catheterisation and improved methods of radiography pulmonary hypertension has been recognised as a not uncommon disorder resulting from mitral disease and other causes. The greatly thickened pulmonary arteries associated with this condition are of interest. It was at first thought that these changes were permanent, and in extreme cases they may be so, but there is now evidence that if the pulmonary hypertension is relieved, and has not been too prolonged and too severe, the vascular changes regress. Similar changes have been produced by experimental pulmonary hypertension (e.g. by repeated small air embolisms) and also have disappeared after some months (Wright 1962). The changes appear to be a consequence rather than a primary cause of the condition. Secondly, pulmonary hypertension has developed at high altitude both in normal man (Peñaloza et al. 1962) and in cattle (brisket disease; Grover and Reeves 1962), and exceptionally large rises in pulmonary arterial pressure (up to 165/96 mm. Hg) may occur during exercise (Vogel et al. 1962). Thirdly when an adult lung is collapsed, perceptible cyanosis is unusual, because of pulmonary vasoconstriction in the unventilated lobes (Barer 1963). The first two of these observations show that extreme pulmonary vasoconstriction may occur in an expanded adult lung, the third might provide an analogy to the vasconstriction in fœtal lungs.

If we now turn to the detailed mechanisms by which pulmonary vasoconstriction is effected in the adult, the evidence cannot be regarded as wholly conclusive. Ventilation of isolated perfused lungs with low O_2 mixtures caused vasoconstriction (Duke and Lee 1963). This is an observation of particular interest to respiratory physiologists, for it could provide a basis for the local regulation of blood flow within the lung, according to whether a group of alveoli were expanded or not. The mechanisms by which local hypoxia causes pulmonary vasoconstriction is uncertain. The fact that a local effect of O_2 lack has been demonstrated does not preclude the probability that in vivo reflex effects or hormone liberation into the bloodstream also play a part. Daly and Daly (1959) have shown that hypoxic stimulation of the perfused carotid bodies in the adult dog causes reflex pulmonary vasoconstriction, but the effect is not large. Injection of catecholamines also can cause pulmonary vasoconstriction, but the effect is smaller than that on the systemic circulation. It is likely that in vivo several different mechanisms summate to produce vasoconstriction in the lungs.

Changes in the pulmonary circulation at birth. In fœtal lambs delivered by cæsarean section under general anæsthesia, and with the chest open to give direct access to the left lung, there was a large fall in pulmonary vascular resistance on positive pressure ventilation with air, O_2 or N_2, but not on expansion with saline (Dawes, Mott, Widdicombe and Wyatt 1953). Ventilation of the isolated lungs of fœtal lambs, perfused with blood from a pump, also caused a large fall in vascular resistance, which was greater when the ventilating gas was air rather than N_2 (Born, Dawes and Mott 1955). Hence some of the vasodilatation observed in vivo must have been due to a local effect of gaseous expansion of the lungs, possibly in part mechanical, but also in part due to O_2, as in adult lungs. The mechanical effect of rhythmic expansion of the lungs could result either in uncoiling or dilatation of twisted or compressed vessels in the collapsed condition (an hypothesis favoured by Reynolds 1956), or in vivo it could cause reflex effects by stimulation of sensory receptors in the thoracic viscera. Similarly changes in alveolar and arterial gas tensions could have an action in vivo both locally upon the pulmonary vessels themselves and systemically on the arterial chemoreceptors and the brain, which could modify the resistance of the pulmonary circulation by nervous reflexes or by release of hormones into the blood stream.

Experiments on fœtal lambs, designed for other purposes, raised the possibility that under some conditions pulmonary blood flow might be large even before ventilation. To test this hypothesis experiments were done on fœtal lambs, still attached by an intact umbilical cord to the mother, in which the lungs were not expanded (Dawes and Mott 1962). Injection of small doses of acetylcholine or histamine into the left pulmonary artery caused as large an increase in blood flow as subsequent ventilation of the lungs (Fig. 2). Raising the O_2-content of the fœtal arterial blood (by giving the mother 100% O_2 in place of air to breathe) caused pulmonary vasodilatation, while hypoxæmia caused vasoconstriction. Asphyxia, caused by

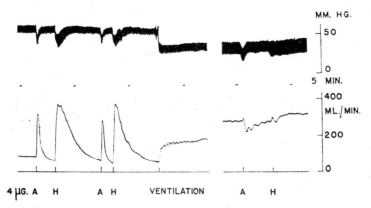

FIG. 2. Mature fœtal lamb. Before ventilation injection of 4 µg. acetylcholine (A) or histamine (H) into the left pulmonary artery caused a great increase of flow (below) and a fall in pressure (above). Ventilation of the lungs caused a more gradual but equal increase in flow, after which acetylcholine and histamine no longer caused significant vasodilatation (Dawes 1962b).

occlusion of the umbilical cord for 2 minutes, caused extreme pulmonary vasoconstriction and a large fall in flow in spite of a rise in blood pressure (Fig. 3). And a brief period of ischæmia (caused by occluding the left pulmonary artery) produced reactive hyperæmia subsequently. There was therefore no doubt that in the mature fœtus the vessels of the unexpanded lung were very reactive. The high vascular resistance usually observed must have been due more to maintained tone rather than to contortion of the blood vessels.

Meanwhile Cook et al. (1963), who had started out to study the effect of underventilation in the newborn lamb, observed that addition of CO_2 to the ventilating gas caused pulmonary vasoconstriction. They also noted that static gaseous inflation of the lung (as compared with rhythmic ventilation) only caused very slight vasodilatation. It was clearly necessary to find out to what extent the O_2- and CO_2-contents of the ventilating gas, and the mechanical effect of gaseous expansion with a gas mixture which did not alter the arterial P_{CO_2} or P_{O_2}, each altered pulmonary vascular resistance, and whether these effects were additive.

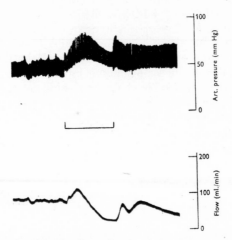

FIG. 3. Mature fœtal lamb. Records of arterial pressure (above) and of flow (below) in loop supplying left pulmonary artery. During the signal mark the fœtus was asphyxiated by occlusion of the umbilical cord for 1¼ minutes, which caused intense pulmonary vasoconstriction (Dawes and Mott 1962).

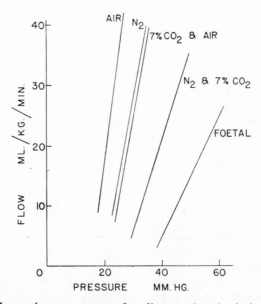

FIG. 4. Mean pulmonary pressure-flow diagrams for 7 lambs in the fœtal condition, and after ventilation with different gas mixtures (Cassin, Dawes, Mott, Ross and Strang 1964).

Experiments carried out for this purpose showed that there was a "mechanical" effect of rhythmic positive pressure ventilation of the lungs irrespective of any change in arterial blood gas tension (Cassin, Dawes, Mott, Ross and Strang 1964). (The word mechanical is used here solely to denote that the effect cannot be attributed to a change in arterial or alveolar gas tension; the mechanism is not known.) Fig. 4 shows that ventilation with 7% CO_2 in N_2 caused pulmonary vasodilatation, as indicated by a higher flow at the same pressure. When this gas was replaced by N_2 alone there was a further vasodilatation, and when it was replaced by air there was a yet further

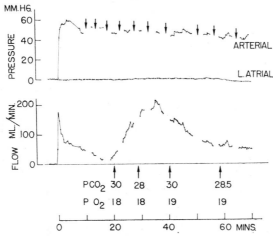

FIG. 5. Mature fœtal lamb. The left pulmonary artery was cannulated at time zero. After the first rapid increase in flow there was a period of vasoconstriction followed, after 20 mins, by considerable vasodilatation with no appreciable change in arterial P_{CO_2} or P_{O_2} (Cassin, Dawes, Mott, Ross and Strang 1964).

vasodilatation. The addition of 7% CO_2 to the ventilating gas mixture caused about the same degree of vasoconstriction whether in the presence or absence of O_2. It was concluded that all three factors, a rise in arterial P_{O_2}, a fall in P_{CO_2} and rhythmical ventilation of the lungs contributed to the pulmonary vasodilatation observed on ventilation of the lungs with air. Ventilation of the right lung only, sufficient to cause a fall in arterial P_{CO_2} and a rise in P_{O_2}, produced an equivalent vasodilatation in the *unventilated* left lung. This effect was therefore independent of changes in alveolar gas tension. Conversely asphyxia had caused vasoconstriction in the unventilated lung (Fig. 3).

During earlier experiments, and also in those just described, a number of instances of unexplained vasodilatation were observed in lungs which had not been ventilated. An example is shown in Fig. 5. These incidents were not accompanied by any significant change in arterial P_{O_2} or P_{CO_2} and the increase in flow sometimes approximated to that on subsequent ventilation of the lungs. The only predisposing factor was that the arterial pressure tended to be higher in these lambs. It is evident that fœtal pulmonary blood flow may be larger than previously supposed.

The experiments so far described were all on mature fœtal lambs, within 10 days of term. The same methods for measuring pulmonary blood flow and vascular resistance were also applied to immature fœtal lambs of 75–91 days gestational age (term is 147 days). In these immature fœtuses the lungs cannot be expanded by gaseous inflation because the alveoli are still solid (Fauré-Fremiet and Dragoiu 1923, Born, Dawes and Mott 1955). The vascular resistance of the lung was less than half that of mature fœtal lambs, whether expressed in terms of total body or lung weight (Cassin, Dawes and Ross 1964). As in mature lambs, so in these immature fœtuses injection of acetylcholine and histamine caused pulmonary vasodilatation, and nor-adrenaline and adrenaline caused (predominantly) vasoconstriction. As-phyxia (produced by occlusion of the umbilical cord for 2 minutes) led to extreme pulmonary vasoconstriction (as in Fig. 3); this was abolished by giving dibenamine, which blocked the vasoconstrictor action of adrenaline and noradrenaline. Injection of dibenamine caused profound vasodilatation.

These observations on immature fœtal lambs demonstrate that some of the mechanisms which regulate the pulmonary circulation are functional before the fœtus is viable. They lend further support to the view that there may be circumstances in which pulmonary flow is relatively greater than was supposed (since mean vascular resistance was so much less in immature fœtuses). And they indicate one of the effector mechanisms (release of catecholamines) by which the pulmonary vascular resistance may be regulated.

To summarise these observations, the following changes cause pulmonary vasodilatation:

1. A rise in arterial P_{O_2}.
2. A fall in arterial P_{CO_2}.
3. Rhythmic ventilation of the lungs.
4. An unknown factor or factors (Fig. 5).

The effect of O_2 is, in part at least, local upon the lungs themselves. Ventilation with N_2 alone also causes vasodilatation in isolated fœtal lungs, but it is uncertain to what extent this is due to a mechanical effect or to a lowering of P_{CO_2}. Part, perhaps a large part, of these effects can be attributed to an effector mechanism which involves release of catecholamines. The part played by afferent sensory mechanisms (e.g. the systemic arterial chemoreceptors) and the brain has yet to be investigated.

Conclusions. The lungs fare particularly badly during acute asphyxia because they are then supplied with less blood containing less oxygen, and if this process is carried too far it might entail tissue damage. This might partly explain why the incidence of respiratory distress is so high in lambs (Dawes, Mott and Stafford 1960) and rhesus monkeys (Dawes, Mott, Shelley and Stafford 1963) which have been asphyxiated after delivery by cæsarean section; the incidence was almost 50% in monkeys (Adamsons, Behrman, Dawes, James and Koford 1964). Rabbits delivered from mothers subjected to previous hypoxia also showed a high incidence of respiratory difficulties during the first 6 hours after delivery (J. A. Davis, unpublished).

In the newborn partial asphyxia causes a rise in vascular resistance both in a lung which is unventilated and in one which is ventilated. The ventilated lung, or portions which are well ventilated but not overdistended, will have a greater blood supply in so far as the mechanical and gaseous effects of ventilation are local. Although there is certainly a local effect (e.g. that of O_2) it is not yet possible to express this quantitatively, and hence to calculate the proportion of blood which might be expected to pass through unventilated areas of lung when only part is expanded.

We may, however, consider in general terms what must happen to an infant with respiratory distress, in which only part of the lung is expanded and the systemic arterial blood is not wholly saturated with O_2 as a result of right-to-left shunts (whether these are intra- or extra-pulmonary). If pulmonary vascular resistance is not too high, flow through the ductus arteriosus will be predominantly left-to-right, and the recirculation of partly oxygenated blood through the ventilated areas of the lung will allow more O_2 to be taken up, so long as the functional alveoli have some diffusion capacity to spare (Dawes, Mott and Widdicombe 1955). This phenomenon is of greater value as the O_2-content of the arterial blood is lowered. But with increasing asphyxia pulmonary vascular resistance will increase, and the shunt through the ductus may then become predominantly right-to-left. Exposure of newborn mongol infants to 10% or 15% O_2 in N_2 for 6 minutes caused a fall in systemic arterial pressure and a rise in pulmonary arterial pressure sufficient to reverse the direction of blood flow through the ductus arteriosus (James and Rowe 1957).

In newborn animals and human infants the walls of the pulmonary arteries are thicker and more muscular than in adults (Edwards 1959). They become thinner during the first few weeks from birth when the pulmonary arterial pressure has fallen. The increased thickness may result from the higher pulmonary arterial pressure, as in adults. In the newborn the pulmonary vessels do not show the extreme gnarling and tortuosity which are found in adults after prolonged pulmonary hypertension. Whatever the cause of the difference in histological appearance the pulmonary blood vessels appear to react differently, both quantitatively and qualitatively, from those of adults. This is suggested by the extreme degree of vasoconstriction usually seen on administration of adrenaline or noradrenaline to fœtal lambs, and in the extreme vasodilatation caused by histamine. In the adult lung sympathetic amines have little vasoconstrictor effect, and histamine usually causes vasoconstriction.

The Closure of the Fœtal Vascular Channels

The foramen ovale. The mechanism of closure of the foramen ovale has already been described (Dawes 1958). Functional closure results from an immediate fall in inferior vena caval pressure (because umbilical flow is interrupted when the cord is occluded) and a rise in left atrial pressure (because pulmonary blood flow is increased). There is also a further gradual increase in left atrial pressure as compared with right atrial pressure over several weeks after birth (van Harreveld and Russell 1956).

The first experimental observations on the time of functional closure were carried out by Barclay and Franklin (1938) using cinéangiography, and suggested that the foramen ovale was functionally patent for some days from birth. Further cinéangiographic observations, also on lambs, suggested that this conclusion was mistaken (Barclay, Franklin and Prichard 1944, Barcroft 1947). Barcroft, Kramer and Millikan (1939) found that the arterial O_2-saturation rose very rapidly after birth, a fact which was regarded as "inconsistent with the short-circuiting of any amount of blood through the foramen ovale so great as to be physiologically important." More recent observations, using dye dilution methods in unanæsthetised newborn lambs, have shown a small right-to-left shunt through the foramen ovale up to the fifth day from birth (Condorelli, Dagianti, Polosa and Guiliano 1957, Stahlmann, Merril and Le Quire 1962). And in human infants Lind and Wegelius (1954) reached the same conclusion. In normal infants it is likely that this shunt is so small as to be of little physiological importance, but in infants with cyanosis, respiratory distress or cardiac failure it might well be of practical significance (see p. 64).

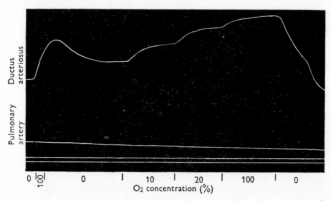

FIG. 6. Isolated strips of sheep fœtus ductus arteriosus and pulmonary artery suspended in warm Tyrode solution. Increasing concentrations of O_2 in the gas mixture bubbled through the solution caused progressive contraction of the ductus arteriosus only. Time marker, 1 min. (Kovalčík 1964).

The ductus arteriosus. The ductus arteriosus constricts when the arterial P_{O_2} is raised (Kennedy and Clark 1941, Born, Dawes, Mott and Rennick 1956). This effect appeared to be on the muscle of the ductus itself, since it was observed not only after destruction of the nervous system, but also in an isolated heart-ductus preparation supplied with blood from an artificial lung. This conclusion has been confirmed by Kovalčík (1963) who has demonstrated that strips and rings of ductus arteriosus from fœtal lambs and guinea-pigs, suspended in an isolated organ bath, progressively contract as the P_{O_2} of the gas bubbling through the solution is progressively increased (Fig. 6). The illustration shows that the contraction is slow as compared with many other types of smooth muscle. Sympathetic amines such as noradrenaline also cause constriction of the ductus arteriosus, but the effect of O_2 persists when the action of noradrenaline has been blocked by drugs. It also persists after administration of 4–20 mM cyanide, a concentration which could be expected to block cytochrome oxidase and which very greatly reduces the O_2-consumption of the isolated ductus arteriosus. The mechanism by which a rise in P_{O_2} causes constriction is still obscure. Isolated strips of aorta and pulmonary artery, prepared from the same animals adjacent to the ductus arteriosus, did not respond to variations in P_{O_2}, nor did strips of umbilical or coronary artery.

While these observations provide a rational basis for the normal mechanism of closure of the ductus, we are still as far as ever from understanding why it sometimes fails to close after birth. This could be due to a failure in development of the proper mechanism. It has also been suggested that failure to close is associated with prolonged hypoxæmia after birth (Record and McKeown 1953, Alzamora *et al.* 1953). This explanation requires that the normal mechanism which is present at birth but inoperative because of hypoxæmia, must become deranged during the period of hypoxæmia, so that it is inadequate to cause closure when a normal arterial P_{O_2} is attained. Far from being a sufficient explanation, this hypothesis merely substitutes a different problem.

During the past 10 years evidence has accumulated to support the view that, in the human infant as in animals, the ductus arteriosus is often patent for up to a few days from birth. The cardiac murmur from the ductus, which is such a prominent feature of large newborn animals such as the lamb, calf and foal, was not heard in the newborn monkey which weighs only about 500 g. at birth and has a high heart rate. In newborn piglets a continuous murmur could sometimes be detected within the pulmonary trunk while nothing was heard externally (Burnard 1963). In human infants Burnard (1958) often found a transient pansystolic or crescendo systolic murmur which was attributed to flow through a constricted ductus arteriosus; more recent evidence suggests that it could also be due to mitral regurgitation (Burnard, 1963), possibly as a result of asphyxia and cardiac dilatation. In small newborn animals and human infants, which have a lower blood pressure than large farm animals, the physical conditions may not be present for the development of sufficient turbulence to generate a loud widely conducted murmur, even though the ductus is only partly constricted.

Asphyxia at Birth

Anærobic glycolysis. It is well known that fœtuses or newborn animals of many species are able to survive in the absence of oxygen for a much longer period of time than adults. The tolerance of newborn animals to asphyxia or anoxia is inversely related both to their maturity at birth and to the environmental temperature (Edwards 1824, Mott 1961). Thus at room temperature newborn rats deprived of O_2 continue to gasp for 50 minutes, kittens and puppies 23–25 minutes, rabbits 17 minutes, guinea-pigs 7 minutes (Fazekas, Alexander and Himwich 1941) and mature fœtal lambs 6 minutes (Dawes, Jacobson *et al.* 1963). While adult rats survive breathing nitrogen for only 3 minutes, newborn rats survive for 28 minutes on the average in a neutral thermal environment (35–36°C), and for an hour at 20–22°C (Fig. 7; Stafford and Weatherall 1960).

Under anærobic conditions the tissues continue to obtain energy from carbohydrate, but not from fat. Glucose or glycogen is converted to lactic acid, providing that there are adequate supplies of glucose available and that the enzymes can continue to function. The injection of sodium iodacetate or fluoride, both of which inhibit glycolytic enzymes, reduces the survival times of newborn rats in nitrogen to that of adult rats (Himwich, Bernstein, Herrlich, Chesler and Fazekas 1942). The survival time of newborn rats in nitrogen is also reduced by measures which decrease the carbohydrate reserves, such as administration of insulin (Himwich *et al.* 1942, Himwich, Fazekas and Homburger 1943, Hicks 1953) or fasting (Stafford and Weatherall 1960). Administration of glucose in hypoglycæmia increases survival

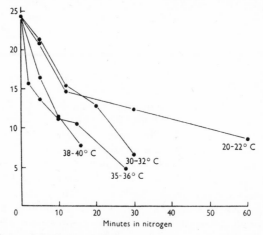

Fig. 7. Rates of depletion of total carbohydrate in the hearts of newborn rats exposed to nitrogen at different environmental temperatures. Each point is the mean of 2–4 observations. The last point is at the mean time to last breath (Stafford and Weatherall 1960).

time. It is therefore tolerably certain that the ability of the newborn animal to survive prolonged O_2 lack is dependent on the supply of energy by glycolysis. The amount of energy which can be made available by breakdown of carbohydrate to lactic acid is small, only one-fifth to one-seventh that yielded when the same quantity of carbohydrate is converted to carbon dioxide and water.

We now have to consider how it is that immature animals survive asphyxia so much longer than adults. This phenomenon is not necessarily related to a change which occurs at birth. Thus the fœtal lamb loses its ability to survive prolonged asphyxia during the last half of gestation, before birth (Dawes, Mott and Shelley 1959), while the rat loses it during the first 2–3 weeks after birth (Fazekas *et al.* 1941). Reiss (1931) suggested that immature animals might have a greater ability to glycolyse anærobically, but subsequent observations did not confirm this hypothesis either on tissue slices or *in vivo*. Chesler and Himwich (1944) observed that the *in vitro* rate of oxidative metabolism in rat brain increased with age more rapidly than anærobic glycolysis, leaving an increasing hypothetical energy deficit. But oxidative metabolism did not start to increase until 10 days after birth, by which time survival had already decreased from 50 to 10 minutes (at room temperature).

Some other explanation was needed, and further experiments were begun as a consequence of writing a chapter for the second edition of this book (Dawes 1958).

Cardiac carbohydrate and asphyxia.   Experiments on fœtal lambs during the second half of gestation showed that there was a direct correlation between the carbohydrate concentration in the cardiac ventricles and the ability of the cardiovascular system to withstand asphyxia (Dawes, Mott and Shelley 1959). The cardiac carbohydrate is high in young fœtuses or newborn

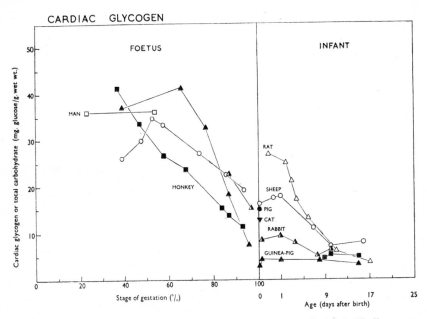

Fig. 8. Cardiac glycogen in different species before and after birth (Shelley 1961).

animals and falls with increasing age (Fig. 8). This is also true for human infants when account is taken of the effect of asphyxia in depleting the cardiac carbohydrate stores; the cardiac carbohydrate concentration has exceeded 40 mg./g. when rapid delivery unaccompanied by asphyxia has been followed by sudden death from other causes (Shelley 1964). In newborn rats, rabbits and guinea-pigs (Dawes, Mott and Shelley 1959, Stafford and Weatherall 1960) and fœtal monkeys (Dawes, Jacobson, Mott and Shelley 1960) there was also a direct relation between the initial cardiac carbohydrate concentration and the time to last gasp during exposure to nitrogen or asphyxia (e.g. Fig. 9).

In order to examine whether this relation between the initial cardiac carbohydrate and the duration of gasping in anoxia was causal or coincidental, the effect on the cardiac carbohydrate of manœuvres which were known to alter the duration of gasping was investigated. In newborn rats exposed to nitrogen the cardiac carbohydrate fell more rapidly at higher environmental temperatures (Fig. 7; Stafford and Weatherall 1960). Fasting, or previous anoxia also reduced both the cardiac carbohydrate concentration and the survival time in nitrogen in the same proportion. Changes in the carbohydrate concentrations of the brain (always very low) the blood, liver, kidney, lung and skeletal muscle during asphyxia or anoxia bore no relation to survival time in lambs, monkeys or rats. We may therefore suppose that the maintenance of the circulation is of primary importance for the continuation of gasping during asphyxia or anoxia at birth, and that this is dependent on the glycogen concentration in the cardiac ventricles.

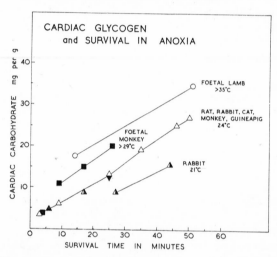

FIG. 9. The figure shows the linear relation between survival time during anoxia and cardiac carbohydrate concentration at a given environmental temperature.

Before this proposition is considered further we must ask why the glycogen concentration is so large in the hearts of immature animals, and why it falls with increasing age. Although much work has been devoted to analysis of the biochemical mechanisms of glycogen breakdown and synthesis *in vitro*, and although it is evident that the glycogen concentration at any given time must represent the net effect of these processes, the deciding factors *in vivo* are uncertain. We can only speculate that the work of the heart, relative to its size, may increase with growth. We do not know how cardiac output changes during the period in question, but we do know that in all the species for which there is information available (lamb, monkey, rabbit and rat) the blood pressure increases rapidly as the cardiac carbohydrate concentration falls.

Arterial pH during asphyxia. In fœtal monkeys during total asphyxia the time to the last gasp was decreased by interruption of the circulation (Dawes, Jacobson, Mott and Shelley 1959). This adds additional weight to the conclusion that the maintenance or failure of the circulation may be a limiting factor to respiratory activity during asphyxia. The circulation cannot be important as a means of distributing oxygen, for the oxygen in the bloodstream is almost wholly exhausted within 2–3 minutes of tying the umbilical cord if no breath is taken. The brain has very small glycogen reserves, and it might be dependent on the blood for its supply of glucose, or for removing the acid products of glycolysis.

Infusion of alkali (sodium carbonate or Tris, tris-hydroxymethylaminomethane, THAM) together with glucose into asphyxiated immature fœtal lambs, in concentrations sufficient to maintain the arterial pH and to raise the blood glucose, maintained the heart rate and blood pressure and the rate of glycolysis (as measured by the rate of accumulation of blood and tissue lactate) for much longer than in untreated lambs (Dawes, Mott, Shelley and Stafford 1963). Under anærobic conditions mammalian tissues gradually lose the ability to concentrate potassium within cells and to extrude sodium. The rate of rise in plasma potassium during asphyxia was reduced by infusion of alkali and glucose. Infusion of glucose alone was without effect, while infusion of glucose with saline, or of sodium carbonate alone caused a more rapid failure of the circulation. The rate of rise of blood lactate was greatest when the arterial pH was maintained above 7·3 and the blood glucose above 200 mg./100 ml. Bicarbonate was too weak an alkali for practical use. It was concluded that in immature lambs both the fall in pH and hypoglycæmia could limit circulatory efficiency.

Further experiments, in fœtal lambs and rhesus monkeys delivered by cæsarean section under local anæsthesia, showed that infusion of alkali and glucose during asphyxia not only maintained the circulation but prolonged the duration of gasping and greatly facilitated resuscitation (Dawes, Jacobson, Mott, Shelley and Stafford 1963). But before discussing these observations the natural history of asphyxia at birth in fœtuses delivered under local anæsthesia must be described.

The natural history of asphyxia and resuscitation at birth. When a mature fœtal monkey is delivered without general anæsthesia within 10 days of term, the umbilical cord is tied, and it is prevented from inhaling air by placing a small bag containing saline over its head, a characteristic series of events takes place (Dawes, Jacobson, Mott, Shelley and Stafford 1963, Adamsons, Behrman, Dawes, Dawkins, James and Ross 1963, Adamsons, Behrman, Dawes, James and Koford 1964). Within 15–30 secs. of dividing the cord rapid *rhythmic* respiratory efforts begin; these are interrupted after 1–1·8 minutes by a convulsion or series of clonic movements followed by a period of apnœa (*primary apnœa*) lasting for 30–60 sec. The monkey then begins to gasp, and the rate of gasping rises to 3–8/min. after 6–7 min. asphyxia (Fig. 10). There is little change in rate, though the gasps gradually become weaker up to the last gasp which, at an environmental temperature of 30°C, occurs after a mean of 8·5 min. from tying the cord (range 6·7–10·1 min. S.E. ± 0·20 min., in 21 monkeys). There then follows *secondary apnœa*, and, if resuscitation is not begun within a few minutes, death.

The foregoing account only applies to monkeys which are in reasonable condition on delivery, that is with an umbilical arterial pH of 7·3 or more. Asphyxia before delivery reduces the arterial pH and changes the course of events. When the arterial pH on delivery is less than 7·1 there is no initial period of rhythmic respiratory efforts and gasping starts sooner and ceases earlier than in monkeys in good condition. When the arterial pH is less than

6·8 on delivery there may be no gasps at all. General anæsthesia lengthens each part of the cycle of events; what is particularly important from a practical point of view is that the duration of the *primary apnœa* may be greatly extended. For instance in a monkey delivered under light pento-barbitone primary apnœa lasted $7\frac{1}{2}$ minutes, and the last gasp was not taken until $17\frac{1}{2}$ minutes after tying the cord. Although general anæsthesia prolongs the duration of gasping it does not improve the chance of ultimate survival.

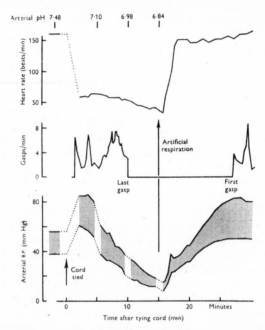

Fig. 10. Mature fœtal monkey, delivered by cæsarean section and asphyxi-ated by tying the cord and preventing breathing. Artificial ventilation with O_2 was begun after 15 minutes (Dawes, Jacobson, Mott, Shelley and Stafford 1963).

When the umbilical cord is tied the heart rate falls precipitously, recovers slightly and then subsides gradually over the next 10 minutes (Fig. 10). In the ECG irregularities of rhythm are seen only occasionally, though there are large changes in the QRS and T complexes. The blood pressure rises at first and falls to its initial level after 5 minutes; in monkeys which are already asphyxiated on delivery the rise in arterial pressure is small or absent. The blood lactate concentration rises considerably but the blood glucose changes very little. The plasma potassium rises abruptly by nearly 2 mEq./l. in the first 5 minutes of asphyxia. The arterial pH falls to about 6·95 in 5 minutes and to 6·7 in 15 minutes while the P_{CO_2} rises to 150–200 mm. Hg, and there is an increase in the plasma CO_2 concentration which may be as much as threefold. The newly delivered monkey is small (450–550 g. at term) and its fur is wet. Its rectal temperature falls by 2–3°C during a 10–15 minute period of asphyxia, partly because of reduced heat production, but mainly because of evaporative heat loss. Monkeys (and even lambs) which are not asphyxiated also cool on delivery.

If the rubber bag is removed from the head of an asphyxiated monkey before the last gasp, the monkey will usually recover spontaneously. Sometimes (after more than 8 minutes asphyxia) the gasps are too weak to expand the lungs adequately and rapidly enough. If the monkey was no longer gasping, or if its gasps were inadequate (in that the heart did not accelerate within 30 seconds), resuscitation was performed by positive pressure ventilation with 100% O_2 through an endotracheal tube. The primary object of resuscitation is to raise the arterial P_{O_2} and to lower the P_{CO_2} as rapidly as possible. Asphyxia causes extreme pulmonary vasoconstriction (see above, p. 7) and it is now evident that to relieve this vasoconstriction it is necessary to raise the *arterial* P_{O_2} and lower the P_{CO_2}. Consequently 100% O_2 only is used to give as large a P_{O_2} and P_{CO_2} gradient across the lungs as possible. Experience has also shown that it is very easy to underventilate asphyxiated fœtal monkeys and lambs. The initial pressure required to expand the lungs is high (35–40 mm. Hg) because of surface tension forces, and it is often necessary to maintain these pressures for several minutes to achieve adequate ventilation. Even in the hands of practised operators doing several resuscitations a week the need was sometimes underestimated. The best possible criterion of efficient resuscitation is given by simultaneous measurement of O_2-consumption. In monkeys which had been asphyxiated for 10 minutes, resuscitation by artificial ventilation with 100% O_2 (accompanied by cardiac massage if necessary) did not cause an immediate rise in O_2-consumption up to the level normal for a newborn monkey. There was usually an interval of up to 2 minutes during which O_2-consumption was only a third or less of normal. Partial asphyxia therefore continues for a short while after resuscitation is begun, even when the lungs are well ventilated.

In some lambs and monkeys asphyxiated for 10–15 minutes the circulation had failed to such an extent that positive pressure ventilation alone was inadequate to ensure rapid recovery. There is ample evidence that enduring asphyxia, partial or complete, increases the degree of brain damage and it is therefore essential to have some simple guide as to the efficacy of resuscitation. The criterion adopted was that the heart should have accelerated within 30 seconds of beginning ventilation. Experience showed that if it did not accelerate at once, then recovery would be very slow and stormy, usually with a fatal outcome, unless the heart was massaged. External cardiac massage was applied by lateral compression of the thoracic cage for 5–10 seconds while ventilation was temporarily interrupted. Two or three periods of cardiac massage never failed to cause recovery even after 15 minutes asphyxia, and also in two monkeys in which the heart stopped beating (for up to $4\frac{1}{2}$ minutes). Cardiac massage was required in 14 monkeys, in all of which the arterial blood pressure at the onset of resuscitation was less than 20 mm. Hg.

After resuscitation by ventilation with O_2 (and cardiac massage where necessary) the heart rate and blood pressure rise rapidly (Fig. 10). There is an interval between the onset of resuscitation and the first gasp which bears a linear relation to the duration of asphyxia (Fig. 11). The regression of time

to first gasp on duration of asphyxia intercepts the abscissa close to the time
to last gasp (Fig. 11, - - -). Hence had resuscitation been started at the last
gasp the monkey would have gone on gasping without interruption. For
each minute's asphyxia after that, there is an interval of almost 2 minutes
until the start of gasping, and of more than 4 minutes until the onset of
spontaneous rhythmic breathing (Fig. 11, ———). It was usually possible to
stop artificial ventilation within a few minutes of the establishment of
spontaneous breathing, although additional O_2 was almost always required
for some while, particularly in premature monkeys. The facts illustrated in
Fig. 11 emphasize, if any emphasis be needed, the importance of early and
adequate resuscitation.

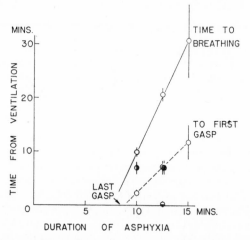

FIG. 11. Observations on the mean time from ventilation to the first gasp
(- - -) and to rhythmic breathing (———) in groups each of 5–6 foetal rhesus
monkeys asphyxiated for 10, 12·5 or 15 min. under standard conditions
without treatment (○). The mean time, to first gasp (◖) and to rhythmic
breathing (●) is also shown for monkeys asphyxiated for 12·5 min. and
treated by infusion of alkali and glucose for 4 min., beginning 6·5 min.
after the onset of asphyxia. The mean time to rhythmic breathing (◑) is
also shown for monkeys asphyxiated for 10 min. and treated by infusion
of alkali and glucose at the onset of ventilation (Adamsons, Behrman,
Dawes, James and Koford 1964). The vertical lines indicate S.E.

Treatment of birth asphyxia with alkali and glucose. Infusion of alkali and
glucose in lambs and monkeys asphyxiated for 10–15 minutes on delivery
facilitated resuscitation and reduced the time from beginning resuscitation
to the first gasp and to the onset of spontaneous breathing. The best results
were obtained when the alkali was infused intravenously (into a femoral or
umbilical vein) either throughout asphyxia, or from 6½ minutes after tying
the cord (Fig. 11, ◖, ●). There was still a beneficial effect, though smaller,
when the infusion was begun at the same time as beginning artificial ventilation (Fig. 11, ◑). When the infusion was begun during asphyxia, the duration of gasping was prolonged and cardiac massage was not required. When
the infusion was begun at the same time as ventilation, cardiac massage was
sometimes needed, but in all instances the rate of O_2-consumption rose more

rapidly than in monkeys which were resuscitated without an infusion, and spontaneous breathing was established more quickly. The beneficial effect when the infusion was started with ventilation is attributed, firstly to enhanced glycolysis in the heart and brain (since asphyxia is not at once relieved), and secondly to the more rapid fall in arterial P_{CO_2} which might be expected to accelerate pulmonary vasodilatation. It is possible that the Bohr effect (the shift in the O_2 dissociation curve with pH) may make a minor contribution.

In asphyxiated monkeys which are adequately ventilated without an infusion the arterial P_{CO_2} falls to normal values within 8 minutes. To obtain a real advantage, therefore, alkali must be administered rapidly, over not more than 4 minutes. Sodium bicarbonate is too weak and sodium carbonate too caustic for practical use. A solution of $0.5\ M$ Tris (tris-hydroxymethylaminomethane, THAM) with $0.3\ M$ glucose proved effective and not toxic: 6 ml. were given to monkeys weighing about 400–500 g. to raise the arterial pH from about 6.8 to 7.4. The solution is strongly hyperosmolar and caused a large fall in hæmatocrit; this is a necessary consequence of having to provide a large quantity of base to neutralize the circulating fixed acids. It was concluded that there is a case established for a cautious trial of this method of treatment in severely asphyxiated infants, in addition to artificial ventilation with $100\%\ O_2$.

The conclusion that infusion of alkali and glucose during asphyxia was of real benefit has been confirmed by the observation that it reduced the incidence and the extent of permanent brain damage (Dawes, Hibbard and Windle 1964). Thirteen monkeys asphyxiated at birth for 12.5 min. were killed $1\frac{1}{2}$–2 months later. Of 5 which received no infusion all had severe and widespread lesions in the brain-stem on histological examination, and one had gross neurological signs (spastic paralysis of the upper limbs). Of the 8 which had received infusions of glucose and alkali, 2 had no lesions and the remainder had subtotal lesions of the nucleus of the inferior colliculus alone.

Other clinical implications. The differences between these animal experiments and asphyxiated human infants at birth are threefold. We know precisely how long the animals have been asphyxiated and in what condition they were beforehand, they have received no general anæsthetic or drugs which might modify respiration, and it is permissible to take greater risks with them than with human infants. Nevertheless it is reasonable to draw some inferences.

The natural physiological history of asphyxia at birth explains why some infants, who neither breathe nor gasp on delivery, start to gasp after an interval of several minutes, either spontaneously or in response to stimuli, such as slapping, cold or injection of analeptics. These infants are in the stage of *primary apnœa* (as defined above), which can be long. More rarely an infant may be delivered in the stage of *secondary apnœa* and so far as we know in these circumstances only artificial ventilation, with cardiac massage if necessary, will save its life.

Can we then distinguish between primary and secondary apnœa? In animal experiments, *when the animal was in good physiological condition before the onset of asphyxia*, this was possible. During the stage of primary apnœa the pulse rate is higher, the blood pressure is raised and the pulse strong, the skin is blue rather than white, and the arterial pH exceeds 7·0. In secondary apnœa the pulse is slow and weak, even barely perceptible, the skin is grey or white and the pH less than 6·9. However these criteria become blurred and of little value when the animal is already in poor condition before delivery, due to repeated episodes of mild asphyxia, or from depressant drugs. The heart only recovers its glycogen stores over a period of hours after asphyxia, so that the effect of short episodes of partial asphyxia *in utero* can be cumulative. In practice then, if there is any doubt about an infant's condition, it is better to treat it as if it were in secondary apnœa, and to proceed at once with artificial ventilation.

The time element can be crucial. Asphyxia at birth causes cerebral damage in experimental animals (Ranck and Windle 1959). Many monkeys which have been asphyxiated to beyond the last gasp and then resuscitated have feeding difficulties, defects of locomotion and spastic paralysis of their extremities subsequently; their brains show a variety of widespread lesions at necropsy. The time interval between a period of asphyxia which causes no perceptible damage and that which causes extensive damage is no more than 2–3 minutes. Every minute of delay in starting adequate ventilation may delay the establishment of breathing fourfold (Fig. 11). If this is true of human babies as it is of monkeys, then not only can there be no justification in delay in treating the baby which is limp, with a slow heart rate and does not breathe within a minute; but before using new drugs in the treatment of birth asphyxia in human babies, far more rigorous and practical tests are needed in *newborn animals* than have hitherto been used. The fact that a drug can increase the rate or depth of breathing in a newborn human infant or animal which is well supplied with oxygen does not mean that it will be effective, or better than other methods, in asphyxia at birth. It should not be used in human infants until it has been shown to be more effective in animals.

Temperature Regulation and the Metabolic Response to Cold

Adaptation to cold in the newborn. Newborn animals, being smaller than adults of the same species, have a larger surface to body weight ratio, and hence a greater physical problem in maintaining their body temperature. When they are exposed to cold there is almost always a fall in rectal temperature, and this is accompanied by an immediate increase in O_2-consumption. The increase is small and difficult to measure in newborn rats but is larger in newborn rabbits, kittens, puppies, guinea-pigs, piglets, lambs and monkeys. Fig. 12 illustrates the effect of exposing newborn rats, rabbits and monkeys to cold. Newborn rats weigh about 5 g., and rabbits about 50 g. and the critical temperature (above which O_2-consumption is minimal) usually exceeds 35°C. O_2-consumption is 15–20 ml./kg.min. in a neutral thermal environment (i.e. when minimal) and increases considerably on exposure to cold. Newborn monkeys weigh about 500 g., the critical temperature is 35°C and O_2-consumption in a neutral thermal environment is 9–10 ml/kg. min. at birth. Newborn human babies weigh more and the critical temperature (32–35°C) and O_2-consumption in a neutral thermal environment (about

5 ml./kg.min.) are less. The smaller the animal, the larger is the rate of O_2-consumption in a neutral thermal environment, the higher the critical temperature, and the greater the relative increase in metabolic rate in response to a given decrease in environmental temperature. These phenomena are attributable to the relatively large surface area from which heat is lost in small animals. When newborn animals are exposed to environmental temperatures of 37·5–38°C or more, their rectal temperature and respiration rate increase, they become restless and O_2-consumption begins to rise sharply (Fig. 12).

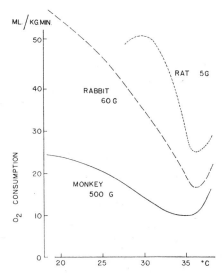

Fig. 12. To show the increase in O_2-consumption on exposing newborn animals of different species to a cold environment.

The changes in (minimal) O_2-consumption in a neutral thermal environment after birth are complicated. In some species, such as the lamb (Dawes and Mott 1959b) there is a more than twofold increase during the first 24 hours. Probably the same rapid increase occurs in the goat (Barcroft, Flexner and McClurkin 1934) and the piglet (Mount 1959). All three species are well developed at birth. In the rhesus monkey, O_2-consumption in a neutral thermal environment increases twofold during the first 2–3 weeks from birth (Dawes, Jacobson, Mott and Shelley 1960) even when the monkey is reared in an incubator at 35°C from within an hour or two of delivery (Dawes 1961). It is probable that there is also a small increase soon after birth in the rat (Taylor 1960) but not in the rabbit or kitten (Scopes and Tizard 1963). Information about the human infant is not easy to interpret. If we include premature deliveries there is some increase in O_2-consumption at the neutral environmental temperature shortly after birth. If premature deliveries are excluded there is an increase, but it reaches a peak only 2–3 weeks after delivery (Brück 1961). Thus in several species there is an increase in minimal O_2-consumption with increasing age from birth, but this increase takes place over different periods of time and the reasons for it and the mechanisms involved are not known.

With increasing age and growth in any one species the critical temperature falls (from about 35°C) and the region of thermal neutrality widens. The maximum rate of O_2-consumption on exposure to cold (expressed in ml./kg. min.) increases after birth in spite of an increase in body weight. This change is particularly striking in the rat (Fig. 13) and has also been seen in puppies (Gelineo 1957, McIntyre and Ederstrom 1958) and monkeys (Dawes, Jacobson, Mott and Shelley 1960) as well as in human infants (Brück, Brück and Lemtis 1958).

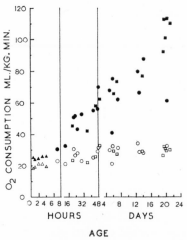

Fig. 13. The minimal (open symbols) rate of O_2-consumption at the neutral temperature and the maximal rate (closed symbols) in a cool environment has been plotted for rats of different ages, before suckling (triangles) and placed in a respirator together (circles) or separated by partitions (squares) (Taylor 1960).

Sympathetic amines and heat production. Considerable attention has recently been given to the mechanism of the remarkable metabolic response to cold in newborn animals (Fig. 12). There is no doubt that this is responsible for considerable heat production, since when it is impaired or absent, in animals under anæsthesia (Dawes and Mestyán 1963) or in human infants with cerebral damage the control of body temperature on exposure to cold is reduced or lost. Increased muscular tone or shivering only contributes in part to the rise in O_2-consumption on exposure to cold. Large increases in O_2-consumption are not usually accompanied by visible shivering, and administration of gallamine (a neuromuscular blocking agent) to newborn rabbits exposed to cold did not reduce the increased rate of O_2-consumption (Dawes and Mestyán 1963). This is not to say that shivering makes no contribution whatsoever (see below), but that some other mechanism must exist.

For many years the effect of sympathetic amines in increasing heat production and O_2-consumption in adult animals has been discussed as a possible factor in thermoregulation. In normal adult animals noradrenaline has little effect on O_2-consumption, but adrenaline causes an increase. Rats acclimatised to cold have an increased ability to produce heat without shivering (Cottle and Carlson 1956) and this has been attributed to release of noradrenaline (Leduc 1961). Moore and Underwood (1963) showed that noradrenaline injected subcutaneously in very large doses into newborn kittens caused a large increase in O_2-consumption. Experiments on human infants (Karlberg, Moore and Oliver 1962)and newborn kittens and rabbits (Scopes and Tizard 1963) have shown that intravenous infusions of small doses of noradrenaline (0·5 μg. or less /kg.min.) cause a rise in O_2-consumption. However, in newborn animals an infusion of about 2 μg./kg.min. noradrenaline is required to mimic the actual metabolic response to cold (Dawes and Mestyán 1963). This is a large amount by adult standards.

Moore and Underwood stated that adrenaline had little effect on O_2-consumption in newborn kittens. Scopes and Tizard (1963) found that intravenous infusions of adrenaline raised O_2-consumption in kittens, but that it was less active than noradrenaline. Direct comparison of the effect of intravenous infusions showed that adrenaline was as active as noradrenaline in the anæsthetised newborn guinea-pig, and half as active in the rabbit (Dawes and Mestyán 1963). The effect of adrenaline therefore cannot be discounted. The only other sympathomimetic amine which has been identified in mammalian tissues (in very small amounts) is isoprenaline, which is as active as noradrenaline in increasing O_2-consumption in the rabbit. A particularly striking feature of the phenomenon is that with increasing age from birth the activity of noradrenaline in causing an increase in O_2-consumption decreases, both relative to the activity of adrenaline and absolutely in kittens and rabbits (Moore and Underwood 1963, Scopes and Tizard 1963). This suggests that the newborn animal has some special propensity for responding to noradrenaline, which is not normally present in the adult.

The next question is whether evidence can be adduced to prove that the metabolic response to cold in newborn animals is due to secretion of catecholamines. Moore and Underwood (1962) injected a ganglion-blocking agent, hexamethonium, into newborn kittens and puppies, found that this abolished the metabolic response to cold and attributed it to interruption of the secretion of noradrenaline. However in newborn guinea-pigs and rabbits hexamethonium did not always abolish the metabolic response to cold, although it was then much reduced (Dawes and Mestyán 1963). Interpretation of these observations is complicated by the fact that administration of hexamethonium to newborn rabbits causes a fall of blood pressure due not merely to peripheral vasodilatation but also to a decrease in cardiac output. Indeed any procedure which causes a fall of blood pressure in newborn guinea-pigs or rabbits also causes a substantial fall in O_2-consumption in a cold environment. Hence the fact that hexamethonium reduces the metabolic response to cold does not constitute positive evidence for the view that this response is due to secretion of catecholamines; the observation is only consistent with the hypothesis.

Another method of attack on the problem has been to measure the urinary output of noradrenaline (Lind, quoted by Scopes and Tizard 1963) or degradation products of catecholamines such as vanillyl mandelic acid (Sandler,

Ruthven, Normand and Moore 1961). Their excretion is increased on exposing newborn human infants to a cool environment, but this does not necessarily
implicate catecholamines in the primary mechanism by which more heat is
produced. When an animal is exposed to cold and O_2-consumption increases,
there is a rise of blood pressure, and probably a redistribution and increase
of cardiac output, as well as an increase in respiratory activity. Similar
changes must be supposed to occur in newborn human infants and would be
expected to involve increased sympathetic activity in themselves. We have
to distinguish between the mechanism by which O_2-consumption is primarily
regulated, and the secondary changes which ensue as a consequence.

A further advance has been made by the use of a new type of catecholamine
blocking agent named pronethalol. Agents such as ergotoxine and dibenamine
block the vasoconstrictor action and many other effects of catecholamines,
but do not modify their vasodilator, cardio-accelerator or metabolic effects.
Pronethalol does not block the vasoconstrictor action, but reduces or abolishes
the vasodilator and cardio-accelerator effects, and also the hyperglycæmia
and mobilisation of free fatty acids. Hull (1964) found that injection of
pronethalol into newborn rabbits abolished the effect of noradrenaline
infusions in increasing O_2-consumption, without altering the increase on
exposure to cold. Therefore the metabolic response to cold cannot be due to
secretion of noradrenaline into the blood stream in this species. It could
still be due to liberation of noradrenaline at the end-organ in a situation to
which pronethalol cannot penetrate. Pronethalol had less effect on the
action of adrenaline.

Brown fat. An approach from another point of view has thrown new light
on the subject. During experiments on newborn rabbits Dawkins and Hull
(1964) observed that there was a pad of brown fat (about 5% of body weight)
encircling the neck and stretching down either side of the spine between
the shoulder blades. This brown fat shrank during the first 7 days after birth
as a result of lipid depletion and was then gradually replaced with white fat.
The brown fat was abundantly supplied with nerves and blood vessels and
had a very high rate of O_2-consumption *in vitro*. On exposure to cold, or on
intravenous administration of noradrenaline, the temperature close to the
brown fat pad (measured by a subcutaneous thermocouple) rose as compared
with rectal temperature or with a subcutaneous thermocouple not in proximity to the brown fat pad. There was no significant increase in plasma free
fatty acids, but a large rise in plasma glycerol. These observations suggest
that at least part of the increased heat production takes place in brown fat,
which may be regarded almost as a tissue specialised for the purpose and
developed in proximity to the thorax and great vessels. Brown fat also
appears in hibernating and cold adapted animals. It is present in many, but
not all, species at birth.

More work is needed, both on the rabbit and on other species, before we
can properly evaluate the significance of these findings. It is interesting to
note how well they could explain some observations which are otherwise
puzzling. For instance, the disappearance of brown fat in the rabbit during
the first few weeks from birth might be related to the very rapid fall in the
response to noradrenaline infusions observed by Scopes and Tizard (1963).

The rat is born with little fat of any kind, although it has large carbohydrate stores (see below); at birth the metabolic response to cold is small (Fig. 13). Within the next few days it receives large quantities of fat in its milk, its carbohydrate reserves are decreased and yet the metabolic response to cold increases greatly in size.

Hypoxia, shivering and the metabolic response to cold. When normal newborn and young animals are exposed to acute moderate hypoxia (e.g. 10% O_2) in a neutral thermal environment, there is usually no change in O_2-consumption (kitten, Hill 1959, rabbit, Adamsons 1959, rhesus monkey, Dawes,

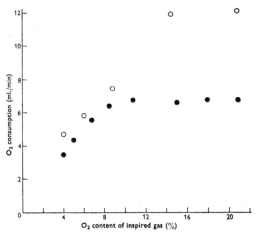

FIG. 14. Rabbit, 20 days of age. The rate of O_2-consumption has been plotted against the O_2-content of the inspired air in the neutral environment (●) and in the cold (○) (Adamsons 1959).

Jacobson, Mott and Shelley 1960). More severe hypoxia (e.g. 8% O_2) causes a fall in O_2-consumption even in a neutral thermal environment (Fig. 14, ●). When young animals are exposed to a cool environment, in which O_2 consumption is raised while breathing air, even moderate acute hypoxia causes an immediate fall in O_2-consumption and in rectal temperature (Fig. 14, ○). This phenomenon is not peculiar to the newborn as it has also been seen in adult rats and guinea-pigs.

The fall in O_2-consumption during acute hypoxia in a cool environment could be due either to a deficiency in O_2-uptake and distribution, as a result of the reduced P_{O_2} gradient from inspired air to the tissues, or to a specific effect of hypoxæmia, on the systemic arterial chemoreceptors or the brain for instance. In newborn lambs exposure to cold causes perceptible shivering, even under anæsthesia, and this shivering is abolished by hypoxia. In 1958 von Euler and Söderberg found that an intravenous injection of lobeline arrested shivering in cats, and suggested that this could be due to excitation of arterial chemoreceptors. Mott (1963) has confirmed the hypothesis that chemoreceptor stimulation temporarily abolishes shivering. Hence the abolition of shivering in the lamb by hypoxia is probably due to chemoreceptor stimulation. However, in many newborn animals, as already mentioned, exposure to cold often causes a large increase in O_2-consumption without perceptible shivering, and Blatteis (1963) has shown that in these circumstances, in newborn rabbits, hypoxia still causes an immediate fall in consumption even when the afferent nerves from the arterial chemoreceptors have been cut.

The possibility that the effect of hypoxia is partly due to a deficiency in O_2-uptake and distribution is supported by the fact that hypoxia reduces the increase in O_2-consumption caused by administration of noradrenaline even with intravenous infusions in a neutral thermal environment (Scopes and Tizard 1963). Exposure to large concentrations of CO_2 decreased the rise in rectal temperature on administration of noradrenaline. The fact that both a fall in P_{O_2} and a rise in P_{CO_2} cause pulmonary vasoconstriction in the newborn has already been mentioned, but it is not known whether this is sufficiently great to reduce cardiac output and hence explain the phenomenon.

All the observations described in the last three paragraphs relate to the immediate effect of hypoxia on O_2-consumption in the cold. It might then be supposed that animals born at high altitude, in colder conditions and with a lower environmental P_{O_2}, than at sea level, would be at a disadvantage. This is probably true, yet Blatteis (1964) found no difference between the O_2-consumption of animals of several species born at high altitude in the Peruvian Andes and of those born in Lima at sea level. While hypoxia always caused an *immediate* fall in the O_2-consumption of newborn rabbits in a cold environment, when the exposure was continued the rate of O_2-consumption rose considerably over the next four hours; this rise was usually accompanied by the appearance of visible shivering. It is evident that newborn animals can adapt themselves to cold and hypoxia, but the extent to which this is possible needs measurement. Brück, Adams and Brück (1962) showed that young infants with chronic hypoxæmia (mainly due to cardiac malformations) could also respond to cold by an increase in O_2-consumption. Some species, such as the pig, are known to be particularly susceptible to cold exposure during the first week or two after birth under natural conditions. They are relatively small, have little thermal insulation and limited metabolic reserves (McCance and Widdowson 1959, Mount 1959). Most newborn animals and human infants survive because they are reared in favourable conditions (e.g. nests, burrows or bassinettes).

Carbohydrate and Fat Metabolism

Glycogen reserves. The changes in cardiac glycogen before and after birth have already been described (Fig. 8). Even more remarkable and rapid changes occur in liver glycogen. Fig. 15 shows that there is little glycogen in the liver early in gestation (Shelley 1961). But towards term there is a rise, more gradual in those species with a longer period of gestation (man 280 days; rhesus monkey 168 days) and more abrupt in those with a shorter gestation (rat 22 days; rabbit 31 days) to reach up to twice the normal adult concentration (of 40–60 mg./g.) at term. At birth the liver glycogen starts to fall very rapidly and usually reaches 10% or less of its initial value within a few hours. The level remains low for some days and only recovers over a period of 2–3 weeks even when suckling has been established within a few hours of birth. In the fœtus the blood glucose concentration is less than that of its mother but related to it, rising and falling as it rises and falls. After birth the animal is dependent on a limited supply of carbohydrate in the milk and on gluconeogenesis.

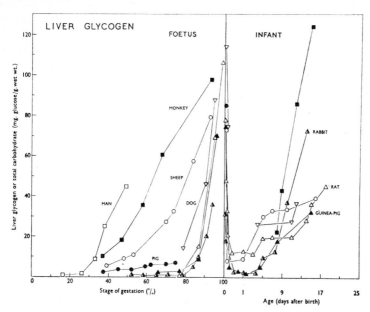

FIG. 15. Liver glycogen in different species before and after birth (Shelley 1961).

Large amounts of glycogen also accumulate in the skeletal muscles during gestation (Fig. 16). The concentration at term is greater in species with a longer period of gestation, which are born in a more mature condition and are more capable of vigorous muscular activity. Whereas newborn piglets have more than 70 mg./g., newborn rats have less than 13 mg./g. In all the species investigated the muscle glycogen at birth is on average at least twice the adult concentration, and falls to or below the adult value within 1–3 days. The greater the activity of the species at birth, the more rapid is the fall of muscle glycogen; it is slowest in the rat. The changes in the glycogen content of individual groups of muscles also is related to their activity after birth. Thus in monkeys suffering from severe respiratory distress the glycogen reserves of the diaphragm are almost wholly exhausted (Dawes, Jacobson, Mott, Shelley and Stafford 1963); the same is true of newborn human infants (Shelley 1964).

Large changes occur in the glycogen content of the lung during gestation. The concentration is low early in gestation. It rises to a peak of 15–35 mg./g., varying with different species. The peak is reached about halfway through gestation in those with long gestation periods, but only towards the end of gestation in the rabbit (31 days at term). The glycogen is concentrated in the alveolar epithelium of the fœtal lung, in which the concentration has been calculated to reach 75–78 mg./g. (Fauré-Fremiet and Dragoiu 1923). The fall in lung glycogen is associated with the loss of this epithelium, and coincides with the time at which the lungs can first be expanded.

Compared with the heart, liver, skeletal muscles and lungs the carbohydrate reserves of the brain are very small during fœtal life and after birth, 0·2–1·6 mg./g. Those of other fœtal tissues are intermediate, and the changes during gestation and at birth are not of immediate interest. In some species, such as the rabbit, the placenta contains large quantities of glycogen during the early part of gestation, but the significance of this is not known.

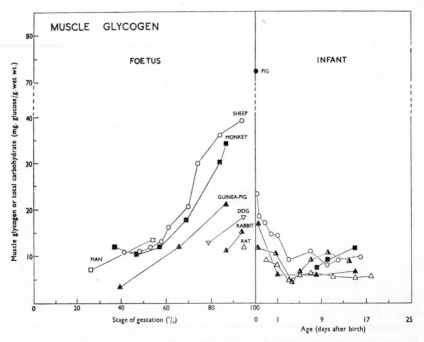

FIG. 16. Skeletal muscle glycogen in different species before and after birth (Shelley 1961).

Glycogen mobilisation and use. The large reserves of glycogen which are present in different tissues at different periods of gestation are ready sources of energy. In some tissues, such as the skeletal muscle, lung or kidney the glycogen is not mobilised to blood glucose during asphyxia. The glycogen in the liver is released during acute asphyxia or after birth, but the evidence available at present suggests that the mechanisms which control its release in the fœtus and newborn animal are less swift and precise than those in the adult. Thus administration of large doses of adrenaline or noradrenaline to fœtal lambs only caused a slow small rise in blood glucose; the same is true in the immediate newborn period, and also on injection of glucagon (Dawkins 1963). In newborn animals the blood glucose is often considerably lower than in adults of the same species, and it falls to negligible values in the terminal stages of the respiratory distress syndrome in lambs and monkeys.

A remarkable feature is the lack of pathognomonic signs of hypoglycæmia. (see also Chapter 5, p. 112, and Chapter 6, p. 139). Convulsive episodes are uncommon; the usual picture is that of extreme lethargy passing into a condition in which the animal cannot be aroused, and finally respiratory failure. We therefore have two questions to answer, why is the control of the blood sugar so imperfect in the newborn animal? and why does hypoglycæmia not produce symptoms as in the adult?

There is in late fœtal life a deficiency in one of the hepatic enzymes, glucose-6-phosphatase, which is concerned in glycogen mobilisation, but its activity increases by as much as thirtyfold soon after birth (Dawkins 1961). Enzyme deficiency does not explain the imperfect control of the blood sugar in the newborn.

Fat. The part played by fat in the metabolism of the newborn has received less attention (except in Czechoslovakia), probably because of the misconception that there is so little fat present at birth that it is negligible as an energy source. Yet human infants can survive without food for 5–6 days from birth and the carbohydrate reserves are clearly insufficient alone to provide the energy which must have been used. There is a large species variation, both in the ability to survive without food and in body fat content. In newborn piglets which are starved, 80% of the solids metabolised are carbohydrate (McCance and Widdowson 1959), but the pig seems to be a special case among large farm animals (Goodwin 1957). An abrupt rise in plasma free fatty acids has been demonstrated in the lamb and human infant at birth (Van Duyne and Havel 1959, Van Duyne, Parker, Havel and Holm 1960). In species such as the rabbit, guinea-pig and coypu the resources of fat are not inconsiderable and brown fat seems to be particularly important, (p. 26). During starvation infant rats use proportionately more fat than do older ones or adults (Hahn, Koldovský, Melichar and Novák 1961). In young rats reared in the cold little fat is laid down in the skin as compared with rats raised at 33°C (Vacek, Hahn and Koldovský 1961); this is just the opposite to what happens in the adult, and was attributed to the preferential use of fat in the food as an energy source. The magnitude and nature of the fat supply to the young rat during the weaning period has a considerable effect on its future growth (Hahn and Koldovský 1961). These and other observations have suggested that at birth the infant, which was formerly supplied with carbohydrate from its mother, now must turn over to the use of fat supplied in the milk as its major source of energy.

Conclusion

In the selection of material for a chapter of this kind, personal prejudices and interests play a large part. The topics chosen and the observations used to illustrate them are only a part of the very wide advances which are now being made in the physiology of late fœtal and early neonatal life. One of the objects of this chapter has been to justify by specific illustration, the conclusion that the general physiology of the newborn infant is in many important details different from that of the adult. The transition from fœtal life to independent existence is abrupt but the consequences persist for several weeks. Even at the end of that time we have an infant which is grossly different from an adult, smaller, less active, growing more rapidly and dependent on others for its food and warmth. So it should not be surprising that its physiological behaviour is different. Yet the infant is made of the same stuff as the adult, its fundamental physiology is the same, its enzymes are the same (though some may differ in concentration) and the differences in structure are in quantity rather than in quality. So it is with the differences in physiological mechanisms, which are truly quantitative variations on the adult pattern, though often of so large a degree as to appear to have a distinctive character.

REFERENCES

ADAMSONS, K. (1959) Breathing and the thermal environment in young rabbits. *J. Physiol.* **149**, 144

ADAMSONS, K., BEHRMAN, R. E., DAWES, G. S., DAWKINS, M. J. R., JAMES, L. S., ROSS, B. B. (1963) The treatment of acidosis with alkali and glucose during asphyxia in fœtal rhesus monkeys. *J. Physiol.* **169**, 679

ADAMSONS, K., BEHRMAN, R. E., DAWES, G. S., JAMES, L. S., KOFORD, C. B. (1964) Resuscitation by positive pressure ventilation and tris-hydroxymethylaminomethane of rhesus monkeys asphyxiated at birth. *J. Pediat.* (in press).

ALZAMORA, V., ROTTA, A., BATTILANA, G., ABUGATTAS, R., RUBIO, C., BOURONCLE, J., ZAPATA, C., SANTA-MARIÁ, E., BINDER, T., SUBIRIA, R., PAREDES, D., PANDO, B., GRAHAM, G. G. (1953) On the possible influence of great altitudes on the determination of certain cardiovascular anomalies. *Pediatrics*, **12**, 259

BARCLAY, A. E., FRANKLIN, K. J. (1938) The time of functional closure of the foramen ovale in the lamb. *J. Physiol.* **94**, 256

BARCLAY, A. E., FRANKLIN, K. J., PRICHARD, M. M. L. (1944) *The Foetal Circulation and Cardiovascular System, and the Changes that they Undergo at Birth.* Blackwell, Oxford

BARCROFT, J. (1946) *Researches on Prenatal Life.* Blackwell, Oxford

BARCROFT, J., FLEXNER, L. B., MCCLURKIN, T. (1934) The output of the fœtal heart in the goat. *J. Physiol.* **82**, 498

BARCROFT, J., KRAMER, K., MILLIKAN, G. A. (1939) The oxygen in the carotid blood at birth. *J. Physiol.* **105**, 22P

BARER, G. R. (1963) The circulation through collapsed adult lungs. *J. Physiol.* **168**, 10P

BLATTEIS, C. M. (1964) Hypoxia and the metabolic response to cold in new-born rabbits. *J. Physiol.* **172**, 358

BORN, G. V. R., DAWES, G. S., MOTT, J. C. (1955) The viability of premature lambs. *J. Physiol.* **130**, 191

BORN, G. V. R., DAWES, G. S., MOTT, J. C., RENNICK, B. R. (1956) Constriction of the ductus arteriosus caused by oxygen and by asphyxia in new-born lambs. *J. Physiol.* **132**, 304

BRÜCK, K. (1961) Temperature regulation in the newborn infant. *Biol. neonatorum.* **3**, 65

BRÜCK, K., ADAMS, F. H., BRÜCK, M. (1962) Temperature regulation in infants with chronic hypoxemia. *Pediatrics*, **30**, 350

BRÜCK, K., BRÜCK, M., LEMTIS, H. (1958) Thermoregulatorische Veränderungen des Energiestoffwechsels bei reifen Neugeborenen. *Pflüg.Arch. ges. Physiol.* **267**, 382

BURNARD, E. D. (1958) A murmur from the ductus arteriosus in the newborn baby. *Brit. med. J.* **1**, 806

BURNARD, E. D. (1963) Respiratory and cardiovascular changes in the immediate neonatal period, in *Modern Trends in Reproductive Physiology*—Carey, H. M., Butterworths, London

CASSIN, S., DAWES, G. S., MOTT, J. C., ROSS, B. B., STRANG, L. B. (1964) The vascular resistance of the fœtal and newly ventilated lung of the lamb. *J. Physiol.* **171**, 61.

CASSIN, S., DAWES, G. S., ROSS, B. B. (1964) Pulmonary blood flow and vascular resistance in immature fœtal lambs. *J. Physiol.* **171**, 80.

CHESLER, A., HIMWICH, H. E. (1944) Comparative studies of the rates of oxidation and glycolysis in the cerebral cortex and brain stem of the rat. *Amer. J. Physiol.* **141**, 513.

CONDORELLI, M., DAGIANTI, A., POLOSA, C., GUILIANO, G. (1957) Sulla persistenza di un fisiologico corto circuito attraverso il forame ovale nei primi giorni della vita extra uterina. *Atti Soc. ital. Cardiol.* XIX Congresso. **2**, 165

COOK, C. D., DRINKER, P. A., JACOBSON, H. N., LEVISON, H., STRANG, L. B. (1963) Control of pulmonary blood flow in the fœtal and newly born rabbit. *J. Physiol* **169**, 10

COTTLE, W. H., CARLSON, L. D. (1956) Regulation of heat production in cold adapted rats. *Proc. Soc. exp. Biol., N.Y.* **92**, 845

CROSS, K. W., KLAUS, M., TOOLEY, W. H., WEISSER, K. (1960) The response of the newborn baby to inflation of the lungs. *J. Physiol.* **151**, 551

CROSS, K. W., OPPÉ, T. E. (1952) The effect of inhalation of high and low concentrations of oxygen on the respiration of the premature infant. *J. Physiol.* **117**, 38.

CROSS, K. W., TIZARD, J. P. M., TRYTHALL, D. A. H. (1958) The gaseous metabolism of the newborn infant breathing 15% oxygen. *Acta pædiat.* **47**, 217

DALY, I. DE B., DALY, M. DE B. (1959) The effects of stimulation of the carotid body chemoreceptors on the pulmonary vascular bed in the dog: the "vasosensory controlled perfused living animal" preparation. *J. Physiol.* **148**, 201

DAWES, G. S. (1958) Changes in the circulation at birth and the effects of asphyxia, in *Recent Advances in Pœdiatrics*, 2nd Ed. ed. Gairdner, D., Churchill, London, p. 1

DAWES, G. S. (1961) Oxygen consumption and hypoxia in the newborn animal, in *Somatic Stability in the Newly Born, Ciba Foundation Symposium*, ed. Wolstenholme, G. E. W., O'Connor, M., Churchill, London

DAWES, G. S. (1962a) The umbilical circulation. *Amer. J. Obst. Gynec.* **84**, 1634

DAWES, G. S. (1962b) Vasodilatation in the unexpanded fœtal lung. *Med. thorac.* **19**, 153

DAWES, G. S., HIBBARD, E., WINDLE, W. F. (1964) Asphyxia at birth and brain damage. *J. Pediat.* (in press)

DAWES, G. S., JACOBSON, H. N., MOTT, J. C., SHELLEY, H. J., STAFFORD, A. (1963) The treatment of asphyxiated, mature fœtal lambs and rhesus monkeys with intravenous glucose and sodium carbonate. *J. Physiol.* **169**, 167

DAWES, G. S., MESTYÁN, G. (1963) Changes in the oxygen consumption of new-born guinea-pigs and rabbits on exposure to cold. *J. Physiol.* **168**, 22

DAWES, G. S., MOTT, J. C. (1959a) Reflex respiratory activity in the new-born rabbit. *J. Physiol.* **145**, 85

DAWES, G. S., MOTT, J. C. (1959b) The increase in oxygen consumption of the lamb after birth. *J. Physiol,* **146**, 295

DAWES, G. S., MOTT, J. C. (1962) The vascular tone of the fœtal lung. *J. Physiol.* **164**, 465

DAWES, G. S., MOTT, J. C. (1964) Changes in O_2 distribution and consumption in fœtal lambs with variations in umbilical blood flow. *J. Physiol.* **170**, 524

DAWES, G. S., MOTT, J. C., SHELLEY, H. J. (1959) The importance of cardiac glycogen for the maintenance of life in fœtal lambs and new-born animals during anoxia. *J. Physiol.* **146**, 516

DAWES, G. S., MOTT, J. C., STAFFORD, A. (1960) Prolongation of survival in the anoxic fœtal lamb. *J. Physiol.* **153**, 16P

DAWES, G. S., MOTT, J. C., WIDDICOMBE, J. G. (1955) Patency of the ductus arteriosus in newborn lambs and its physiological consequences. *J. Physiol.* **128**, 361

DAWES, G. S., MOTT, J. C., WIDDICOMBE, J. G., WYATT, D. G. (1953) Changes in the lungs of the newborn lamb. *J. Physiol.* **121**, 141

DAWKINS, M. J. R. (1963) Glycogen synthesis and breakdown in rat liver at birth. *Quart. J. exp. Physiol.* **48**, 265

DAWKINS, M. J. R., HULL, D. (1964) Brown fat and the response of the new-born rabbit to cold. *J. Physiol.* **172**, 216.

DUKE, H. N., LEE, G. DE J. (1963) The regulation of blood flow through the lungs. *Brit. med. Bull.* **19**, 71

VAN DUYNE, C. M., HAVEL, R. J. (1959) Plasma unesterified fatty acids concentration in fetal and neonatal life. *Proc. Soc. exp. Biol. N.Y.* **102**, 599

VAN DUYNE, C. M., PARKER, H. R., HAVEL, R. J., HOLM, L. W. (1960) Free fatty acid in serum of sheep. *Amer. J. Physiol.* **199**, 987

EDWARDS, J. E. (1959) Classification of pulmonary hypertension and anatomy of the postnatal and fetal pulmonary vascular bed, in *Pulmonary Circulation*, ed. Adams, W., Veith, I. Grune & Stratton, New York

EDWARDS, W. F. (1824) *De l'influence des agens physiques sur la vie*. Paris, Crochard

VON EULER, C., SÖDERBERG, V. (1958) Coordinated changes in temperature thresholds for thermoregulatory reflexes. *Acta physiol. Scand.* **42**, 112

VON EULER, U. S., LILJESTRAND, G. (1946) Observations on the pulmonary arterial blood pressure in the cat. *Acta physiol. Scand.* **12**, 301

FAURÉ-FREMIET, E., DRAGOIU, J. (1923) Le développement du poumon fœtal chez le mouton. *Arch. Anat. micr.* **19**, 411

FAZEKAS, J. F., ALEXANDER, F. A. D., HIMWICH, H. E. (1941) Tolerance of the newborn to anoxia. *Amer. J. Physiol.* **134**, 281

GELINEO, S. (1957) Développement ontogénétique de la thermorégulation chez le chien. *Bull. Acad. serbe. Sci.* **18**, 97

GOODWIN, R. F. W. (1957) The relationship between the concentration of blood sugar and some vital bodily functions in the new-born pig. *J. Physiol.* **136**, 208

GROVER, R. F., REEVES, J. T. (1962) Experimental induction of pulmonary hypertension in normal steers at high altitude. *Med. thorac.* **19**, 351

HAHN, P., KOLDOVSKÝ, O. (1961) The effect of individual nutrients on growth and carbohydrate formation in rats of different ages. *Physiol. Bohemoslov.* **10**, 481

HAHN, P., KOLDOVSKÝ, O., MELICHAR, V., NOVÁK, M. (1961) Quantitative and qualitative aspects of energy metabolism during postnatal development of the rat. *The Development of Homeostasis.* Publishing house of the Czechoslovak Academy of Sciences, Praha, p. 141

HICKS, S. P. (1953) Developmental brain metabolism. Effects of cortisone, anoxia, fluoroacetate, radiation, insulin and other inhibitors on the embryo, newborn and adult. *Arch. Path.* (*Lab. Med.*) **55**, 302

VAN HARREVELD, A., RUSSELL, F. E. (1956) Postnatal development of a left-right atrial pressure gradient. *Amer. J. Physiol.* **186**, 521

HILL, J. (1959) The oxygen consumption of new-born and adult mammals. Its dependence on the oxygen tension in the inspired air and on the environmental temperature. *J. Physiol.* **149**, 346

HIMWICH, H. E., BERNSTEIN, A. O., HERRLICH, H., CHESLER, A., FAZEKAS, J. F. (1942) Mechanisms for the maintenance of life in the newborn during anoxia. *Amer. J. Physiol.* **135**, 387

HIMWICH, F. E., FAZEKAS, J. F., HOMBURGER, E. (1943) Effect of hypoglycemia and anoxia on the survival period of infant and adult rats and cats. *Endocrinology* **33**, 96

HUGGETT, A. ST. G. (1927) Fœtal blood-gas tensions and gas transfusion through the placenta of the goat. *J. Physiol.* **62**, 373

HULL, D. (1964) Pronethacol and O_2 consumption in the newborn rabbit. *J. Physiol.* **173**, 13

JAMES, L. S., ROWE, R. D. (1957) The pattern of response of pulmonary and systemic arterial pressures in newborn and older children to short periods of hypoxia. *J. Pediat.* **51**, 5

KARLBERG, P., MOORE, R. E., OLIVER, T. K. (1962) The thermogenic response of the newborn infant to noradrenaline. *Acta pœdiat.* **51**, 284

KENNEDY, J. A., CLARK, S. L. (1941) Observations on the ductus arteriosus of the guinea-pig in relation to its method of closure. *Anat. Rec.* **79**, 349

KOVALČÍK, V. (1963) The response of the isolated ductus arteriosus to oxygen and anoxia. *J. Physiol.* **169**, 185

LEDUC, J. (1961) Catecholamines production and release in exposure and acclimation to cold. *Acta physiol scand.* **53**, Suppl. 183, 101

LIM, K. T., SNYDER, F. F. (1945) The effect of respiratory stimulants in the newborn infant. *Amer. J. Obstet. Gynec.* **50**, 146

LIND, J., WEGELIUS, C. (1954) Human fetal circulation: changes in the cardiovascular system at birth and disturbances in the post-natal closure of the foramen ovale and ductus arteriosus. *Cold Spr. Harb. Symp. quant. Biol.* **19**, 109

McCANCE, R. A., WIDDOWSON, E. M. (1959) The effect of lowering the ambient temperature on the metabolism of the new-born pig. *J. Physiol.* **147**, 124

McINTYRE, D. G., EDERSTOM, H. E. (1958) Metabolic factors in the development of homeothermy in dogs. *Amer. J. Physiol.* **194**, 293

MOORE, R. E., UNDERWOOD, M. (1962) Hexamethonium, hypoxia and heat production in new-born and infant kittens and puppies. *J. Physiol.* **161**, 30

MOORE, R. E., UNDERWOOD, M. (1963) The thermogenic effects of noradrenaline. in new-born and infant kittens and other small mammals. A possible hormonal mechanism in the control of heat production. *J. Physiol.* **168**, 290

MOTT, J. C. (1961) The ability of young mammals to withstand total oxygen lack. *Brit. med. Bull.* **17**, 144

MOTT, J. C. (1963) The effects of pressoreceptor and chemoreceptor stimulation on shivering. *J. Physiol.* **166**, 563

MOUNT, L. E. (1959) The metabolic rate of the new-born piglet in relation to environmental temperature and to age. *J. Physiol.* **147**, 333

PEÑALOZA, D., SIME, F., BANCHERO, N., GAMBOA, R. (1962) Pulmonary hypertension in healthy man born and living at high altitudes. *Med. thorac.* **19**, 257

RANCK, J. B., WINDLE, W. F. (1959) Brain damage in the monkey, Macaca mulatta, by asphyxia neonatorum. *Exp. Neurol.* **1**, 130

RECORD, R. G., McKEOWN, T. (1953) Observations relating to the ætiology of patent ductus arteriosus. *Brit. Heart J.* **4**, 376

REISS, M. (1931) Das Verhalten des Stoffwechsels bei der Erstickung neugeborener Ratten und Mäuse. *Z. ges. exp. Med.* **79**, 345

REYNOLDS, S. R. M. (1956) The fetal and neonatal pulmonary vasculature in the guinea pig in relation to hemodynamic changes at birth. *Amer. J. Anat.* **98**, 97

SANDLER, M., RUTHVEN, C. R. J. NORMAND, K. S., MOORE, R. E.   (1961) Environmental temperature and urinary excretion of 3-methoxy-4-hydroxymandelic acid in the new-born. *Lancet*, **280**, 485

SCOPES, J. W., TIZARD, J. P. M. (1963). The effect of intravenous noradrenaline on the oxygen consumption of new-born mammals. *J. Physiol.* **165**, 305

SHELLEY, H. J. (1961) Glycogen reserves and their changes at birth and in anoxia. *Brit. med. Bull.* **17**, 137

SHELLEY, H. J. (1964) Carbohydrate reserves in the newborn infant. *Brit. med. J.* **1**, 273

STAFFORD, A., WEATHERALL, J. A. (1960) The survival of young rats in nitrogen. *J. Physiol.* **153**, 457

STAHLMAN, M. T., MERRIL, R. E., LeQUIRE, V. S. (1962) Cardiovascular adjustments in normal newborn lambs. *Amer. J. Dis Child.* **104**, 360

TAYLOR, P. M. (1960) O$_2$ consumption in new-born rats. *J. Physiol.* **154**, 153

VACEK, Z., HAHN, P., KOLDOVSKÝ, O. (1961) The effect of rearing infant rats at three environmental temperatures on the structure of some of their organs. *J. Anat.* **95**, 210

VOGEL, J. H. K., WEAVER, W. F., ROSE, R. L., BLOUNT, S. G., GROVER, R. F. (1962) Pulmonary hypertension on exertion in normal man living at 10,150 feet (Leadville, Colorado). *Med. thorac.* **19**, 269

WINDLE, W. F. (1940) *The Physiology of the Fetus.* Saunders, Philadelphia

WRIGHT, R. W. (1962) Experimental pulmonary hypertension produced by recurrent air emboli. *Med. thorac.* **19**, 231

Figures 3–7, 10, 13, 14 are taken by permission from the *Journal of Physiology* and Figures 8, 15, 16 from *British Medical Bulletin*.

CHAPTER 2

RESPIRATORY AND CIRCULATORY ADAPTATION IN THE NEWBORN INFANT WITH PARTICULAR REFERENCE TO THE IMMEDIATE POSTNATAL PERIOD*

PETTER KARLBERG AND OLOV CELANDER

THE most urgent and therefore also the most critical adaptive changes after birth are those involved in the shift of gaseous exchange from the transplacental to the pulmonary route, a transition which has to be carried out by the newborn baby within a very brief period. Normally, it does this with marvellous facility—to the onlooker the baby just starts breathing, and the fact that its colour rapidly becomes pink is ample evidence that its circulation is now diverted to the new source for gaseous exchange. Failures are frequent, however, and still dominate early neonatal deaths. Such failures may arise from a variety of conditions and may proceed on quite different time scales, although in the long run they all have in common a "strangling" effect upon tissue metabolism.

In this chapter will be described how this crucial adaptation of the newborn baby is carried through and maintained; and also some of the risks that the baby may meet, but still succeed in overcoming, by physiological reserve mechanisms not normally called upon.

The Establishment of Pulmonary Gaseous Exchange

By the end of the neonatal period respiratory function, its mechanics, and its control by the central nervous system are all essentially the same as in the adult. The lungs are well aerated. The functional residual volume (of air left in his lungs at the end of normal expiration) is around 100 ml. (Geubelle, Karlberg, Kock, Lind, Wallgren and Wegelius 1959). The relative ratios of the various pulmonary volumes are essentially the same as those in the adult (Cook, Barrie and Avery 1960). The baby also needs about the same negative intrathoracic pressure change on inspiration (4–5 cm. H_2O). In pulmonary gas exchange the baby is about as successful in oxygen uptake, relative to the magnitude of ventilation, as the adult (Cook, Cherry, O'Brien Karlberg and Smith 1955). The functional demand, in terms of oxygen uptake, is however larger in relation to body size than in the adult. The baby's need for an increased pulmonary ventilation is mainly reflected as an increased rate of breathing, the relation between tidal volume and alveolar ventilation being adjusted in an economical way as later in life (Cook,

* This chapter should be read in conjunction with the previous one by G. S. Dawes, as the two chapters complement one another, with a good deal of common ground which is approached from two different standpoints—that of an experimental physiologist and that of a physiologically-minded clinician.—Editor

Sutherland, Segal, Cherry, Mead, McIlroy and Smith 1957). Although the baby has a considerable respiratory reserve, it seems as if this is smaller than in the adult.

In the uterus the fœtus is under a higher pressure than atmospheric. The pressure may increase further during uterine contractions but this can have little effect on the fœtus, so long as no part of the fœtus is in contact with the outside world. At the passage through the birth canal there may be a considerable compression of the thoracic cage (Borell and Fernström 1962), and as soon as the upper airways of the child come into contact with the outside this compression tends to express amniotic fluid. As the thoracic cage passes through, its elastic recoil will draw air into the upper airways and may also expand the lungs to some extent (Karlberg, Adams, Geubelle and Wallgren 1962). True aeration does not occur by this passive mechanism but it may be facilitated.

In the establishment of respiration the following vital steps have to be considered.

1. The lungs must become aerated, after which a certain amount of air will be left in the lungs, forming the residual capacity.

2. Alveolar ventilation must be initiated and maintained at a level corresponding to the metabolic demands of the body tissues. In this context the *distribution* of air amongst the alveoli is as important as the total amount of air inhaled or expelled at each breath.

3. Gas molecules must be able to diffuse through the separating membranes and fluid layers separated alveolar air from the interior of the red cells in the pulmonary capillaries. The rate of this movement of gas molecules mainly depends on the partial pressures, on the total alveolar-capillary surface area, and on the thickness of the separating layers (probably also on the surface area of the erythrocytes passing through the capillaries).

4. Pulmonary blood flow must be established at a rate which corresponds to the alveolar ventilation. Here also the *distribution* of blood flow is important, as well as the amount of blood diverted to the lungs per unit time.

5. Blood gas transport in the systemic circulation in terms of blood flow rates must be adjusted to the metabolic demands of the tissues.

All these steps in the uptake of O_2 and elimination of CO_2 are closely inter-related, although it is convenient to discuss them separately.

Aeration of the Lungs

Although expansion of the lungs may be prepared for by the events consequent on the passage through the birth canal, and probably also by those occurring in the upper airways just afterwards (Bosma, Lind and Grentz 1959), normal aeration of the lungs is entirely dependent on the first few breaths, initiated in the brain stem respiratory centres. The inspiratory muscle (mainly the diaphragm) must overcome, (1) the increasing elastic tension of expanding tissues involved, (2) the friction from flow of air and liquid through tubes of small calibres and from tissue movements, and (3) the cohesive forces developing at gas-liquid interphases in the air passages.

Fig. 1 shows three ciné-radiographs of the lungs and the thorax before and during the first breath (Geubelle, Karlberg, Koch, Lind, Wallgren and Wegelius

1959, Fawcitt, Lind and Wegelius 1960). It is evident from studies of this type that the aeration of the lungs is largely a consequence of the very first breath. This aeration is affected by the forceful contraction of the inspiratory muscles, mainly the diaphragm. Simultaneous recordings of the volume changes thus obtained, and the necessary intrathoracic pressure forces behind them, are illustrated in Fig. 2. The first prominent change after full delivery is the rapid development of a negative pressure. About 0·02 seconds later this pressure is translated into a considerable increase in the volume of the air spaces. Although individual variations are considerable, some common features are present. First, it is obvious that quite large pressure forces are operating. During inspiration there is a negative or "sucking" pressure of 20–70 cm. H_2O. In most instances this is followed by a positive pressure wave caused by an active expiration through partially obstructed upper airways; this positive-pressure may facilitate absorption of amniotic fluid by the pulmonary circulation. Frequently these pressure differences between inspiration and expiration exceed 100 cm. H_2O. The tidal volume of the first breath varies considerably, with a range of 20–80 ml., which means that it is some 2–3 times greater than an ordinary breath such as will be taken during quiet breathing later (20–25 ml.), but is smaller than the vital capacity, as measured by a forceful cry (120–150 ml.). It is also apparent from Fig. 2 that a large fraction of the first breath has remained in the lungs as a residual volume of air.

The resistance to aeration (or alternatively the readiness of the lungs to expand upon the first breath) is illustrated by the respiratory loops shown in Fig. 3, where the actual volume measured is plotted against a simultaneous recording of pressure (see also Chapter 3, p. 60). Although with such respiratory loops it is possible to calculate the increase in lung volume per unit increase in distending pressure, to give the distensibility or *compliance* of the structures involved, such measurements of lung compliance cannot be directly compared with the situation in older infants or adults, since lung compliance is related to the size of the individual. They are useful, however, in studying changes in the mechanics of aeration over a short period of time, such as the neonatal period (Karlberg and Koch 1962).

Here also we meet a great deal of individual variation. The upper loop in Fig. 3 represents one type, which shows what might be anticipated. There is no important volume change until a considerable pressure force has been developed; once such a force is operating, the "critical opening pressure" is overcome, air rushes into the air passages and lung volume rapidly increases. At the end of the first expiration a considerable fraction of this air is retained in the lungs as the residual capacity.

The situation illustrated in the lower loop of Fig. 3 is different. A large inspiratory volume change is here seen in response to a fairly low expanding pressure with no marked "opening pressure". Another difference is the fact that the lung volume at the end of expiration returns almost to the initial level. Thus the aeration of the lungs by the first breath is here much "easier" than in the first case. In those cases where aeration during the first breath has been "easy" there has always been a rapid expiratory volume change immediately before, suggesting a relationship to events preceding the first

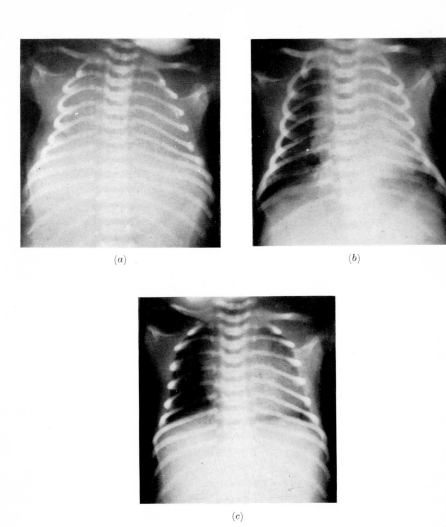

(a) (b)

(c)

Fig. 1 (a, b, c). Ciné-radiographs of the first breath; 2/3 seconds between each exposure (Karlberg 1960).

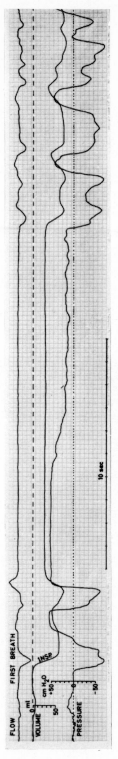

Fig. 2. Intrathoracic volume and pressure changes at initiation of breathing (Karlberg, Cherry, Escardo and Koch 1962).

breath. It seems that in these cases thoracic compression during delivery, followed by elastic recoil, has had a significant effect on amniotic fluid drainage (Karlberg, Adams, Geubelle and Wallgren 1962).

The total residual volume at the end of the first breath is ordinarily about 50–80 ml., i.e. about half that when aeration of the lungs is complete.

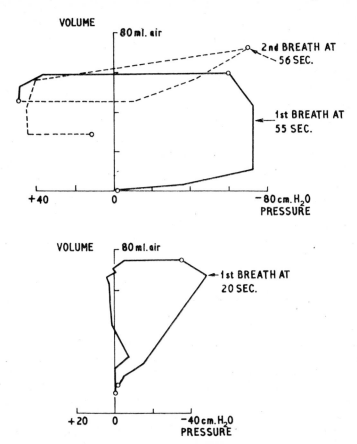

FIG. 3. Respiratory loops of the first breaths in two normal babies, showing widely differing patterns (see text) (Geubelle, Karlberg, Koch, Lind, Wallgren and Wegelius 1959).

During the following 10–20 minutes the functional residual capacity increases further, reaching about three-quarters that at final aeration. This means that the aeration of the lungs is established in the main very rapidly after birth. Ciné-radiographic studies have also shown that this rapid aeration is both even and stable, a phenomenon which is understandable in the light of our knowledge of the surface active material lining the alveolar walls (see Chapter 3, p. 67).

Although it is true that the first breath could be described as a forceful one, somewhat excessive emphasis has been placed on the forces necessary for the initiation of breathing, compared with the forces which may be operating in other types of respiratory activity. The mechanical work of respiration can be estimated if the volume change is related to the pressure change (see p. 60). Such measurements made later on in the neonatal period have shown that the respiratory work (in relation to inspiratory volume change) of the first few breaths is about equal to that during forceful crying later (Karlberg, Cherry, Escardo and Koch 1962). It has also been observed that a baby with a pleural drain after a thoracic operation, is capable of "sucking" pressures in the drain exceeding 100 cm. H_2O.

The Release of Respiration and Maintenance of Ventilation

The strong inspiratory efforts at the initiation of breathing and the further rhythmic activities of the ventilatory muscles are entirely dependent upon the brain-stem respiratory centres. Many years ago Barcroft and co-workers concluded that the release of breathing in the newborn is due to both sensory nervous stimuli and blood chemical changes. Work on man has clearly established that there is no one chemical or nervous stimulus to breathing. The ability of the brain-stem respiratory neurones to discharge is certainly dependent upon a large number of different influences. One group of such influences, converging upon the brain-stem centre, is nervous in origin. It has been shown by Burns (1963) that the excitability of the respiratory neurones is largely maintained by the non-specific impulse-traffic through the formatio reticularis, in which area the respiratory neurones are situated. Observations on adults during exercise indicate that the amount of outgoing impulse-traffic from the central nervous system relaying over the reticular formation also has such an "arousal" effect on the respiratory centres. Other studies performed on man (Bellville 1963) show that the responsiveness of the respiratory centre to CO_2 is greatly influenced by the state of wakefulness. Considering these mechanisms, there is probably no situation in human life in which there is a more sudden and dramatic change of sensory and motor impulse-traffic through the brain-stem than at birth itself. Before birth there is no effect of gravity, no thermal load, no light, and also the movements of the body are largely restricted. At birth all these types of non-specific nervous activities must increase immensely.

The situation in the brain-stem chemosensitive neurones and in the peripheral chemoreceptors before birth is difficult to ascertain. However, even if the O_2-saturation of blood coming from the placenta should be nearly complete, some mixing with systemic venous blood with a low O_2-tension seems inevitable before placental blood reaches the chemosensitive areas. On the other hand, there is little evidence to suggest that the foetal state is one of acidosis. Avery (1963, and unpublished) has suggested the importance of rhythmic changes in the CO_2-tension during breathing as a stimulus to respiration, so that the absence of such pulsatile changes during foetal life, when there is a steady release of CO_2 through the placenta, may be of significance.

To sum up, it seems that before birth the sum of all excitatory stimuli (nervous and chemical) is not high enough to bring the "central excitatory state" of respiratory brain-stem neurones to the point of spontaneous discharge.

We have already stressed the situation at birth whereby the sudden showers of excitatory impulses from non-respiratory sources probably exert a prominent "arousal" effect on the respiratory centres. What happens to the chemical stimuli in the circulating blood during the brief transitional period from a transplacental to an adequate pulmonary gaseous exchange? Certainly at the outset the situation at chemosensitive areas can differ little from that in the blood which flows from the placenta shortly after birth. From measurements of blood drawn from the umbilical vein a few seconds after birth, it appears that the CO_2-tension is normal or near normal, but that there is a more or less pronounced non-respiratory "metabolic" acidosis. O_2-tension is in the region of 35–40 mm.Hg (James and Burnard 1961, Rooth and Sjöstedt 1962, Wulf 1962, Engström, Karlberg, Rooth and Tunell 1964).

What is the situation in the respiratory centres? Probably, the O_2-transport to the centres is diminished by the trauma of birth. This may be one reason why the neurones in general do not immediately respond to a CO_2-tension, which later is fully capable of maintaining respiratory activity.

In a recent study (Engström, Karlberg, Rooth and Tunell 1964, Tunell, Engström, Karlberg and Moore, unpublished) the blood chemical changes in the arterial side of the systemic circulation have been followed by serial sampling during the first hour of life. The data thus obtained have been correlated with measurements of ventilation (Fig. 4). They confirm that arterial blood (below the ductus arteriosus) is hypoxic at birth. The O_2-saturation at the first sampling varies from 10 to 35%. CO_2-tension varies within wide limits. One important feature, however, is that during the first few minutes after birth CO_2-tension tends to increase further. The possibility that the child is subjected to some degree of hypoxia with disturbance of tissue metabolism is substantiated by a further lowering of the buffering power of blood, expressed as a negative *base excess*. The sum of hydrogen ion accumulation from respiratory and non-respiratory sources brings the pH to a low value.

Hypoxia of all degrees is believed to act depressively on the respiratory brain stem centres, but this is counteracted by the hypoxic drive of the chemoreceptors in the aortic arch and carotid bodies. The latter influence, combines with the excitatory effect of CO_2 (or hydrogen ion?) accumulation in the brain-stem, so that the arousal effect of sensory stimuli from non-respiratory sources is able to overcome the central depression of hypoxia and to bring the inspiratory neurones in the brain-stem to the point of extensive discharge. Previous assumptions from clinical impressions that the baby can initiate breathing without making use of these chemical stimuli are probably not correct. In the studies of blood chemistry referred to the changes described were observed in many cases before the first breath was taken.

Following the first breath the respiratory pattern tends for a time to be that of a succession of irregular single breaths. It looks as if further acidotic changes must occur before continuous regular breathing takes over. Following the first few breaths CO_2 may accumulate further, or a further accumulation of CO_2 may just be prevented. In spite of this, the hydrogen ion concentration increases further, and it appears as if the start of regular respiration

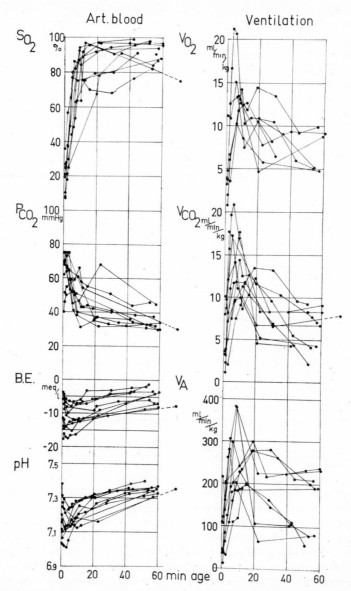

FIG. 4. Repeated sampling of arterial blood and ventilatory data during the first hour of life. Arterial O_2-saturation, P_{CO_2}, base excess, and pH; the volume of O_2 taken up, the volume of CO_2 excreted, and the volume of alveolar ventilation are shown.

with medium tidal volume does not in general occur unless the acidity of the blood has reached a level between pH $7 \cdot 2$–$7 \cdot 1$.

Another interesting observation in these studies has been the relation between O_2-tension in arterial blood and the point where the falling buffer base begins to rise. Or to stress the point—at what O_2-tension does "necro-chemistry" turn into "biochemistry"? It has been found that as long as O_2-tension is below about 35–40 mm.Hg, available buffer base gradually declines, whereas above this level buffer base gradually returns to normal values irrespective of how long after birth this change may take place. Repair of the metabolic acidosis takes a considerable time, and is in general not completed within the first hour of life.

Measurements of ventilatory data such as O_2 uptake and CO_2 elimination show that pulmonary ventilation rapidly becomes effective for gas exchange. During the first few minutes the ventilatory performance of the lungs rapidly increases and during the first 20 minutes most of the accumulated CO_2 is being blown off and the oxygen debt resulting from birth is being repaid.

At this stage an entirely new situation exists as to the chemical control of respiration. The newborn baby now has a high level of arterial O_2. The responsiveness of the respiratory centres to CO_2 and other possible influences is thereby raised, and regular breathing continues despite a falling CO_2-tension, until a new steady state is established via the feed-back system by means of which the blood gases control the magnitude of ventilation.

One may speculate further that the first breath, once elicited, will have such an effect on CO_2 elimination (due to the sudden aeration of the lungs), that in the respiratory centre there will be a rapid decrease in CO_2-tension to a sub-threshold level. CO_2 soon re-accumulates to provide excitation, but only to initiate a type of respiration which is not effective enough in terms of O_2 uptake either to provide sufficient O_2 to the centre, or to relieve the depression of tissue metabolism. Thus metabolic acidosis increases further, the sum of "chemical" stimuli is kept high and regular breathing is triggered off. O_2 uptake now becomes more effective, and the O_2-tension at the respiratory centre increases. The previous depression is relieved and the centre continues to discharge, despite a decrease in CO_2-tension and other "chemical" stimuli.

The variable degree of metabolic acidosis at birth may be one reason for the great variation in the pattern of establishment of breathing. Three types of situation may be considered.

Firstly, in a baby born by elective cæsarean section, the apnœic period often noted after the first one or two breaths may be explained by the presence of a normal P_{CO_2}, and the absence of any considerable metabolic acidosis. There are thus insufficient chemical stimuli coming to the respiratory centre to trigger off breathing, and some delay is required for them to build up. Clinically, therefore, the temporary apnœic phase may engender an alarm which is groundless.

Secondly, during a spontaneous delivery where there has been some complication causing impaired fœtal gas exchange, the fœtus develops both a metabolic and a respiratory acidosis. In spite of a low P_{O_2}, the chemical stimuli will be considerable, so that the baby may well start to breathe regularly immediately after birth. Clinically, such a baby may be assessed as in good condition, yet may run into difficulties later on account of the metabolic acidosis.

Finally, in a baby with a much more severe degree of hypoxia, hypercapnia and metabolic acidosis, the chemical milieu is too deranged for breathing to be initiated, and the baby will deteriorate further during apnœa. This situation requires active interference, such as positive pressure breathing.

Gas Diffusion in the Lungs

Practically nothing is known about this in the first few minutes of life and the following speculations are entirely based upon the morphological background for diffusion and the clinical impressions from everyday neonatal problems.

The capacity of the lungs for gas diffusion depends amongst other things on the magnitude of the total alveolar-capillary surface area, the thickness and properties of the separating fluids and membranes, and upon the partial pressures of the gases on each side. The quantity and the quality of the functioning alveolar-capillary area is one of the factors deciding whether or not the newborn makes the transition from transplacental to pulmonary gas exchange successfully. Maturity of pulmonary structures will effect both. Obviously there must be a critical point where there is simply insufficient area effective for diffusion, while at the same time the need for gaseous exchange is proportionally higher per unit weight the more immature the fœtus is. To this unfavourable situation may be added the lack of surface active material in the alveolar cells of the immature lung (Chapter 3, p. 68) which will further reduce the area available for diffusion. Increased thickness of the alveolar epithelium and capillary endothelium will slow down the diffusion processes. Not only is the diffusion of blood gases impaired under these circumstances, but the transport of amniotic fluid into the pulmonary circulation may also be retarded.

As in all diffusion problems O_2-tension is much more affected than is CO_2-tension, owing to the much more rapid diffusion of CO_2.

Pulmonary Blood Flow

After birth there is an opening up of blood vessels in the lungs and a rapid increase of blood flow to the lungs (see also Chapter 1, p. 6).

It has already been shown (p. 38) that considerable pressure forces are operating in the thoracic cavity at the initiation of breathing. The magnitude of these pressures is striking when compared to pressures within the circulatory system, more especially on the venous side of the systemic circulation. The effect of a sudden negative pressure in the thorax is to suck blood as well as air into the thoracic cavity. Lind and Wegelius (1954) have also shown, by means of ciné-radiology and dye injection into the umbilical vein, that the circulation converts suddenly from the fœtal type via foramen ovale to a pulmonary route during the first inspiration. During inspiration there is a significant decrease in the heart size, while during the following active expiration the heart size increases. The systemic blood pressure shows similar rhythmic fluctuations (Wallgren, Karlberg and Lind 1960). These rhythmic changes during the breathing cycles indicate that the mechanical events associated with the initiation of breathing must have important influences on both the pulmonary and the systemic circulations. These mechanisms have aptly been called the "auxiliary heart."

On the other hand it is also known that the resistance of the pulmonary circulation is largely influenced by local gas tensions in the air passages. Recent studies on newborn lambs (Cook, Drinker, Jacobson, Levison and Strang 1963) have shown a marked fall in the pulmonary vascular resistance upon exposure of the pulmonary vascular bed to a high O_2- or to a low CO_2-tension. In this context it should be recalled that changes in gas tensions in the lung at the first few breaths are more profound than at any later stage, the first gas reaching the alveoli being pure air.

In the sudden aeration of the alveoli which causes the increased pulmonary circulation, it is mechanical factors that seem to play initially the dominant rôle, but changes in gas tensions probably rapidly become important. This part of the subject clearly needs further elucidation.

With the ductus arteriosus still open the pressure difference between the pulmonary artery and the aorta will direct the blood flow through the ductus and will thus also influence the pulmonary blood flow. That the initial drop in pulmonary vascular resistance may take some time is evident from the clinical observation that in newborn infants who are somewhat slow to establish breathing, the skin is often pink in the upper part of the body in contrast to a more or less cyanotic lower part. As respiration improves, this differential cyanosis disappears. Catheterisation studies in newborn infants (Saling 1960) have shown that there is a right-to-left or bidirectional shunt, at least during the first half hour, which later changes to a left-to-right shunt (Adams and Lind 1957, Rudolph, Drorbaugh, Auld, Rudolph, Nadas and Smith 1961, Moss, Emmanouilides and Duffie 1963). There are, however, great individual variations, and the respiratory cycle has a significant influence on such shunts, especially during crying. In general, there is probably during the first few minutes a gradual decrease in pulmonary vascular resistance, coinciding with an increasing aeration of the lungs and improved blood gas conditions.

The magnitude of the pulmonary blood flow also depends on the patency of the ductus arteriosus. Apparently the main cause of the closure of the ductus is the high O_2-tension in arterial blood after breathing has begun, with a purely local myogenic response of the smooth muscle cells in the ductus. When the decrease in pulmonary vascular resistance reaches a certain level, the shunt in the ductus will be predominantly left-to-right. With good arterial O_2-saturation the ductus will constrict gradually, until the shunting of blood either becomes physiologically insignificant or ceases entirely. Moss, Emmanouilides and Duffie (1963) have found this to happen at approximately 15 hours of age, while Jegier, Blankenship and Lind (1963) found it to take several days.

Pulmonary vascular resistance continues to decrease, as indicated by the gradually decreasing pulmonary artery pressure, up to the age of about one week (Rowe and James 1957). Here also there are great individual variations.

There is an associated gradual decrease in the thickness of the muscular coat and elastic fibres of the pulmonary arterioles.

How is the distribution of blood flow within the lungs regulated to match the distribution of alveolar ventilation? That is, what are the mechanisms by which local ventilation to perfusion ratios are adjusted? Since the aeration of alveoli and opening up of corresponding pulmonary capillaries are likely to be caused initially by the same mechanical factor, a gross adaptation in this respect seems possible from mainly mechanical forces. On the other hand, since the over-all pulmonary vascular resistance is known to be sensitive to the composition of alveolar air, the same mechanisms may operate locally, so as to adjust pulmonary blood flow to the prevailing alveolar ventilation. Such a mechanism would tend to direct pulmonary blood flow to areas of good ventilation and prevent blood from reaching areas where little gas exchange is occurring. Probably maldistribution alone, or combined with maldiffusion, is the main disturbance of pulmonary function in the immediate postnatal period.

In this connection there exists a possible physiological "reserve" mechanism. Should oxygenation of the arterial blood be deficient, the ductus arteriosus may not close completely and blood will recirculate into the pulmonary circulation, with several possible consequences. The pressure in the pulmonary artery may remain high, thereby promoting further opening up of pulmonary capillaries; unsaturated blood entering the left atrium has a further chance of picking up more oxygen during the next pulmonary transit. Clinical as well as angiocardiographic evidence indicates that the ductus closure may be delayed in postnatal hypoxic states.

The closure of the foramen ovale is probably simply a consequence of the increase of pulmonary blood flow and the resulting increase in the left atrial pressure relative to the right (see Dawes 1958). It has also been claimed that prominent shunting through the foramen ovale may exist, especially if laboured breathing or crying leads to more pronounced pressure changes within the thorax.

For completeness it may be mentioned that the third shunt during fœtal life, that through the ductus venosus between portal vein and inferior vena cava, seems to have no significance after the placental circulation has ceased (Jegier, Blankenship and Lind 1963).

Gas Transport in the Systemic Circulation

The counterpart to gas exchange in the lungs is a corresponding exchange in the reverse direction in the various parallel coupled circuits in the systemic circulation. Of prime importance is the fact that circulatory stability, in terms of a normal or nearly normal blood pressure, must be maintained to guarantee an adequate pressure head for blood perfusion of the most vital areas, namely the central nervous system and the myocardium. To achieve this, in spite of a perhaps severely depressed cardiac output or an acute loss of circulating blood volume, the body must possess effective control mechanisms over the vascular bed. Various sensory reflex mechanisms converge, once again in the brain-stem, over the vasomotor centre. The main effector mechanism is the sympathetic outflow of vasoconstrictor nerve fibres to all areas. The fact that the newborn infant is able to withstand the dramatic stresses and changes in circulation at birth strongly suggests that these mechanisms are fully active.

Large changes in the blood volume occur during the immediate postnatal period. There is at normal delivery a significant shift of blood from the placenta to the newborn infant, when about a quarter of the final blood volume is transferred to the baby. This seems to take place very rapidly at and after birth, a large proportion of the total being transferred during the first minute of life (Gunther 1957, Secher and Karlberg, 1962, Usher, Shephard and Lind 1963).

In spite of this rapid change in blood volume and the sudden cessation of the placental circulation, the systemic blood pressure is kept surprisingly constant during quiet breathing. The expected rise is barely noticeable in records of arterial blood pressure (Wallgren, Karlberg and Lind 1960, Ashworth and Neligan 1959). After 10–15 minutes there is, however, a gradual decrease in pressure by 10–15 mm.Hg over the following 1–2 hours. On the second or third day the pressure starts to increase again. The pulse rate follows the same pattern (Contis and Lind 1963).

An intriguing adaptive change is the increase in heart size shortly after birth. After about 15 minutes the heart size starts to decrease again, most markedly during the first hours and continuing during the first week of life (Lind and Wegelius 1954, Kjellberg, Rudhe and Zetterström 1954).

Cardiac output in the immediate postnatal period has not been possible to assess. The ability of the myocardium to withstand oxygen lack is related to its glycogen content, as has been convincingly shown in animal experiments. The increase in heart size which normally occurs after birth may be exaggerated by prolonged asphyxia (Burnard and James 1963). It is difficult to say what such cardiac dilatation really means, but it seems likely that it indicates impairment of the working conditions of the heart muscle. Studies on newborn infants in the first days of life have shown that a moderate lowering of oxygen concentration in inspired air down to 12% may cause severe cardiac disturbances (Berg and Celander unpublished). Such observations are illustrated in Fig. 5. Upon gradual lowering the O_2-concentration in inspired air a slight tachycardia was noticed at approximately the level of 14% O_2. A further lowering down to 12% brought about a sudden reduction of heart rate to half the initial figure. This change occurred abruptly and could be explained by a nodal block. One conclusion that may be drawn from this observation is that the performance of the heart can be disturbed by quite a moderate degree of hypoxia.

Quantitative measurements of blood flow rates in parts of the systemic circulation during the immediate postnatal period have shown marked reductions of flow rates in the extremities (for references see Celander and Mårild 1962, a and b). Normally this phase is short, but it may be prolonged for hours or even days in a baby who has had a difficult delivery or who has been asphyxiated at birth. In the case shown in Fig. 6 blood pressure determinations revealed nothing striking; nevertheless, dramatic alterations of peripheral circulation were taking place beneath this "silent surface" of a normal blood pressure level, the rate of blood flow in the foot and calf

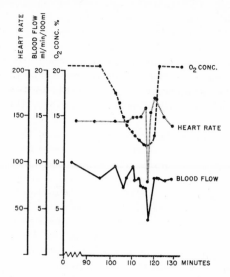

FIG. 5. Changes in heart rate and in peripheral blood flow in response to a gradual lowering of O_2-concentration of inspired air (see text) (Berg, K. and Celander, O., unpublished data).

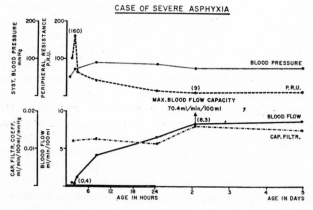

FIG. 6. Peripheral circulation in a newborn baby recovering from severe asphyxia (Berg, K. and Celander, O., unpublished data).

being cut down almost to nil. Calculations of the peripheral resistance in this part of systemic circulation came out at the extraordinarily high level of 160 PRU (peripheral resistance units). Measurements in this baby also illustrate the very wide range of possible flow rates. The rate of blood flow when the baby was in normal condition at the age of two days was around 8 ml./min./100 ml. of tissue. During the first few hours of life it was as low as 0·4 ml./min./100 ml. When the maximal flow capacity was explored by inducing a reactive hyperæmia by a 10 minutes arrest of circulation, the dilated blood vessels of the limb permitted flow rates up to 70 ml./min./100 ml. Measurements of this kind show that, when the child for some reason is incapable of successfully adapting to extra-uterine life, reductions in peripheral circulation must readily lead to further hypoxic damage to the tissues. Mechanisms controlling the vascular bed must, therefore, during these circumstances play an important rôle.

The Metabolic Cost of Extra-uterine Adaptation

In the newborn, energy is needed to maintain basal metabolism and to meet the many new activities such as breathing and the regulation of body temperature on exposure to a colder environment. (A metabolic response to low environmental temperature is already demonstrable in the first hour of life, Brück 1961). During the period of postnatal adaptation the newborn infant has to rely upon his own body reserves, mainly carbohydrate and fat, which can be oxidized with the production of biologically useful energy. Some tissues, such as the brain and the myocardium, are dependent on carbohydrate which they may get from their own sources or from the liver. The fall in blood glucose after birth (see Chapter 5) indicates the difference between the rates at which glucose is added to and removed from the blood. In states of oxygen lack glucose may be oxidised anaerobically, but this pathway is highly uneconomical and only generates about 5% of the potential energy in each glucose molecule. This is clearly an emergency wastage of available fuel.

Free fatty acids (FFA) liberated from depôt fat, probably constitute the second principal transport form of fuel which is available for the metabolic needs of the newborn. If oxygen is available, FFA will enter the tissue cells to be oxidised to CO_2 and water. That fat metabolism has to be increasingly used during the first adaptive period is indicated by the decreasing respiratory quotient during the first days of life. After about the third day, when the food intake has become significant, the RQ begins to rise again (Cross, Tizard and Trythall 1958, for further references see Karlberg 1952).

The liberation of glucose from liver glycogen and of FFA from depôt fat are both known to be influenced by catechol amines, in the newborn predominantly noradrenaline. It is also known that the administration of noradrenaline to a newborn will produce a metabolic response in terms of an increase in O_2-consumption (Karlberg, Moore and Oliver 1962). The physiological significance of these mechanisms is difficult to judge. It is, however, interesting to note that in animal experiments the release of catechol amines from the adrenal medulla is greatly increased in states of severe asphyxia (Celander 1954), although Stern, Leduc and Lind (1964) have not been able to show any significant catecholamine excretion in newborn infants on brief exposures to 10% O_2.

It is obvious from these considerations that energy release will be severely limited by lack of oxygen. If hypoxia is a consequence of pulmonary disorder, it will lead to a further costly expenditure of work from laboured breathing, and a vicious circle is apt to follow, because hypoxia will itself limit the work of respiratory muscles (see Chapter 3, p. 73).

Clinical Appreciation

The underlying cause of neonatal respiratory failure may be: neuro-muscular failure; failure of aeration and alveolar ventilation; failure of pulmonary circulation; or failure of systemic circulation.

Neuromuscular failure. Malformation of the central nervous system or depression from trauma, congenital infection, intra-uterine asphyxia or depressive effects of drugs given to the mother, may all cause central nervous system depression.

Failure of aeration and alveolar ventilation. These may be caused by airway obstruction at any level, and from either intrinsic or extrinsic causes. The commonest clinical condition is failure to drain amniotic fluid contaminated with meconium. Extra-pulmonary space-occupying conditions in the thorax, such as diaphragmatic hernia, pneumothorax or pneumomediastinum, may have similar mechanical consequences.

Failure of pulmonary circulation. Except in transposition of the great vessels or atresia of the pulmonary artery, an inadequate pulmonary circulation is probably rarely the prime cause of respiratory failure. But distur-bances of the pulmonary circulation at capillary level may be commoner than it is now possible to prove, and could be responsible for the respiratory distress syndrome in prematures (see Chapter 3, p. 69).

Failure of systemic circulation. Present methods rarely allow precise diagnoses of cardio-vascular disorders in the immediate postnatal period. While the clinician is often faced with a newborn baby in the state which he recognises as "shock," that is, with hypotension and marked peripheral vasoconstriction, he is unlikely to be in a position to determine whether this state has arisen primarily from disorder of the nervous system, of the circul-atory system, or of the respiratory system.

In Fig. 7 we have tried to illustrate the inter-relationships between the three main systems upon which a successful adaptation at birth must depend. Although one of the systems may have been primarily at fault, depression of the remaining systems must follow and give rise to a state of general depression, rendering elucidation of the original cause often im-possible.

There is no single key which makes it possible to enter into and effectively break the vicious circle illustrated in Fig. 7. At the present time little can be done to improve the responsiveness of the central nervous system, except by restoring respiratory and circulatory functions. Where pulmonary function is at fault, intubation and positive pressure breathing is logical. It is still not possible to assess the value of hypothermia (Westin, Nyberg, Wedenberg and Miller 1962) or the use of buffering substances such as THAM (pp. 21, 76).

The transfusion of arterialised blood is an interesting approach which may prove to be of real value (Westin et al. 1962).

Rapid determinations of blood pH, CO_2-tension and the degree of metabolic acidosis have taken a place as routine procedures. Such determinations, especially when made serially, are valuable in assessing the severity of the condition and the effect of therapeutic measures, and so further the handling of the case. Radiography of heart and lungs similarly provides a most valuable adjunct to the information given by clinical examination. In both chemical and radiological investigations the necessary equipment is twice as valuable if close to the delivery department.

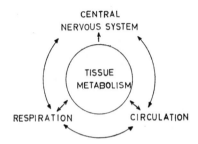

Fig. 7. Possible inter-relationships between central nervous system, respiration, circulation and tissue metabolism.

Conclusion

The present review is concentrated upon recent work in the field of normal neonatal physiology. Much progress has been made during the last decade and more can be expected in the years to come, as research in this field is flourishing at a steadily increasing number of units all over the world. This study of the normal is essential, if we are to understand why and how failures of adaptation occur. Furthermore, the time of fixed regimes and trials has come to an end, to be replaced by more careful and detailed clinical and laboratory study of the individual newborn baby.

REFERENCES

ADAMS, F. H., LIND, J. (1957) Physiologic studies on the cardiovascular status of normal newborn infants (with special references to the ductus arteriosus). *Pediatrics*, **19**, 431

ASHWORTH, A., NELIGAN, G. (1959) Changes in the systolic blood-pressure of normal babies during the first twenty-four hours of life. *Lancet*, **1**, 804

AVERY, M. E. (1963) Transact. Interdisciplinary Conference on Neonatal Respiratory Adaptation. Nat. Inst. Child Health and Human Development, Princeton

BELLVILLE, J. W. (1963) Communication at the 2nd Int. Pharmacological Meeting in Prague

BERG, K., CELANDER, O. Unpublished data

BORELL, U., FERNSTRÖM, I. (1962) The shape of the fœtal chest during its passage through the birth canal. A radiographic study. *Acta obstet. gynec. scand.* **41**, 213

BOSMA, J., LIND, J., GENTZ, N. (1959) Motions of the pharynx associated with initial aeration of the lungs of the newborn infant. *Acta pœdiat. Suppl.* **48**, 117

BRÜCK, K. (1961) Temperature regulation in the newborn infant. *Biol. Neonat.* **3**, 65

BURNARD, E. D., JAMES, S. (1963) Atrial pressures and cardiac size in the newborn infant. Relationships with degree of birth asphyxia and size of placental transfusion. *J. Pediat.* **62**, 815

BURNS, B. D. (1963) The central control of respiratory movements. *Brit. med. Bull.* **19,** 7

CELANDER, O. (1954) The range of control exercised by the "sympathicoadrenal system." A quantitative study on blood vessels and other smooth muscle effectors in the cat. *Acta physiol. scand.* **32,** *Suppl.* 6

CELANDER, O. (1963) Respiration och cirkulation. II. *Svenska Läk.-Tidn.* **60,** 3583

CELANDER, O., MÅRILD, K. (1962) Reactive hyperæmia in the foot and calf of the newborn infant. *Acta pœdiat.* **51,** 544

CELANDER, O., MÅRILD, K. (1962) Regional circulation and capillary filtration in relation to capillary exchange in the foot and calf of the newborn infant. *Acta pœdiat.* **51,** 385

CONTIS, G., LIND, J. (1963) Study of systolic blood pressure, heart rate, body temperature of normal newborn infants through the first week of life. *Acta pœdiat.* **52,** Suppl. 146, 41

COOK, C. D., CHERRY, R. B., O'BRIEN, D., KARLBERG, P. SMITH, C. A. (1955) Studies of respiratory physiology in the newborn infant. I. Observations on normal premature and full-term infants. *J. clin. Invest.* **34,** 975

COOK, C. D., SUTHERLAND, J. M., SEGAL, S., CHERRY, R. B., MEAD, J., McILROY, M. B., SMITH, C. A. (1957) Studies of respiratory physiology in the newborn infant: Measurements of mechanics of respiration. *J. clin. Invest.* **36,** 440

COOK, C. D., BARRIE, H., AVERY, M. E. (1960) Respiration and respiratory problems of the newborn infant. *Advanc. Pediat.* **9,** 11

COOK, C. D., DRINKER, P. A., JACOBSON, H. N., LEVISON, H., STRANG, L. B. (1963) Control of pulmonary blood flow in the fœtal and newly born lamb. *J. Physiol.* **169,** 10

CROSS, K. W., TIZARD, J. P. M., TRYTHALL, D. A. H. (1958) The gaseous metabolism of the newborn infant breathing 15% oxygen. *Acta pœdiat.* **47,** 217

DAWES, G. (1958) Changes in the circulation at birth and the effects of asphyxia, in *Recent Advances in Pœdiatrics,* 2nd Ed., ed. Gairdner, D., Churchill, London, p. 15

ENGSTRÖM, L., KARLBERG, P., ROOTH, G., TUNELL, R. (1964) The onset of respiration. A study of respiration and changes in blood gases and acid base balance (to be published)

FAWCITT, J., LIND, J., WEGELIUS, C. (1960) The first breath. A preliminary communication describing some methods of investigations of the first breath of a baby and the results obtained from them. *Acta pœdiat.* **49,** Suppl. 123

GEUBELLE, F., KARLBERG, P., KOCH, G., LIND, J., WALLGREN, G., WEGELIUS, C. (1959) L'aération du poumon chez le nouveau-né. *Biol. Neonat.* **1,** 169

GUNTHER, M. (1957) The transfer of blood between baby and placenta in the minutes after birth. *Lancet,* **1,** 1277

JAMES, L. S., BURNARD, E. D. (1961) Biochemical changes occurring during asphyxia at birth and some effects on the heart, in *Somatic Stability in the Newly Born (Ciba Found. Symp.)* Churchill, London

JEGIER, W., BLANKENSHIP, W., LIND, J. (1963) Venous pressure in the first hour of life and its relationship to placental transfusion. *Acta pœdiat.* **52,** 485

KARLBERG, P. (1952) Determinations of standard energy metabolism (basal metabolism) in normal infants. *Acta pœdiat.* **41,** Suppl. 89

KARLBERG, P. (1960) The adaptive changes in the immediate postnatal period, with particular reference to respiration. *J. pediat.* **56,** 585

KARLBERG, P., ADAMS, F. H., GEUBELLE, F., WALLGREN, G. (1962) Alteration of the infant's thorax during vaginal delivery. Physiological studies. *Acta obstet. gynec. scand.* **41,** 223

KARLBERG, P., CHERRY, R. B., ESCARDO, F. E., KOCH, G. (1962) Respiratory studies in newborn infants. II. Pulmonary ventilation and mechanism of breathing in the first minutes of life, including the onset of respiration. *Acta pœdiat.* **51,** 121

KARLBERG, P., KOCH, G. (1962) Respiratory studies in newborn infants. III. Development of mechanics of breathing during the first week of life. A longitudinal study. *Acta pœdiat. Suppl.* **135,** 121

KARLBERG, P., MOORE, R. E., OLIVER, T. (1962) The response of the newborn infant to noradrenaline. *Acta pœdiat.* **51,** 284

KJELLBERG, S. R., RUDHE, U., ZETTERSTRÖM, R. (1954) Heart volume variations in neonatal period. I. Normal infants. *Acta pœdiat.* **42,** 173

LIND, J., WEGELIUS, C. (1954) Human fetal circulation: changes in the cardiovascular system at birth and disturbances in the postnatal closure of the foramen ovale and ductus arteriosus. *Cold Spr. Harb. Symp. quant. Biol.* **19,** 109

MOSS, A. J., EMMANOUILIDES, G., DUFFIE, E. R. (1963) Closure of the ductus arteriosus in the newborn infant. *Pediatrics,* **32,** 25

ROOTH, G., SJÖSTEDT, S. (1962) The placental transfer of gaseous and fixed acids. *Arch. Dis. Childh.* **37**, 366

ROWE, R. D., JAMES, L. S. (1957) The normal pulmonary arterial pressure during the first year of life. *J. Pediat.* **51**, 1

RUDOLPH, A. M., DRORBAUGH, J. E., AULD, P. A. M., RUDOLPH, A. J., NADAS, A. S., SMITH, C. A., HUBBELL, J. P. (1961) Studies on the circulation in the neonatal period. The circulation in the respiratory distress syndrome. *Pediatrics*, **27**, 551

SALING, E. (1960) Neue Untersuchungsergebnisse über den Kreislauf des Kindes unmittelbar nach der Geburt. *Arch. Gynäk.* **194**, 287

SECHER, O., KARLBERG, P. (1962) Placental blood-transfusion for newborns delivered by Cæsarean section. *Lancet*, **1**, 1203

STERN, L., LEDUC, J., LIND, J. (1964) Hypoxia as a stimulus to catecholamine excretion in the newborn infant. *Acta pædiat.* **53**, 13

TUNELL, R., ENGSTRÖM, L., KARLBERG, P., MOORE, R. E., unpublished

USHER, R., SHEPHARD, M., LIND, J. (1963) The blood of the newborn infant and placental transfusion. *Acta pædiat.* **52**, 497

WALLGREN, G., KARLBERG, P., LIND, J. (1960) Studies of the circulatory adaptation immediately after birth. *Acta pædiat.* **49**, 843

WESTIN, B., NYBERG, R., WEDENBERG, E., MILLER, J. A. (1962) Hypothermia and transfusion with oxygenated blood in the treatment of asphyxia neonatorum. *Acta pædiat.* **51**, Suppl. 139, 1962

WULF, H. (1962) Der Gasaustausch in der reifen Plazenta des Menschen. *Z. Geburtsh. Gynäk.* **158**, 117

GENERAL REFERENCES

Clinical Physiology (1963) ed. Campbell, C. J. M., Dickinson, C. J., Slater, J. D. H., 2nd Ed., Blackwell, Oxford

Fœtal and Neonatal Pathology (1963) Morrison, J. E., 2nd Ed., Butterworth, London

Fœtal and Neonatal Physiology (1961) *Brit. med. Bull.* **17**, 2

The Physiology of the Newborn Infant (1959) Smith, C. A., Thomas, Springfield

Pulmonary Structure and Function (1962) *Ciba Foundation Symposium*, ed. de Reuck, A. V. S., O'Connor, M., Churchill, London

The Regulation of Human Respiration (1963) ed. Cunningham, D. J. C., Lloyd, B. B., Blackwell, Oxford

Respiratory Physiology (1963) *Brit. med. Bull.*, **19**, (1)

Resuscitation of the Newborn Infant (1960) ed. Abramson, H., Mosby, St. Louis

Somatic Stability in the Newly Born (1961) *Ciba Foundation Symposium*, ed. Wolstenholme, G. E. W., O'Connor, M., Churchill, London

CHAPTER 3

RESPIRATORY DISTRESS IN THE NEWBORN

Douglas Gairdner

The challenging problem of neonatal respiratory distress, with the large contribution this condition makes to neonatal mortality, particularly amongst prematures, continues to exert a fascination for pædiatricians. For some years it could be said that advances remained tantalisingly meagre when set against the intensive research devoted to it in many centres. Recently, however, tangible progress has at last been made in our understanding of the condition, if not as yet in our ability to prevent it. In reviewing present knowledge it is hoped to make clear which facts have been solidly established, and which remain conjectural. The reader should also be reminded of the admirable articles which have been published by James (1959), Silverman (1961), Strang (1963), Stahlman (1964) and Avery (1964).

A brief description of a typical case is as follows. The baby, who is usually premature or the offspring of a diabetic mother, starts to breathe without serious difficulty and within a few minutes has achieved rhythmic breathing and a good colour. Being re-examined some half hour later the breathing now shows undue effort, inspiration involves retraction of the lower ribs and sternum, and expiration is accompanied by a moan. The colour at this stage is still good, and auscultation reveals fairly good air entry without adventitia.

By about 4 hours the signs of respiratory insufficiency are more obvious. The respiratory rate has risen to 80 to 120 and each breath requires an obvious effort. The diaphragm contracts powerfully with a large excursion, but the main effect is merely to cause retraction of the lower ribs and sternum, the actual ventilation achieved, judged by auscultation, being small. (A scheme for scoring such retractions has been given by Silverman and Andersen, 1956.) Fine inspiratory râles are audible over the lungs. Cyanosis is now present, but at this stage can be abolished by raising the ambient O_2 to about 40%.

During the period 12 to 24 hours these signs of respiratory insufficiency may gradually decrease and complete recovery ensue. But all too often the signs become intensified, and in particular cyanosis increases despite raising the O_2 inspired to 80% or more. The baby lies flaccid, inert and unresponsive. Apnœic spells now set in. At first these are brief and breathing can be re-started by any mild stimulus, but soon they last longer and are terminated only with more difficulty, e.g. by intermittent positive pressure applied by mask and bag. Once such apnœic spells have appeared the chances of recovery are small, and death usually occurs on the first or second day. Any baby with the syndrome who survives 72 hours has a good chance of recovering.

54

Definition and Incidence

A serious difficulty lies in the fact that the syndrome is not one which can at present be sharply defined, so that questions such as incidence, mortality, or the efficacy of different treatments cannot be clearly answered.

In 1959 a group of pædiatricians at the IXth International Congress of Pædiatrics at Montreal spent an evening trying to produce an agreed definition of the condition (Rudolph and Smith 1960). This they failed to do, having to be content with a majority decision to give it the non-committal if long-winded title of *idiopathic respiratory distress syndrome of the newborn* (RDS). Because babies that have had respiratory distress and who die within a few days of birth frequently have pulmonary hyaline membrane as a conspicuous feature, the term *hyaline membrane disease* is often applied to the clinical syndrome, whether fatal or not. Finally, *pulmonary syndrome* has also been used to cover those early neonatal deaths where the main pathological finding has been pulmonary hyaline membrane, œdema or intra-alveolar hæmorrhage (Bound, Butler and Spector 1956).

Usher (1961) defined RDS as, "chest retraction, expiratory grunting and decreased air entry on auscultation, present during and persisting beyond the first 3 hours of life, in the absence of coexisting disease." Over a 2-year period in Montreal, Canada, he found 14% of 694 babies of 2·5 kg. and less developed clinical signs of RDS. Miller (1962) defined *severe RDS* as: expiratory grunt present after 1 hour of age; resting respiratory rate above 65 between 1 and 30 hours persisting for more than one observation; an increase in resting respiratory rate between 1 and 30 hours of age of more than 15 per minute over the highest rate recorded during the first hour of life; cyanosis observed beyond the first few minutes after birth. Thus defined his data show that 16% of 976 babies of 1·0–2·5 kg. developed RDS.

The incidence of clinical RDS amongst a series of 381 babies of less than 2·5 kg. in the author's unit was 10%, rather lower than the above figures.

The incidence of the condition may also be assessed in terms of the finding of hyaline membrane in the lungs of those babies that die in the first few days of life. Two complicating factors enter here. Firstly, in many cases necropsy reveals gross cerebral hæmorrhage in addition to pulmonary hyaline membrane. Thus Bound *et al.* (1956) noted that 42% of babies with intra-ventricular hæmorrhage also had hyaline membrane in the lung. Although the clinical course of some babies may strongly suggest that the respiratory illness is primary and the cerebral hæmorrhage is terminal, it is impossible to be sure of the order of events. Secondly, when the hyaline membrane is present in lesser degree, it will be a matter of opinion whether the case should be so classified (Miller and Jennison 1950, Latham, Nesbitt and Anderson 1955).

The incidence of "atelectasis with hyaline membrane" amongst 901 first-week deaths in Great Britain (Perinatal Survey, Butler 1963) was 15%, being second only to congenital malformations as a "cause" of death. (If cases of "atelectasis without hyaline membrane" are added, the incidence of atelectasis, with or without membrane, was 24%.)

The Table shows some published figures for the incidence of hyaline membrane in necropsy material from various centres in Western countries.

In the group below 2·5 kg. the incidence is 4–7% of live births, while in the group above 2·5 kg. the incidence is very low, 0·2% or less.

TABLE

INCIDENCE OF PULMONARY HYALINE MEMBRANE AT NECROPSY IN PREMATURE AND MATURE INFANTS

Author and place	2·5 kg. and below		Above 2·5 kg.
	PHM per 100 neonatal deaths	PHM per 100 live births	PHM per 100 live births
Miller et al. (1950), Kansas, U.S.A.		6·8*	0·2*
Latham et al. (1955), Baltimore, U.S.A.		4·3*	0·1*
Cohen et al. (1960), Buffalo, U.S.A.	27	3·9	0·1
Neligan (1961), Newcastle, England	34	6·5	
Smith (1959), Boston, U.S.A.	41	5·8	

* As recalculated by Cohen et al. (1960).

It was formerly often alleged that RDS was notably infrequent in under-developed countries, but this is not the case. Webb et al. (1962) in South India found the incidence of hyaline membrane in necropsy material to be 7–10% of liveborn premature babies, allowing for the fact that the figure for birth weight defining prematurity must be set lower in India than in Western countries. This is a higher incidence than is shown in the Table for centres in the U.K. and U.S.A., and it was concluded that the incidence of hyaline membrane is in fact somewhat higher amongst prematures in South India. (This paper gives a useful account of the possible pitfalls when comparing figures of this kind from different centres.)

Necropsy data from centres in Lebanon (Younozai 1962), Thailand (Rosahn and Sheanakul 1961), Singapore (Sivanesan 1961) and Hawaii (Chuang 1962) leave no doubt that pulmonary hyaline is found with the same order of frequency in these countries as in Western countries. Thus environmental and racial factors are unimportant compared with the basic factor of prematurity.

The question of whether the condition increases in incidence the more immature the baby was considered by Silverman and Silverman (1958), who analysed the fate of 692 babies under 2·0 kg. of whom 197 died in the first 72 hours. Necropsy was carried out in all but 17, and the following figures have been compensated for that fact. Pulmonary hyaline membrane was present in 16% of livebirths of less than 1·0 kg., in 16% of those of 1·0–1·5 kg., and in 9% of those of 1·5–2·0 kg. Quite similar figures were given by Cohen et al. (1960), with rates of 11% for under 1·0 kg., 14% for 1·0–1·5 kg., 7% for 1·5–2·0 kg., and 1·3% for 2·0–2·5 kg. The fact that the incidence in the under 1·0 kg. group is no higher than in the 1·0–1·5 kg. group may well be that so many of the extremely immature babies die within a few hours of birth and before hyaline membrane has had time to form (p. 66). With this proviso, it does appear that the condition, in terms of the necropsy finding of hyaline membrane, has the highest incidence in the lowest weight groups.

If we conclude from the figures quoted that of 100 prematures born, about 6 will be found at necropsy to have pulmonary hyaline membrane, the mortality rate of RDS would be roughly 40%. (This neglects the fact that some clinical cases of RDS that come to necropsy do not show membrane in the lungs.)

This figure accords reasonably well with clinical impressions. At the Cambridge Maternity Hospital during a 2-year period (analysed by Dr. Mary Calladine) there were 381 livebirths under 2·5 kg., 38 (10%) of these developed clinical RDS, which was fatal in 16 (case mortality 42%). In every fatal case the lungs showed profound atelectasis, while in 12 (75%) hyaline membrane was conspicuous as well, and in 2 massive intrapulmonary hæmorrhage dominated the picture. Usher (1963) quotes similar mortality rates of 37% and 42% for two series where the babies with RDS were treated without intravenous bicarbonate, and a mortality rate of 17% when this was used.

Males are much more prone to RDS, the M:F ratio being 2:1 in our series, whether clinical RDS or only fatal cases are considered. Usher (1961) and Miller (1963) noted a similar male preponderance.

Incidence of RDS in babies of diabetic mothers. Although only a small fraction of all cases of RDS fall within this group, the subject is of great theoretical importance, because the babies of diabetic mothers are the only clear-cut group, apart from prematures, with a high incidence of RDS.

The large series collected by Gellis and Hsia (1959) may be quoted as typical. From 934 pregnancies of diabetic mothers there were 104 neonatal deaths. In 73 (70%) of these the only major necropsy finding was "hyaline membrane with or without atelectasis," which completely overshadowed all other causes of death such as congenital defects, intra-cranial bleeding or hypoglycæmia. (Pathological review of the same material by Driscoll, Benirschke and Curtis (1960) gave the somewhat lower figure of 52% for the incidence of hyaline membrane syndrome as the main finding.) 19 of these cases of hyaline membrane were in babies born between 36 and 38 weeks gestation (few were delivered later than this), i.e. at a stage of maturity where non-diabetic pregnancies rarely lead to neonatal deaths from this cause.

As is well known, the babies of diabetic mothers tend to have abnormally high birth weights, yet it is the *less* heavy babies that tend to be affected by RDS. Thus among Farquhar's (1962) series of 205 babies of diabetic mothers the incidence of *clinical RDS with recovery* was 12% for babies of less than 3 kg., against 8% for those over 3 kg. The incidence of *neonatal death* (which in some 50–70% of cases will be associated with pulmonary hyaline membrane) was 14% for babies of less than 3 kg., against 3% for those over 3 kg. The same tendency for the less heavy babies to be affected was equally apparent in those babies that were of 36 weeks or more gestation (see Chapter 6, p. 142).

Thus RDS in the babies of diabetic mothers is exceptional in that many of the affected babies are over 36 weeks gestation and/or over 3 kg. in weight. In all other respects the clinical and pathological features are the same whether the mother is diabetic or not.

Radiology

The characteristic radiological appearance, first described by Donald and Steiner (1953), consists in the early stages of a fine mottling of the lung fields, which coarsens and intensifies as the disease progresses (see Fig. 5, p. 65). With the increasing opacification of the lungs the bronchial tree shows up as an "air bronchogram." Terminally, the lung fields are reduced to a uniform opacity which merges with the heart shadow.

This is the commonest picture seen, but in some clinically typical cases we have observed the opacification of the lungs has had a ground-glass character, rather than the more usual mottling. A ground-glass appearance was also noted by Currafino and Silverman (1957), although Fawcitt (1956) thought this appearance should be differentiated from that of "hyaline membrane disease," and that it implied a better prognosis. Conversely a fine mottling can sometimes be seen in conditions other than RDS; we have seen it, for instance, produced by severe pulmonary congestion in a case of anomalous pulmonary venous drainage.

The limitations of radiology as a diagnostic criterion of this condition were brought out in the prospective study of Bauman and Nadelhaft (1958). A consecutive series of 104 premature babies were radiographed on one or more occasions during the first 72 hours; 35 showed fine mottling (reticulo-granularity), but in only 16 of these were there clinical signs of RDS. Of the remaining 19 with positive radiographs 4 died, but only 1 of these showed hyaline membrane histologically. Finally, 3 babies with clinical signs of RDS had normal radiographs.

Pulmonary Function

Much can be inferred from simple clinical observation. The inspiratory retraction of the lower chest suggests that the lungs are stiff (low compliance), resisting unduly the efforts of the respiratory muscles to expand the thoracic cavity, and so increasing the work of breathing. The cyanosis, persisting in the more severe cases even when high concentrations of O_2 are inspired, implies that the arterial blood stream is receiving large amounts of unoxy-genated blood, i.e. that a large right-to-left shunt is present. Auscultation reveals diminished breath sounds, suggesting that alveolar ventilation is poor, relative to the exaggerated efforts of the respiratory muscles. The expiratory moan (grunt) must involve an increase in expiratory air flow resistance.

The measurement of pulmonary function in these small and gravely ill patients has naturally posed great technical problems, which have proved in part surmountable, notably by the Boston group of workers led by C. A. Smith. Observations have probably often been mainly made, under-standably enough, on the less severe cases, and this point needs to be kept in mind in appreciating published data.

Ventilation. If we compare two newborn babies, one breathless from RDS, the other from cardiac failure due to, say, a coarctation of aorta, the impres-sion is gained that the baby with RDS is achieving relatively little ventilation. Tidal volume is extremely difficult to measure accurately in an ill premature baby, but figures have been given by three sets of workers. Karlberg *et al.* (1954) arrived at the conclusion that tidal volumes in RDS were normal or only slightly reduced. Since these babies breathe at 2 to 3 times normal rates the values for minute volume were much above normal, averaging 170% of normal. Miller, Behrle, Smull and Blim (1957) on the other hand found that a reduction in tidal volume was an important feature in RDS and that the babies studied (none of whom appear to have been severely affected) compensated with increased respiratory rate and so attained fairly normal minute volume. Inspection of the data published more recently by Nelson et al. (1962) shows that their results are rather similar to those of Karlberg et al., with tidal volumes normal or moderately reduced, and minute volumes often above normal.

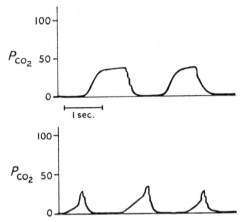

FIG. 1. Mass spectrometer tracings of P_{CO_2} of gas in baby's nostril. *Upper record* from normal baby. In expiration the tracing forms a plateau at a P_{CO_2} of about 40 mm. Hg, after dead space has been washed out and when alveolar air reaches the nostril. *Lower record* from baby with severe RDS: there is no alveolar plateau, the tidal volume being too small to wash out the dead space (Strang 1963).

If babies with *severe* RDS attained near-normal tidal volumes it would be surprising, seeing that CO_2 retention is a prominent feature of such cases (p. 62). Some observations by Strang (1963) strongly point to tidal volume being greatly reduced. A small plastic tube was sited within the baby's nostril, enabling CO_2 to be continuously analysed by a mass spectrometer (Fig. 1). Normally during expiration the first part of the breath clears the dead space, and is followed by alveolar gas with a fairly uniform concentration, so that the last part of expiration is represented by a plateau. If tidal volume is reduced, the length of the plateau is curtailed. In the tracing from the fatal case of RDS illustrated there is no plateau, and in this case the tidal volume was too small to wash out the anatomical dead space completely.

Equally as important as the volume of tidal air is the size of that portion of it which merely serves functionally to ventilate dead space. *Functional dead space* in the normal newborn forms a fraction of 0·25 to 0·5 of tidal volume, according to different observers, while for babies with RDS figures of 0·6–0·7 of tidal volume have been given by Karlberg *et al.* (1954) and Nelson *et al.* (1962). This would imply that only about one-third of the tidal air was utilised for alveolar ventilation. Even this must be a serious under-estimate of the situation, at least in severe RDS, because Fig. 1 shows that in a case such as that illustrated the anatomical dead space actually exceeds tidal volume.

Pressure-volume relations. The nature of the pulmonary disturbance in RDS can be well displayed by tracing the pressure-volume changes during the course of a single breath. Figs. 2 and 3 refer to a pair of twins studied by Dr. K. Weisser (Weisser 1963), one of whom weighed 1·29 kg. and breathed normally (Fig. 2), the other weighed 1·86 kg. and had RDS (Fig. 3) which proved fatal. During inspiration the pressure-volume graph (Fig. 2) follows the course AIB; followed by expiration BEA. AC is the tidal volume, in this

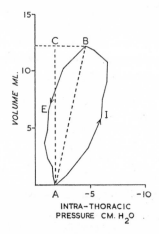

FIG. 2. Pressure-volume changes in single breath of newborn twin (see text).

instance 12·2 ml.; CB is the difference in intrathoracic pressure at the beginning and end of inspiration (Δp), here 2·8 cm. H_2O. Compliance is the ratio of these two, $12·2/2·8 = 4·4$ ml./cm. H_2O, which lies within the normal range.

Fig. 3 shows the respiratory loop of the twin with RDS. The most obvious difference is that while the tidal volume is slightly less (10·5 ml.) the (negative) intrathoracic pressure required to ventilate the lung even to this extent is far greater, Δp having a value of 19·5 cm. H_2O. The ratio of these two, $10·5/19·5 = 0·54$, thus gives a value for compliance which is only 12% of that of the normal twin.

A further conspicuous fact is that during the latter half of expiration the intrathoracic pressure is markedly positive, showing that there is a raised resistance to airflow during *expiration*, which it is tempting to ascribe to partial closure of the glottis, in view of the characteristic expiratory moan.

Since pressure $\times$ volume has the dimensions of work, areas on the pressure-volume diagram can be used to read off the various components of the work of breathing. Pulmonary work is represented by the sum of (i) the work needed to expand the lungs against their elastic tendency to resist—elastic work, area of triangle ABC; (ii) the work needed to move air through air passages during inspiration, area AIB; and (iii) the work needed to move air through air passages during expiration, this being normally largely passive is represented in Fig. 2 only by the small area of AEB which lies to the left of AC. The corresponding area to the left of AC in Fig. 3 is, on the other hand, considerable, so that there is a significant amount of work done in overcoming expiratory flow resistance in RDS.

Inspection of the areas defined in (i), (ii) and (iii) in Figs. 2 and 3 readily shows that the work of breathing is far greater in the twin with RDS. The work done per breath by the affected twin is 3·3 times greater, although the amount of air moved is 14% less than in the normal twin.

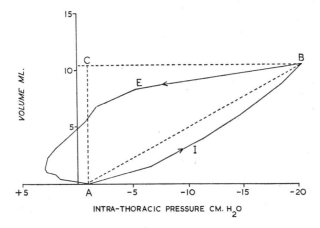

FIG. 3. Pressure-volume changes in single breath of newborn twin with severe RDS (see text). Compared with normal twin (Fig. 2) tidal volume AC is smaller, inspiratory negative pressure CB much larger, giving low compliance.

Figs. 2 and 3 based on data published by Dr K. Weisser (1963) by kind permission.

Much the same results have been obtained by other workers who have measured pressure-volume relations in RDS. Cook *et al.* (1957) and Karlberg *et al.* (1954) found compliance 23% of normal, and respiratory work per minute 4 to 10 times normal. Prod'hom *et al.* (1962) found compliance in the severer cases of RDS 21–29% of normal. These measurements of *dynamic compliance* are also in keeping with the measurements of *static compliance* of excised lungs made by Gribetz, Frank and Avery (1959) (see p. 68). Thus the reduced compliance of the lungs in RDS is a fundamental fact forming the basis of much of the clinical picture observed.

How early is this abnormal compliance recognisable, and is it already apparent in the first breaths? There are as yet no published facts on this important point, but the more carefully these babies are watched from birth, the stronger grows the impression that breathing involves undue effort from the very outset. Compliance, it may therefore be conjectured, is probably abnormal from the very outset.

Whatever may be the state of the lungs in the first minutes after birth, it is a safe assumption that the main cause of the low compliance, once symptoms are apparent, is the collapsed state of many of the alveoli, and the reduced amount of lung tissue capable of expansion. Confirmation of this by demonstrating a low functional residual capacity in RDS has not yet been reported, although it can be inferred from the *post mortem* studies of Gribetz *et al.* (1959).

Blood gas changes. O_2-saturation has been measured serially by means of an ear oximeter (Miller *et al.* 1957), or by sampling aortic blood by means of an in-dwelling catheter in the umbilical artery. If O_2-saturation is measured while the baby inspires either 100% O_2 (Strang and MacLeish 1961, Nelson *et al.* 1963) or any known O_2-concentration over 40–50% (Warley and Gairdner 1962), the amount of right-to-left shunt can be calculated. Expressed as a percentage of the heart output blood which reaches the systemic circulation unoxygenated, right-to-left shunt is known to be about 2% in normal adults; it averaged 20–25% in a series of non-distressed babies of diabetic mothers investigated by Prod'hom *et al.* (1964) on the first day of life.

CO_2-tension should ideally be measured in arterial blood, but "arterialised" skin-prick specimens can give sufficiently accurate results for clinical purposes. The equipment devised by Astrup and co-workers (1960) enables pH, P_{CO_2} and bicarbonate to be measured in a skin-prick sample within a few minutes, and so is ideal for monitoring these variables in babies with RDS.

The respiratory insufficiency in RDS is reflected in both low O_2-saturation and high CO_2-tensions (Blystad 1956, Miller *et al.* 1957). Superimposed on the respiratory acidosis there develops a metabolic acidosis, which, as it tends to run parallel to O_2-unsaturation, is no doubt mainly due to accumulation of metabolites such as lactic and pyruvic acids, resulting from incomplete carbohydrate catabolism (Wang *et al.* 1963). The combination of the respiratory and metabolic acidosis causes the pH to fall below 7·0 in severe cases. Because CO_2-retention and O_2-lack each contribute to the lowering of pH, the latter provides the most useful single measure of the respiratory insufficiency.

Fig. 4 illustrates the characteristic blood gas changes in a severe case of RDS. Respiratory insufficiency was only moderate during the *first day*, so that at this stage O_2-saturation could be maintained at 90–95% while breathing O_2 at 50 to 75% concentration, giving a calculated right-to-left shunt of about 30%. P_{CO_2} remained around 50 mm. Hg; pH was only slightly low, between 7·3 and 7·2. During the *second day* the respiratory insufficiency intensified; O_2-saturation fell to 53% despite raising the O_2 breathed to 90%, giving a value of 69% for the right-to-left shunt. P_{CO_2} rose to 92 mm. Hg. This combination of severe hypoxia plus severe hypercapnia would have resulted in very low values for bicarbonate and for pH, had it not been for the fact that $NaHCO_3$ was infused intravenously. Few babies who develop so extreme a degree of respiratory failure survive, but in this case on the *third day* O_2-saturation and P_{CO_2} moved slightly towards normal, the right-to-left shunt being now less than 50%. Not until the fifth day did this baby cease to be critically ill, when for the first time normal oxygenation while breathing air was achieved.

Oxygen consumption. There are no published data on O_2-consumption by babies with RDS, but the well recognised fact that severely distressed

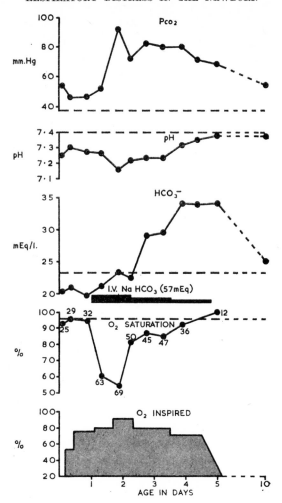

FIG. 4. Severe RDS in a 2·8 kg. baby of a diabetic mother, showing changes in arterial P_{CO_2}, pH, HCO_3^- and O_2-saturation, from birth to 10th day. Normal levels indicated by broken lines. The figures on the O_2-saturation graph give the % right-to-left shunt. Intravenous $NaHCO_3$ was given as shown.

babies tend to maintain a lower body temperature than mildly affected babies (Jonxis et al. 1964) strongly suggests that severe hypoxia prevents O_2-consumption being maintained at a normal level. Furthermore, recent observations (K. W. Cross and June Hill, personal communication) have shown that the O_2-consumption of a cyanosed baby with RDS is increased when the cyanosis is relieved by raising the inspired O_2.

Conclusions. The facts already recounted in this section would be compatible with a situation where in much of the lung there is little gas exchange, with pulmonary blood flow going to non-ventilated alveoli and inspired air going to non-perfused alveoli.

A conspicuous part of the picture in severe cases is the large right-to-left shunt. There are three sites where this shunt might occur, the ductus, the foramen ovale and the lungs. Animal work, discussed in Chapter 1 (p. 10), leads one to expect that pulmonary resistance would be increased by alveolar collapse, by a fall in arterial P_{O_2}, or by a rise in arterial P_{CO_2}, all three of which factors may be prominent in RDS. A raised pulmonary resistance would be reflected in a raised pressure in the pulmonary artery and right ventricle, and would thus favour a right-to-left shunt through the ductus. The only study providing any data on this point is that of Rudolph et al. (1961), who catheterised the heart in 10 cases of severe RDS. They concluded that right ventricular pressure was low rather than high. In all 7 cases where the ductus was successfully catheterised a large left-to-right shunt was noted, while a large right-to-left shunt was present in addition in 1 case only, and a small right-to-left shunt in a further 2 cases.

Equally scanty are the facts bearing on the question of shunts through the foramen ovale in RDS. Rudolph et al. detected a left-to-right shunt at atrial level in 2 of their cases. Stahlman (1964), by dye-dilution methods, has demonstrated large right-to-left shunts through the foramen ovale.

Although therefore a reasonable explanation of the large right-to-left shunt in severe RDS would be that the output from the right heart is diverted away from the lungs and through the fœtal passages, there is as yet no evidence that this actually is the mechanism, or that a substantial shunt does not occur within the lungs, from admixture of blood perfusing collapsed alveoli. (Such intra-pulmonary shunting is known to develop in normal lung, if under-ventilated during general anæsthesia, Bendixen et al. 1963.)

Owing to the greatly increased work of respiration (p. 61) which has to be carried out by muscles progressively impoverished of oxygen, death seems often to be due ultimately to fatigue of the respiratory muscles. In keeping with this clinical impression is the observation by Shelley (1964) that diaphragm muscle from fatal cases of RDS has usually become depleted of all its carbohydrate.

Fluid and Electrolyte Balance

Babies with severe RDS tend to develop pitting œdema of the extremities. Usher (1961) found œdema fluid to have a protein concentration of 1–3% and to be rich in albumen. An increase in leg volume during the first 36 hours is measurable (Sutherland, Oppé, Lucey and Smith 1959), and shows that fluid must be transferred from some other part of the body, since body weight is decreasing during this period. The nature of this fluid shift is obscure. The shift of plasma from the vascular compartment which takes place in the normal baby immediately after birth, substantial though this often is, would not be sufficient to account for a gain in volume of 46 ml. for each leg, the average figure observed by Sutherland et al., nor do premature babies with RDS show a larger post-natal plasma shift than controls (Clark and Gairdner 1960).

The metabolic aspects of RDS were studied by Nicolopoulos and Smith (1961). Babies with RDS tended to show a shift of water from cells into extracellular space, hyperkalæmia and excessive excretion of sodium during the

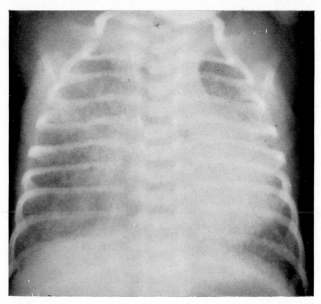

FIG. 5. RDS, first day of life. Cardiac diameter 5·2 cm., cardio-thoracic ratio 0·68.

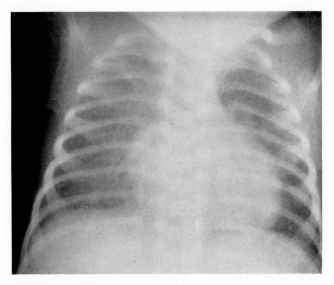

FIG. 6. Same case as Fig. 5, sixth day of life after recovery from RDS. Cardiac diameter 4·5 cm., cardio-thoracic ratio 0·59.

first 48 hours. These changes were not very striking (few of the cases studied were severe) and they could most simply be accounted for on a basis of increased tissue breakdown. Hyperkalæmia was a more prominent finding in the cases studied by Usher (1959, 1961), amongst which were many severe cases. A rise in the serum potassium to 7–9 mEq./l. was common; it was considered to be a consequence of the acidosis, since it could be prevented or reversed if the acidosis was corrected by bicarbonate-glucose infusion.

A rise in serum phosphate and a reciprocal fall in serum calcium was noted by Jonxis et al. (1964).

Cardiovascular Changes

Radiography shows that the heart is enlarged in RDS (Figs. 5, 6) and that its size returns to normal as pulmonary symptoms abate (Burnard 1959b). The enlargement could be due to intra-cardiac or ductal shunts, or to a raised pulmonary vascular resistance. It could also be a consequence of the exaggerated intra-thoracic negative pressure (p. 61) together with a reduction in the volume of the lungs as they collapse.

Rudolph et al. (1961) succeeded in surmounting the formidable technical difficulties involved in studying a series of 10 babies with severe (fatal) RDS by means of cardiac catheterisation. Their studies were particularly directed to the situation at the ductus, where a large left-to-right shunt was recorded in each case. The amount of right-to-left shunting at this site was usually not large.

A systolic murmur frequently becomes audible during some part of the illness, and was thought by Burnard (1959a) to be of ductal origin.

The ECG in RDS has been studied by Usher (1959) and Keith, Braudo and Rowe (1961). The commonest changes are prolongation of PR and QRS, and flattening of T-waves. Usher considered that many of the ECG changes reflected hyperkalæmia; if the acidosis was corrected both the serum potassium level and the ECG tended to return to normal.

Blood pressure was studied by Neligan and Smith (1961), who found that babies with RDS, both prematures and those with diabetic mothers, showed marked hypotension.

Rudolph et al. (1961) discuss the possibility that the respiratory disorder in RDS might be a consequence of a widely patent ductus. To the writer, however, the evidence strongly points to the patency of the ductus, and the other cardiovascular changes noted, being secondary to the pulmonary disorder. It is worth noting that congenital heart defects are surprisingly rarely found in babies with RDS.

Pathology

The only constant finding at necropsy concerns the lungs. These have the consistency of liver, and their airlessness is such that all or nearly all parts sink in water. An additional fact is the *absence* of froth in any fluid which may be in the air passages or be expressible from the lung; the significance of this has only been appreciated in recent years, pointing as it does to the abnormally high surface tension of the fluids concerned.

Histologically, most of the alveolar spaces contain no air, and are often so completely collapsed that their outlines are lost. In contrast to the airless alveoli the terminal air passages (bronchioles and alveolar ducts) are distended with air. The whole presents an irregular pattern, quite different from the regular pattern made by the fluid-filled alveoli of fœtal lung.

The airlessness of the lungs at death contrasts strikingly with the fact that many of these babies have passed through a phase during the first few hours of life where lung aeration and function were fairly good, as judged clinically, radiologically, or in terms of arterial O_2- and CO_2-tension. Clearly therefore the alveoli have been expanded by air, but have subsequently collapsed. This secondary form of atelectasis was first clearly defined by Dr. Edith Potter, who introduced the term *resorption atelectasis* to describe it. In so far as this term may be thought to imply that alveolar collapse follows resorption of gas distal to obstructed airways, and in the light of what is now known about surface tension effects (p. 68), it would be preferable perhaps to use the term *expulsion atelectasis*.

The histological differentiation of primary atelectasis of fœtal lung from expulsion (resorption) atelectasis is usually fairly clear cut, but in the most immature babies may be less so, with both forms being seen in different areas of the same lung.

The electron microscopic appearances have been described by Van Breeman, *et al.* (1957), Campiche *et al.* (1961), Matsumara *et al.* (1962) and Groniowski and Biczyskowa (1963).

In addition to the highly characteristic type of atelectasis, eosinophilic hyaline material is a prominent feature in most cases. It is never found in stillbirths, and rarely in babies that have died earlier than 4 hours. In cases dying early, in the first 12 hours or so, the hyaline material tends to be seen as irregular masses, frequently containing nuclear fragments. Later it is seen plastered onto the walls of the terminal air passages to give the characteristic appearance of a membrane, the thickness of which tends to increase with time (Robertson 1963). The adjacent epithelium often shows focal necrosis. In the occasional case where death is delayed until the fourth or fifth day the hyaline material is broken up and fragments can be seen lying free within the terminal air passages, surrounded by macrophages. It can thus reasonably be surmised that any membrane present is removed by phagocytosis in those cases where recovery takes place (Driscoll *et al.* 1960, Wade-Evans 1962).

The hyaline material consists mainly of protein, which is rich in fibrin. These two conclusions have been established by means of orthodox histology (Wade-Evans 1962), by electron microscopy (Van Breeman, Neustein and Bruns 1957), by enzymatic digestion (Aronson 1961), and by fluorescent antibody technique (Gitlin and Craig 1956, Gajl-Peczalska 1964). The source of this material can scarcely be other than endogenous: liquor amnii does not contain fibrinogen, and evidence of the inhalation of large amounts of blood is not common. The fibrinogen and other protein is in all probabilty, therefore, derived from transudation of plasma. For further discussion see p. 71.

Besides protein the membrane also contains fat and varying amounts of cellular debris.

Although the majority of clinically typical cases of RDS which end fatally do show obvious hyaline membrane, in a minority it is scanty or absent, particularly if death occurs in the first 12 hours (Briggs and Hogg 1958). But whether or not membrane is present, typical expulsion (resorption) atelectasis is nearly always a feature. In addition, hæmorrhage is often present, both interstitial and into the air passages, but leucocytic infiltration is absent, except in a few cases surviving longer than 48 hours.

Surface Tension Factors

Interest in surface tension in neonatal pulmonary problems goes back more than 30 years, for in Farber and Wilson's (1933) classic paper on "Atelectasis of the Newborn," it was noted that when the excised lungs of newborn babies were inflated, expansion required greater pressures initially than subsequently and this was attributed to "cohesion of the bronchiolar and alveolar walls."

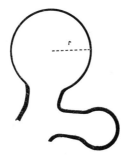

Fig. 7. Diagram of two alveoli with lining surfactant. In the more expanded alveolus the surfactant is represented as stretched and consequently under greater tension (see text).

Gruenwald (1947) noted that expansion of excised lungs of newborns required lower pressure with saline than with air, and postulated with great prescience that "surface-active substances reduce the pressure necessary for aeration." Only in the last few years, however, has the subject been opened up by the development of techniques for measuring the properties of surface-active agents present in the lung. The reader who may have difficulty in resuscitating his schooldays physics is referred to the admirably lucid expositions by Avery (1962) and Clements (1962).

In Fig. 7 each alveolus is imagined as spherical* and lined by a thin layer of fluid. Two opposing forces act on it, (i) the intrathoracic pressure, as measured for instance in the pleural space, which at the end of expiration has a value of about -5 cm. H_2O ($= 5000$ dynes/cm.); and (ii) the pressure (P) within the alveolus caused by the surface tension (T) of the liquid layer, tending to contract the alveolus and to expel air. According to the LaPlace formula, $P = 2T/r$, r being the radius of the sphere. If at the end of expiration the system is to remain in equilibrium, then these two opposing forces must be equal. Taking the radius of curvature of an alveolus as 0·005 cm., the LaPlace formula gives a value for T of about 10 dynes/cm. This is about one-fifth the value of T for plasma and one-seventh the value of T for saline, so that were the alveoli to be moistened by any ordinary biological fluid,

* The validity of taking this or alternative models for the purpose of calculating lung surface tension effects is discussed by Clements *et al.* (1958).

surface tension forces would be so large that alveoli would tend to collapse on expiration. This reasoning leads then to the conclusion that the surface tension of the alveolar lining film must be far lower than that of other biological fluids.

When two alveoli of different sizes are in communication as in Fig. 7 the LaPlace formula shows that if the smaller has half the radius of the larger, the pressure within it will be twice as high. Therefore the tendency will be for the smaller alveolus to expel air into the larger. This will be so whatever the surface tension of the fluid, although the actual pressure difference between the two alveoli will depend on the value for the surface tension. Thus stability of a system of inter-connecting alveoli requires that the surface tension of the lining layer must not be constant (as it is for most fluids) but must diminish as the area of the film contracts, and increase as the film is stretched. Under these circumstances the pressure within the alveolus need not differ much in alveoli of different sizes.

It can be predicted therefore, that not only must the surface tension of the fluid lining the alveolus be much lower than that of other biological fluids, but it must also vary with the area of the film.

The presence in normal lung of a surface agent with strikingly low surface tension was first ingeniously demonstrated by Pattle in 1955, when studying the properties of bubbles in fluid squeezed or washed out of lungs. He found the surface agent to be a lipoprotein (Pattle and Thomas 1961). Clements, Brown and Johnson (1958) showed that it had the additional property of a changing surface tension as the area of film changed. When the film was stretched the tension was relatively high, 40 dynes/cm., which is near that of plasma; but when the film contracted the tension fell to 10 dynes/cm.or less, in good agreement with the values predicted on theoretical grounds (p. 67).

These facts were applied to the problem of RDS by Avery and Mead, (1959). They examined the washings from pieces of lung from 47 infants both still and live births, comparing their surface tension with the material obtained from older children and adults. The material from the lungs of infants over 1·2 kg. had a low surface tension, comparable to older children and adults, with the exception of 9 cases where the lungs contained hyaline membrane; in each of these the surface tension was high. High values were also obtained from a further 9 cases with weights less than 1·2 kg. and also from a stillborn infant of a diabetic mother. Avery and Mead suggested that in the absence of normal surfactant the alveoli tended to collapse at the end of expiration, and that many of the clinical and pathological features of RDS could be explained on this basis.

Subsequent work has brought supporting evidence to these ideas. Gribetz, Frank and Avery (1959) studied the pressure-volume characteristics of excised lungs containing hyaline membrane. They were grossly altered, the lungs requiring extraordinarily high pressures (80 cm. H_2O) to expand them, while on deflation they retained very little air, in keeping with the low compliance and the (surmised) low functional residual capacity obtaining during life (p. 62). (It seems generally agreed that the distensibility of excised lungs examined within a day or two of death is similar to that which existed shortly before death, see McIlroy and Christie 1952.) Gruenwald *et al.* (1962) found a correlation between such abnormal pressure-volume relations in lungs with hyaline membrane and the absence of a low surface tension in extracts. Pattle, Claireaux, Davies and Cameron (1962) studied 6 fatal cases of RDS (5 with hyaline membrane, 1 without) and found in all that the lungs were both unable to retain air after inflation, and lacked the low surface tension agent.

The facts so far known about lung surfactant could imply that the substance is deficient in immature fœtuses, and that a baby born with such a deficiency develops RDS. Since survival beyond 48–72 hours usually spells recovery, it would seem that the deficiency is made good within this time. A developmental immaturity of this kind, if it existed, would provide an analogous situation to the deficiency of glucuronyl transferase in premature babies during the first days of life, which is responsible for the hyperbilirubinæmia of these babies.

A second possibility is that the lung surfactant is destroyed by some other substance. However Pattle *et al.* (1962) found that lung washings from cases of RDS did not interfere with active material prepared from normal lung; nor did either blood or liquor amnii, substances which might be inhaled by the fœtus.

A third possibility is that the production of lung surfactant might be dependent upon the proper oxygenation of the lung epithelium. According to this hypothesis the lack of lung surfactant in babies with RDS could be a consequence of some prenatal hypoxic episode (p. 70). In this connection, the possible rôle of disturbance of the pulmonary circulation is raised by a recent case report by Bozic (1963), describing a remarkable "experiment of Nature."

A 2·4 kg. baby, which died on the third day, was found at necropsy to have complete atelectasis with some hyaline membrane formation affecting all the lobes of both lungs, with the sole exception of the left lower lobe. In this lobe, in striking contrast to the rest of the lung, the alveoli were completely expanded: the blood supply to this lobe came from three aberrant arteries coming off the aorta.

Doubtless evidence will presently emerge which will make clear which of these possible mechanisms operate.

Pregnancy and Parturition

It now seems almost certain that the final pathway in the production of RDS must be a failure of the surface tension-reducing system in the lungs— the "anti-atelectasis factor" (J. A. Clements), but as yet we do not know whether this is primary or secondary. Is this in essence a matter of functional immaturity (see above), or of some environmental factor acting on the fœtus during pregnancy or parturition, such as diabetes, ante-partum hæmorrhage, asphyxia, or cæsarean section ?

Maternal diabetes. The strikingly high incidence of RDS amongst these babies (p. 57) allows two kinds of explanation. In many ways these babies, despite their size, behave like prematures (see Chapter 6), and one might therefore regard their predisposition to RDS as merely one aspect of this fact.

Or, since the lung surfactant is a lipoprotein and deranged lipid metabolism is one aspect of the diabetic state, the abnormal metabolism of the mother might interfere with the formation by the fœtal lung of surfactant.

Maternal bleeding. This was present in 30% of the large series of hyaline membrane deaths analysed by Cohen *et al.* (1960), placenta prævia being particularly common. In a personal series of 82 cases of RDS maternal bleeding was present in 30% of clinical cases, and in 29% of fatal cases. Placenta prævia and "unexplained ante-partum hæmorrhage" were responsible for most of the cases of maternal bleeding, with pre-eclamptic toxæmia noticeably infrequent, considering the frequency with which toxæmia and prematurity coexist. The high incidence of maternal bleeding in premature deliveries generally makes it hard to decide whether or not such bleeding is in any way causally related to the production of RDS. Cohen *et al.* (1960) thought that maternal bleeding might only be important in so far as it was associated with fœtal asphyxia, and that it was this that predisposed to the development of RDS after birth.

Delay in onset of breathing. Since delay in breathing at birth is often a sign of a preceding fœtal asphyxia, if the latter does predispose to RDS we might expect to find that babies with RDS had often had delayed onset of breathing. Using the Apgar scoring for assessing a series of premature babies one minute after delivery, James (1959) found that many cases of RDS fell into the group with low Apgar scores of 6 (out of 10) or less. His data show that this was so in 61% of the babies that developed clinical RDS, and in 70% of those that died with hyaline membrane. The interpretation of these figures is made difficult by the fact that presumably many of the more immature babies were amongst the group with low Apgar scores. In Miller's (1962, 1963) series of RDS babies, for example, those with apnœa at birth were more likely to develop *severe* disease, but the incidence was again highest in the smallest babies.

Twins and triplets. Usher (1961) noted among 50 sets of twins where both were live born and both weighed less than 2·5 kg., that in 7 sets both twins had RDS, and in 4 sets only one of the pair. There were two sets of triplets and all the babies were affected. In the author's series there were two sets of triplets, and again all the babies were affected. In one of these sets the first baby (a female with achondroplasia) survived, while the second and third babies (males, probably uniovular) died. In the other set all 3 babies survived; the first baby (binovular female) being less severely affected than the second and third (uniovular females).

Other observations on RDS in twins are to be found in papers by Rogers and Gruenwald (1956), Silverman (1957), Crosse (1957) and Weisser (1963).

It seems that if one of a set of twins or triplets has RDS, the other babies are more likely than not to have RDS also, but little can be gleaned from the available facts about the significance of prenatal factors in RDS.

Cæsarean section. There is no evidence that cæsarean delivery *per se* affects the incidence of RDS or its severity, if account is taken of the obstetric cause for which section is done* (Craig and Fraser 1957, Strang, Anderson and Platt 1957, Cohen *et al.* 1960).

* For a contrary view, however, see recent paper by Usher *et al.* (*Amer. J. Obstet. Gynec.* 1964, **88**, 806).

Hyaline Membrane

The almost hypnotic attraction that the membranes have for long exerted upon workers in this field has in the past distracted attention from the alveolar collapse, which, as has been emphasised in this chapter and as Gruenwald (1952) has long maintained, is the more fundamental and constant lesion (p. 66). The part played by membrane in the pulmonary disorder is still not clear. Craig, Fenton and Gitlin (1958) injected excised lungs with latex and thought that the membranes mechanically blocked the entrance to alveoli, although actual plugging of air passages in this way is only occasionally to be observed histologically. Since membrane tends to line alveolar ducts and terminal bronchioles, one might expect it to increase inspiratory air flow resistance, but this is not usually increased in RDS. (This can be inferred, for instance, from Fig. 3, p. 61, where the inspiratory loop AIB is of normal "fatness.")

The origin of the eosinophilic material as a transudate from the pulmonary vessels has already been referred to (p. 66). The most obvious factor in RDS favouring the passage of fluid from pulmonary vessels to air spaces is the abnormally high (negative) intra-thoracic pressure (p. 60). Transudation might be expected to occur if the osmotic pressure exerted by the plasma proteins (P_P) was exceeded by the sum of the (negative) intra-alveolar pressure (P_A), plus the pulmonary capillary pressure (P_C). In an adult the following values obtain; $P_P = 25$ mm. Hg, $P_A = 4$ mm. Hg and $P_C = 7$ mm. Hg.

In the baby with RDS these values can be assessed as follows. P_P must be considerably less than the adult value of 25 mm. Hg, because the concentration of plasma protein is relatively low in the premature baby (Fraillon 1962); a value of 15–20 mm. Hg can be presumed. P_A can be calculated to be about -15 mm. Hg (-20 cm. H_2O) by applying the LaPlace formula, assuming a radius of curvature of an air space of 0·005 cm., and a lining layer surface tension of 50 dynes/cm. as for plasma. This calculated pressure of -20 cm. H_2O is also of the same order as the observed inspiratory intra-thoracic pressure in cases of RDS (see Fig. 3). The value of P_C, the pulmonary capillary pressure in babies with RDS, is not known, but it would not need to be very high, it could be argued, for P_P to be exceeded by $P_A + P_C$.

Damage to the endothelial lining of pulmonary capillaries, such as might be caused by anoxia, would favour protein transudation, and a general thickening of the capillary endothelium was noted in electron microscopic studies of lungs with hyaline membrane by Campiche, Prod'hom and Gautier (1961).

Up to a point, therefore, hyaline membrane might plausibly be explained as a form of pulmonary œdema. Pulmonary œdema fluid, irrespective of cause, generally has a high protein content (Cameron 1948), but it remains to be explained how fibrinogen comes to be changed to fibrin and the proteins to condense to form membrane. However hyaline membrane is not unique to the newborn infant's lung, for it also occurs in the adult lung (though not with complete atelectasis) in a wide variety of conditions, such as epidemic influenza, rheumatic fever, mustard gas poisoning and after irradiation (for references see Lancet 1962).

RDS and Pulmonary Hyaline Membrane in Experimental Animals

The clinical and pathological picture seen in babies with RDS has not been observed to occur naturally in any other species. Until recently efforts have been mainly directed towards reproducing in animals' lungs the histological picture seen in babies that have died of RDS. By exposing animals to a variety of insults, eosinophilic material has been produced in lungs, with a distribution sometimes reminiscent of that seen in babies (for references see Berfenstam, Edlund and Zettergren 1958). The measures adopted have all been such as to cause severe congestion or œdema of the lungs, and to this extent the observations have lent some support to the idea that a transudate of plasma is the source of hyaline membrane. The measures used have included vagotomy, exposure to an irritant gas such as 100% O_2, or the injection of α-naphthyl-thiourea. In addition it has often been found necessary to instill into the trachea a substance such as meconium, mucus, plasma or concentrated liquor amnii (Carone and Spector 1960). Although such drastic insults have sometimes succeeded in producing membrane, the typical atelectasis has not been convincingly produced.

Only when a means becomes available for reproducing the essential features of the disease in an experimental animal, will the way be opened for a study of such factors as may operate prenatally on the fœtus and lead to the development of RDS.

Prevention

Any measures which reduce the incidence of prematurity are likely to reduce the number of deaths from RDS, but apart from this little can be done at present. The question whether the *placental transfusion* should be promoted or withheld in these babies, or whether indeed it affects the issue at all, remains still unanswered (British Medical Journal 1964). Earlier reports that serum albumen, given intravenously to premature babies soon after birth, reduced mortality from RDS have not been confirmed (Fraillon 1962).

Treatment

Replacement of the missing lung surfactant would seem to be the logical approach to treatment. Until this becomes feasible, treatment can do no more than tide the baby over the first few days of life, on the assumption that survival beyond 2 or 3 days is likely to spell recovery.

Environment. Reference has already been made (p. 63) to the low heat production and consequent tendency to hypothermia of these babies. The series of carefully controlled studies made by Silverman (1959) and that of Jolly and co-workers (1962) suggest that the baby probably fares best in an environment such that its body temperature is maintained near 37°C, although this is far from having been proven. Hypothermia together with chlorpromazine was at one time recommended (Lacomme 1954, Rossier, Michelin and Holm 1954). In order to maintain the smallest babies near 37°C the environmental temperature may need to be as high as 34°C (94°F), which is close to the *neutral temperature* of the baby of about 1 kg. (Hill 1961, and personal communication). High humidity will cut down water losses from skin and lungs, and will therefore have an effect in reducing evaporative heat losses, and so enable the baby to maintain heat in a slightly cooler atmosphere than would otherwise be the case. It is doubtful, however, whether this effect is of practical importance. Aerosol mists, with or without a detergent, have not improved survival rates (Silverman and Andersen 1955, 1956). A moderate humidity around 65%, such as has been conventional in many premature nurseries in the past, is probably sound practice.

Oxygen. The principles governing the proper use of oxygen in RDS have been discussed by Warley and Gairdner (1962). The aim should be to achieve a high-normal arterial saturation of 95–98%, corresponding to a P_{O_2} of about 100 mm. Hg. In view of the large right-to-left shunt in severe cases (p. 64) this is often impossible to attain, even when the baby inspires near-100% O_2 (see Fig. 4, p. 63).

Following the general recognition in about 1954 that the indiscriminate and prolonged exposure of premature babies to high O_2-concentrations often led to retrolental fibroplasia, there was a widespread reluctance to use higher concentrations than 40% under any circumstances. This was irrational, and may have even led to some increase in the losses from RDS (Avery and Oppenheimer 1960). We have found that central cyanosis in these babies is only detectable when arterial saturation has fallen to about 85%, so that significant hypoxia can exist in the absence of cyanosis. A working rule is that where there is distress O_2 should be given at one-quarter higher concentration than the minimum needed to abolish cyanosis. Thus if cyanosis is absent in air, O_2 at about 25% should be given; if cyanosis is abolished by 60% O_2, then 75% should be given. High concentrations of O_2 will only be needed for a few days in any event, so that the risk of eye damage by using somewhat higher concentrations than may be strictly necessary must be small.

The possibility of irritation of the lung by high ($> 70\%$) concentrations of O_2 is harder to exclude altogether. Warley and Gairdner concluded that there was certainly no evidence of RDS being so caused (as has sometimes been suggested), and that any possible effects of O_2 on the lung do not outweigh the sound reasons that exist for using O_2 in the amounts necessary to oxygenate the distressed baby adequately. Whether or not hyperbaric O_2 has any place in this context is not known.

With most incubators it is difficult to maintain O_2-concentrations much over about 40% unless very high flow rates are used. A transparent plastic hood (Fig. 9) enables high concentrations to be used with low flow rates. Furthermore the chest and abdomen may be examined, and blood samples taken without lowering of the O_2-level. Needless to say, O_2 as a potent substance having toxic effects from overdosage, should be metered in terms of concentration, not of flow rates.

Assisted ventilation. Owing to the increased work of breathing (p. 61) which has to be carried out by muscles progressively impoverished of oxygen, death seems often to be due ultimately to fatigue of respiratory muscles. In keeping with this clinical impression is the observation by Shelley (1964) that diaphragm muscle from fatal cases of RDS has usually become depleted of all its carbohydrate.

Mechanical ventilation is a logical approach to the problem therefore, and was pioneered by Donald and Lord (1953) and by Benson *et al.* (1958). Manual ventilation by means of a rubber bag is effective for short periods, but for long periods it is desirable to employ a mechanical respirator which allows the inflating pressure (or volume) to be regulated, and the inspired gas to be humidified. An endotracheal tube is tolerated for surprisingly long periods by the newborn baby, and is far simpler than a tracheostomy, although the latter is favoured by Heese, Wittman and Malan (1963), and for periods longer than 36–72 hrs. by Delivoria-Papadopoulos and Swyer (1964). A tank-type respirator is preferred by Stahlman (1964), whose article should be consulted for a detailed description of the intensive measures employed in her unit.

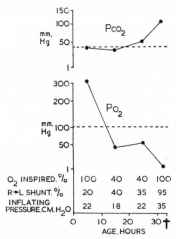

FIG. 8. Severe respiratory failure in a newborn premature treated by mechanical respiration, using intermittent positive pressure with an endotracheal tube. Before starting mechanical respiration at 4 hours the baby was moribund, deeply cyanosed and breathing only in gasps. The measurements of arterial P_{CO_2} and P_{O_2} (plotted logarithmically) were made from 1 hour after the start of mechanical respiration. 40% O_2 was inspired for most of the time, but arterial P_{O_2} remained no higher than 40–50 mm. Hg, indicating a large right-to-left shunt as shown; terminally (1 hour before death) this shunt became total.

A typical situation is as follows. A baby is in terminal respiratory failure with cyanosis, apnoeic spells, and a rapidly rising P_{CO_2}. On starting mechanical ventilation there is a gratifying effect at first, cyanosis disappears and the P_{CO_2}, which may have risen to well over 100 mm. Hg, is rapidly brought to a normal value within an hour or so. After a period of perhaps 6 hours it is noted that in order to expand the chest adequately an increasingly high inflating pressure has to be applied, and there is also increasing difficulty in maintaining oxygenation, despite raising the concentration of O_2 in the inspired gas. The stage is eventually reached, after perhaps 24 hours, where even an inflating pressure of 40 cm. H_2O or more fails to expand the lungs, and cyanosis becomes gross even with 100% O_2. In Fig. 8 data are shown for one such case, and it will be noted that there was less success in maintaining adequate oxygenation than in clearing CO_2, an indication that under these

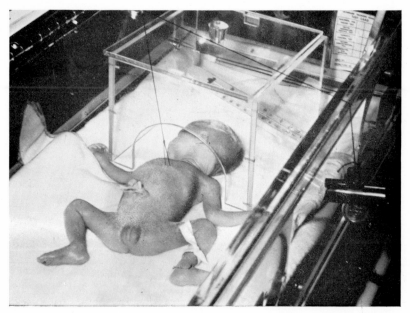

Fig. 9. To show: (1) hood facilitating the use of high concentrations of oxygen: (2) sternal traction; the baby's weight was 950 g. and the traction 50 g.

artificial conditions also, right-to-left shunting of blood is an important fact in RDS (p. 64).

The paucity of reports of mechanical ventilation in babies with RDS probably reflects the generally disappointing results obtained, although Stahlman mentions 11 survivors out of 25 initially moribund babies.

Sternal traction. Effective ventilation requires that the thoracic cage shall be rigid. If it is more compliant than the lungs, then diaphragmatic contractions will tend to cause collapse of the thorax rather than expansion of the lungs. In RDS the thorax of the premature baby is weak and the lungs abnormally stiff, hence the typical indrawing of ribs and sternum. If this is marked it is logical to counter it by fixing the sternum. This can be done by passing a ligature round the xiphisternum and applying traction (Fig. 9). For this purpose the thread may be taken through a hole in the roof of the incubator and attached to a suitable weight; 5–10% of the baby's weight is usually needed to stabilise the sternum, a useful demonstration of the magnitude of the forces being exerted by the respiratory muscles in distressed babies. On applying traction the exaggerated diaphragmatic excursion can be seen to shorten. There is no evidence that the tidal volume increases, but it seems likely that the same tidal volume at least is achieved with a less wasteful effort on the part of the hard pressed respiratory muscles.

Correction of acidosis. On the view that many important metabolic processes break down if the pH departs far from normal (the retention of potassium within the cell is an example), it seems logical to compensate acidosis, whether metabolic or respiratory. As the blood sugar often tends to be low in distressed babies, Usher (1959, 1963) proposed that a combination of $NaHCO_3$ and glucose should be infused intravenously. It was also noted by Dawes, Mott, Shelley and Stafford (1963) that lambs subjected to asphyxia at birth survived much longer if the blood pH was maintained near normal by intravenous infusion of a base—Na_2CO_3 or THAM (p. 76)—plus glucose, but not by the use of base or glucose alone.

The following concentrations of $NaHCO_3$ have been found satisfactory, based on the pH of arterial or "arterialised" skin-prick blood; the concentrations are rather higher than those recommended by Usher (1963) and aim at correcting the acidosis more quickly. The different solutions can be conveniently made up from 5% $NaHCO_3$ by suitable dilution with glucose solutions, such that the final glucose concentration is about 10%. About 65 ml./kg. 24 hrs. is given by scalp vein drip.

pH of blood	Sodium bicarbonate infusion		
	Conc. mEq./l	*Conc. %*	*Dilution of 5% solution*
Below 7·3	100	0·84	1 to 5
Below 7·2	150	1·3	1 to 3
Below 7·1	200	1·7	1 to 2
Below 7·0	300	2·5	1 to 1

The blood pH is checked two or three times in the 24 hours and the amount of bicarbonate given adjusted accordingly, so that in effect the baby is titrated to a pH of between 7·3 and 7·4. Rapid estimations of pH on skin-prick blood have been made possible by the Astrup equipment.

A different scheme has been used by Hutchison *et al.* (1962), who injected into the umbilical vein via an in-dwelling catheter an 8·4% $NaHCO_3$ solution (1000 mEq./l.) in successive amounts, calculated on a basis of the "base excess" as measured in the blood, and the estimated deficit of base in the extracellular fluid. (In view of recent reports that exchange transfusion via the umbilical vein has been succeeded by portal vein thrombosis, it would seem preferable to avoid giving strongly hypertonic or alkaline solutions by this route.)

An alternative base is tris-(hydroxymethyl)-amino-methane (Kaplan, Fox and Clark 1962). THAM acts as an acceptor of hydrogen ions, e.g. in the case of carbonic acid,

$$(CH_3OH)_3 . C . NH_2 + H_2CO_3 \rightarrow (CH_3OH)_3 . C . NH_3^+ + HCO_3^-$$

The use of THAM has two theoretical advantages over $NaHCO_3$: the body sodium is not increased, and the carbonic acid (P_{CO_2}) is reduced. These advantages are partially offset by the disadvantages of the strong alkalinity of solutions of THAM (pH about 10·4). The unbuffered solution cannot be given into a small vein, but has been given into the umbilical vein, although the caveat mentioned above equally applies. Jonxis, Troelstra, Visser and van der Vlugt (1964) used THAM in 0·3 M (3·6%) solution, giving 6 ml./hr. in amounts of about 6–12 ml. Hutchison *et al.* (1964) were unimpressed by their experience with THAM in 26 cases.

Antibiotics. In some centres a distressed newborn is routinely given an antibiotic, on the grounds that it is difficult to exclude a prenatally acquired infection. In the author's unit this has never been the practice, even when manipulations such as the use of in-dwelling arterial catheters have been employed; antibiotics are only given when there is some pointer in the history, or a blood culture (freely taken and reported within 12–24 hours) proves positive. During a 2-year period when in every neonatal death cultures were made *post mortem* from blood, lung and spleen (R. L. Edwards unpublished) no evidence appeared that this conservative policy had resulted in death from unsuspected bacterial infection. Such controlled trials as have been made (Burns *et al.* 1959) give further weight to the view that antibiotics should not be used routinely.

Results of treatment. In Fig. 10 are shown the mortality rates for premature babies of 1·0–2·0 kg. born at Cambridge Maternity Hospital over a 10-year period. The majority of fatal cases of RDS will fall within this 1·0–2·0 kg. group, while an important fraction of all the deaths in the lower part of this weight range, 1·0–1·5 kg., will be caused by RDS. The introduction of an effective treatment for RDS might therefore be expected to show up as a decided fall in mortality rate in either or both of these groups.

At the beginning of 1961 intensive efforts were instituted to treat babies with RDS using intravenous bicarbonate-glucose and high-concentration O_2 according to the principles described, so that the last of the five 2-year periods shown in Fig. 10 covers the period when more active measures were employed. In the 1·0–2·0 kg. group there was a steady fall in mortality rates until the last 2-year period 1961–2, when the figure was unchanged from the previous 2-year period. In the 1·0–1·5 kg. group the mortality rate maintained a steady rate of fall throughout the decade. Our mortality figures therefore fail to show clear-cut change from the trends of the eight years preceding the use of more active treatment. Usher (1963), however, considered that the use of bicarbonate-glucose solutions intravenously had

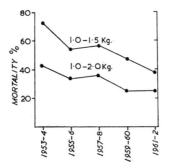

Fig. 10. Neonatal mortality rates for 482 premature babies of 1·0–2·0 kg., including 154 babies of 1·0–1·5 kg., born at Cambridge Maternity Hospital over a 10-year period. More active measures of treating RDS were employed in the last 2-year period 1961–62.

resulted in a large reduction in premature mortality rates, although his figures for a controlled series of babies with RDS just failed to achieve statistical significance. Little effect resulted from his use of such treatment in babies less than 1·5 kg.

It is the writer's impression that active measures will turn the scale between death or survival in a small minority of cases, while a much larger group will either be so severely affected that present methods of treatment are without avail, or so mildly affected that they will recover with conventional care.

REFERENCES

Aronson, N. (1961) Studies on hyaline membranes. *Pediatrics,* **27,** 567
Astrup, P., Jørgensen, K., Andersen, O. S., Engel, K. (1960) The acid-base metabolism: a new approach. *Lancet,* **1,** 1035
Avery, M. E. (1962) The alveolar lining layer. *Pediatrics,* **30,** 324
Avery, M. E. (1964) *The Lung and its Disorders in the Newborn Infant.* Saunders, Philadelphia
Avery, M. E., Mead, J. (1959) Surface properties in relation to atelectasis and hyaline membrane disease. *Amer. J. Dis. Child.* **97,** 517
Avery, M. E., Oppenheimer, E. H. (1960) Increase in mortality from hyaline membrane disease. *J. Pediat.* **57,** 553
Bauman, W. A., Nadelhaft, J. (1958) Chest radiography of prematures. A planned study of 104 patients including clinico-pathologic correlation of the respiratory distress syndrome. *Pediatrics,* **21,** 813
Bendixen, H. H., Hedley-White, J., Laver, M. B. (1963) Impaired oxygenation in surgical patients during general anæsthesia with controlled ventilation: a concept of atelectasis. *New Engl. J. Med.* **269,** 991
Benson, F., Celander, O., Haglund, G., Nilsson, L., Paulsen, L., Renck, L. (1958) Positive-pressure respirator treatment of severe pulmonary insufficiency in the newborn infant. *Acta anaesth. scand.* **2,** 37
Berfenstam, R., Edlund, T., Zettergren, L. (1958) The hyaline membrane disease; a review of earlier clinical and experimental findings and some studies on the pathogenesis of hyaline membrane in O_2-intoxicated rabbits. *Acta pædiat.* **47,** 82

BLYSTAD, W. (1956) Blood gas determinations on premature infants. II—Investigations of premature infants with early neonatal dyspnœa (the hyaline membrane syndrome). *Acta pœdiat.* **45**, 103

BOUND, J. P., BUTLER, N. R., SPECTOR, W. G. (1956) Classification and causes of perinatal mortality. *Brit. med. J.* **2**, 1191

BOZIC, C. (1963) Pulmonary hyaline membranes and vascular anomalies of the lung. *Pediatrics*, **32**, 1094

BRIGGS, J. N., HOGG, G. (1958) Perinatal pulmonary pathology. *Pediatrics*, **22**, 41

BRITISH MEDICAL JOURNAL (1964) Respiratory distress syndrome (Annotation), **1**, 70

BURNARD, E. D. (1959a) The cardiac murmur in relation to symptoms in the newborn. *Brit. med. J.* **1**, 134

BURNARD, E. D. (1959b) Changes in heart size in the dyspnœic newborn baby. *Brit. med. J.* **1**, 1494

BURNS, R. E., HODGMAN, J. E., CASS, A. B. (1959) Fatal circulatory collapse in premature infants receiving chloromphenicol. *New Engl. J. Med.* **261**, 26

BUTLER, N. (1963) Complications of birth asphyxia, with special reference to resuscitation; in *The Obstetrician, Anœsthetist and the Pœdiatrician.* Pergamon Press, London

CAMERON, G. R. (1948) Pulmonary œdema. *Brit. med. J.* **1**, 965

CAMPICHE, M., PROD'HOM, S., GAUTIER, A. (1961) Etude au microscope électronique du poumon de prématurés morts en détresse respiratoire. *Ann. pœdiat.* (Basel) **196**, 81

CARONE, F. A., SPECTOR, W. G. (1960) The interaction of plasma proteins and mucoid substances in the pathogenesis of pulmonary hyaline membranes. *J. Path. Bact.* **80**, 63

CHUANG, K. A. (1962) Pulmonary hyaline membrane disease in Hawaii. *Amer. J. Dis. Child.* **103**, 718

CLARK, A. C. L., GAIRDNER, D. (1960) Postnatal plasma shift in premature infants. *Arch. Dis. Childh.* **35**, 352

CLEMENTS, J. A. (1962) Surface tension in the lungs. *Scientific American*, **207**, 120

CLEMENTS, J. A., BROWN, E. S., JOHNSON, R. P. (1958) Pulmonary surface tension and the mucous lining of the lungs: some theoretical considerations. *J. appl. Physiol.* **12**, 262

COHEN, M. M., WEINTRAUB, D. H., LILIENFELD, A. M. (1960) The relationship of pulmonary hyaline membrane to certain factors in pregnancy and delivery. *Pediatrics*, **26**, 42

COOK, C. D., SUTHERLAND, J. M., SEGAL, S., CHERRY, R. B., MEAD, J., MCILROY, M. B., SMITH, C. A. (1957) Studies of respiratory physiology in the newborn infant. Measurements of mechanics of respiration. *J. clin. Invest.* **36**, 440

CRAIG, J., FRASER, M. S. (1957) The respiratory difficulties of Cæsarean babies. *Ann. Pœdiat. Fenn.* **13**, 143

CRAIG, J. M., FENTON, K., GITLIN, D. (1958) Obstructive factors in the pulmonary hyaline membrane syndrome in asphyxia of the newborn. *Pediatrics*, **22**, 847

CROSSE, V. M. (1957) Atelectasis with hyaline membrane. *Ann. Pœdiat. Fenn.* **3**, 153

CURRARINO, G., SILVERMAN, F. N. (1957) Rœntgen diagnosis of pulmonary disease of the newborn infant. *Pediat. Clin. N. Amer.* **4**, 27

DAWES, G. S., MOTT, J. C., SHELLEY, H. J., STAFFORD, A. (1963) The prolongation of survival time in asphyxiated immature fœtal lambs. *J. physiol.* **168**, 43

DELIVORIA-PAPADOPOULOS, M., SWYER, P. (1964) Assisted ventilation in terminal hyaline membrane disease. *Arch. Dis. Childh.* (In press)

DONALD, I., LORD, J. (1953) Augmented respiration; studies in atelectasis neonatorum. *Lancet*, **1**, 9.

DONALD, I., STEINER, R. E. (1953) Radiography in the diagnosis of hyaline membrane. *Lancet*, **2**, 846

DRISCOLL, S. A., BENIRSCHKE, K., CURTIS, G. W. (1960) Neonatal deaths among infants of diabetic mothers. *Amer. J. Dis. Child.* **100**, 818

FARBER, S., WILSON, J. L. (1933) Atelectasis of newborn, study and critical review. *Amer. J. Dis. Child.* **46**, 572

FARQUHAR, J. W. (1962) Birth weight and the survival of babies of diabetic women. *Arch. Dis. Childh.* **37**, 321

FAWCITT, J. (1956) Radiological findings in the lungs of premature infants. *Arch. Dis. Childh.* **31**, 119

FRAILLON, J. M. G. (1962) The relationship between serum protein levels and hyaline membrane disease in premature babies. *Med. J. Austr.* **2**, 941

GAJL-PECZALSKA, K. (1964) Plasma protein composition of hyaline membrane in the newborn as studied by immunofluoresence. *Arch. Dis. Childh.* **29**, 226

GELLIS, S., HSIA, D. Y-Y. (1959) The infant of the diabetic mother. *Amer. J. Dis. Child.* **97**, 1

GITLIN, D., CRAIG, J. M. (1956) Nature of hyaline membrane in asphyxia of the newborn. *Pediatrics*, **17**, 64

GRIBETZ, I., FRANK, N. R., AVERY, M. E. (1959) Static volume-pressure relations of excised lungs of infants with hyaline membrane disease, newborn and stillborn infants. *J. clin. Invest.* **38**, 2168

GRONIOWSKI, J., BICZYSKOWA, W. (1963) The fine structure of the lungs in the course of hyaline membrane disease of the newborn infant. *Biol. neonat.* **5**, 59

GRUENWALD, P. (1947) Surface tension as a factor in the resistance of neonatal lungs to aeration. *Amer. J. Obstet. Gynec.* **53**, 996

GRUENWALD, P. (1952) In Pulmonary Hyaline Membranes. *Rep. 5th Ross Ped. Res. Conference.* M. & R., Columbus, Ohio, p. 70

GRUENWALD, P. (1960) Prenatal origin of the respiratory distress (hyaline membrane) syndrome. *Lancet*, **1**, 231

GRUENWALD, P., JOHNSON, R. P., HUSTEAD, R. F., CLEMENTS, J. A. (1962) Correlation of mechanical properties of infant lungs with surface activity of extracts. *Proc. Soc. exp. Biol. (N.Y.)* **109**, 369

HEESE, H. DE V., WITTMANN, W., MALAN, A. F. (1963) Management of the respiratory distress syndrome of the newborn with positive-pressure respiration. *S. Afr. med. J.* **37**, 123

HESS, O. W. (1958) Factors influencing perinatal mortality in cesarean section. *Amer. J. Obst. Gynec.* **75**, 376

HILL, J. R. (1961) Reaction of the new-born animal to environmental temperature. *Brit. med. Bull.* **17**, 164

HUTCHISON, J. H., KERR, M. M., MCPHAIL, M. F. M., DOUGLAS, T. A., SMITH, G., NORMAN, J. N., BATES, E. H. (1962) Studies in the treatment of the pulmonary syndrome of the newborn. *Lancet*, **2**, 465

HUTCHISON, J. H., KERR, M. M., DOUGLAS, T. A., INALL, J. A., CROSBIE, J. C. (1964) A therapeutic approach in 100 cases of the respiratory distress syndrome of the new-born infant. *Pediatrics*, **33**, 956

JAMES, L. S. (1959) Physiology of respiration in newborn infants and in the respiratory distress syndrome. *Pediatrics*, **24**, 1069

JOLLY, H., MOLYNEUX, P., NEWELL, D. J. (1962) A controlled study of the effect of temperature in premature babies. *Pediatrics*, **60**, 889

JONXIS, J. H. P., TROELSTRA, J. A., VISSER, H. K. A., VAN DER VLUGT, J. J. (1964) Treatment of respiratory distress syndrome with THAM, sodium bicarbonate and parathormone. To be published.

KAPLAN, S., FOX, R. P., CLARK, L. C. (1962) Amine buffers in the management of acidosis. *Amer. J. Dis. Child.* **103**, 4

KARLBERG, P., COOK, C. D., O'BRIEN, D., CHERRY, R. B., SMITH, C. A. (1954) Studies of respiratory physiology in the newborn infant. Observations during and after respiratory distress. *Acta pædiat.* **43**, *Suppl.* 100, 397

KEITH, J. D., BRAUDO, M., ROWE, R. D. (1961) The electrocardiogram in the respiratory distress syndrome and related cardiovascular dynamics. *J. Pediat.* **59**, 167

LACOMME, M. (1954) L'hibernation artificielle en pathologie néo-natale. *Sem. Hop. (Paris)* **30**, 153

LANCET (1962) Hyaline-membrane formation in the adult lung (Annotation), **1**, 362

LATHAM, E. F., NESBITT, R. E. L., ANDERSON, G. W. (1955) A clinical pathological study of the newborn lung with hyaline-like membranes. *Bull. Johns Hopk. Hosp.* **96**, 173

MCILROY, M. B., CHRISTIE, R. V. (1959) A post-mortem study of the viscoelestic pro-perties of the lungs in emphysema. *Thorax*, **7**, 295

MATSUMURA, T., ONISHI, I., MASUDA, T., YOMURA, W. (1962) Electronmicroscopic observations on the development of alveolar structures with special reference to the cause of respiratory distress in premature infants. *Ann. pœdiat. jap.* **8**, 72

MILLER, H. C. (1962) Respiratory distress syndrome of newborn infants. I. Diagnosis and incidence. II. Pathogenesis. *J. Pediat.* **61**, 2, 9

MILLER, H. C. (1963) Respiratory distress syndrome of newborn infants. III. Statistical evaluation of factors possibly affecting survival of premature infants. *Pediatrics*, **31**, 573

MILLER, H. C., JENNISON, M. A. (1950) Study of pulmonary hyaline-like material in 4,117 consecutive births. *Pediatrics*, **5**, 7

MILLER, H. C., BEHRLE, F. C., SMULL, N. W., BLIM, R. D. (1957) Studies of respiratory insufficiency in newborn infants. II. Correlation of hydrogen-ion concentration, CO_2 tension and oxygen saturation of blood with trend of respiratory rates. *Pediatrics*, **19**, 387

NELIGAN, G. A. (1961) quoted by Webb *et al.* (1962)

NELIGAN, G. A., SMITH, C. A. (1960) The blood pressure of newborn infants in asphyxial states and in hyaline membrane disease. *Pediatrics*, **26**, 735

NELSON, W. M., PROD'HOM, L. S., CHERRY, M. A., LIPSITZ, P. J., SMITH, C. A. (1962) Pulmonary function in the newborn infant. II. Perfusion-estimation by analysis of the arterial-alveolar CO_2 difference. *Pediatrics*, **30**, 975

NELSON, W. M., PROD'HOM, L. S., CHERRY, R. B., LIPSITZ, P. J., SMITH, C. A. (1963) Pulmonary function in the newborn: the alveolar-arterial oxygen gradient. *J. appl. Physiol.* **18**, 534

NICOLOPOULOS, B. A., SMITH, C. A. (1961) Metabolic aspects of idiopathic respiratory distress (hyaline membrane syndrome) in newborn infants. *Pediatrics*, **28**, 206

PATTLE, R. E. (1955) Properties, function, and origin of the alveolar lining layer. *Nature, Lond.* **175**, 1125

PATTLE, R. E., THOMAS, L. C. (1961) Lipoprotein composition of the film lining in the lung. *Nature, Lond.* **189**, 844

PATTLE, R. E., CLAIREAUX, A. E., DAVIES, P. A., CAMERON, A. H. (1962) Inability to form a lung-lining film as a cause of the respiratory-distress syndrome in the newborn. *Lancet*, **2**, 469

PROD'HOM, L. S., CHERRY, R. B., NELSON, N. M., LEVISON, H., SMITH, C. A. (1962) Oxygen and gas exchange in the lung. *Exhibit at Xth Internat. Congr. Pœdiat., Lisbon.*

PROD'HOM, L. S., LEVISON, H., CHERRY, R. B., DRORBAUGH, J. E., HUBBELL, J. P., SMITH, C. A. (1964) Adjustment of ventilation, intra-pulmonary gas exchange and acid-base balance during the first day of life. *Pediatrics*, **33**, 682

ROBERTSON, B. (1963) Hyaline membranes of the newborn and the presence of other pulmonary lesions. *Acta pœdiat.* **52**, 569

ROGERS, W. S., GRUENWALD, P. (1956) Hyaline membranes in the lungs of premature infants. *Amer. J. Obstet. Gynec.* **71**, 9

ROSAHN, P. D., SHEANAKUL, C. (1961) Hyaline membrane disease of the lungs in Thailand. *Amer. J. Dis. Child.* **102**, 236

ROSSIER, A., MICHELIN, J., HOLM, I. (1954) Essais théapeutique par le 4560 R.P. chez la prématuré. *Sem. hop. (Paris)*, **30**, 166

RUDOLPH, A. M., DRORBAUGH, J. E., AULD, P. A. M., RUDOLPH, A. J., NADAS, A. S., SMITH, C. A., HUBBELL, J. P. (1961) Study on the circulation in the neonatal period. The circulation in the respiratory distress syndrome. *Pediatrics*, **27**, 551

RUDOLPH, A. J., SMITH, C. A. (1960) Idiopathic respiratory distress syndrome of the newborn. An international exploration. *Pediatrics*, **57**, 905

SHELLEY, H. J. (1964) Carbohydrate reserves in the newborn infant. *Brit. med. J.* **1**, 273

SILVERMAN, W. A. (1959) The physical environment and the premature infant. *Pediatrics*, **23**, 166

SILVERMAN, W. A. (1961) *Dunham's Premature Infants.* Hoeber, New York

SILVERMAN, W. A., ANDERSEN, D. H. (1955) Controlled clinical trial of effects of Alevaire mist on premature infants. *J. Amer. med. Ass.* **157**, 1093

SILVERMAN, W. A., ANDERSEN, D. H. (1956) A controlled clinical trial of effects of water mist on obstructive clinical signs, death rate and necropsy findings among premature infants. *Pediatrics*, **17**, 1

SILVERMAN, W. A., SILVERMAN, R. H. (1958) "Incidence" of hyaline membrane in premature infants. *Lancet*, **2**, 588

SIVANESAN, S. (1961) Neonatal pulmonary pathology in Singapore. *J. Pediat.* **59**, 600

SMITH, C. A. (1959) quoted by Webb *et al.* (1962)

STAHLMAN, M. (1964) Treatment of cardiovascular disorders of the newborn. *Pediat. Clin. N. Amer.*, **11**, 363

STRANG, L. B. (1963) Respiratory distress in new-born infants. *Brit. med. Bull.* **19/1**, 45

STRANG, L. B., MACLEISH, M. H. (1961) Ventilatory failure and right-to-left shunt in newborn infants with respiratory distress. *Pediatrics*, **28**, 17

STRANG, L. B., ANDERSON, G. S., PLATT, J. W. (1957) Neonatal death and elective cæsarean section. *Lancet*, **1**, 954

SUTHERLAND, J. M., OPPÉ, T. E., LUCEY, J. F., SMITH, C. A. (1959) Leg volume observed in hyaline membrane disease. *Amer. J. Dis. Child.* **98**, 24

USHER, R. H. (1959) The respiratory distress syndrome of prematurity. I. Changes in potassium in the serum and ECG and effects of therapy. *Pediatrics*, **24**, 562

USHER, R. H. (1961) Clinical investigation of the respiratory distress syndrome of prematurity—Interim report. *N.Y. State J. Med.*, **61**, 1677

USHER, R. H. (1963) Reduction of mortality from respiratory distress syndrome of prematurity with early administration of intravenous glucose and sodium bicarbonate. *Pediatrics*, **32**, 966

VAN BREEMAN, V. L., NEUSTEIN, H. B., BRUNS, P. D. (1957) Pulmonary hyaline membranes studied with the electron microscope. *Amer. J. Path.* **33**, 769

WADE-EVANS, T. (1962) The formation of pulmonary hyaline membranes in the new-born baby. *Arch. Dis. Childh.* **37**, 470

WANG, C. S. C., LEVISON, H., MUIRHEAD, D. M., BOSTON, R. W., SMITH, C. A. (1963) Relationship of blood lactate to acidosis and hypoxia in respiratory distress syndrome. *J. Pediat.* **63**, 732

WARLEY, M. A., GAIRDNER, D. (1962) Respiratory distress syndrome of the newborn—principles in treatment. *Arch. Dis. Childh.* **37**, 455

WEBB, J. K. G., JOHN, T. J., JADHAR, M., GRAHAM, M. D., WALTER, A. (1962) The incidence of hyaline membrane syndrome in South India. *J. Indian ped. Soc.* **1**, 193

WEISSER, K. (1963) Zur Pathophysiologie des "Respiratory Distress Syndrome." *Ann. pœdiat. (Basel)* **200**, 81

YOUNOZAI, M. K. (1962) Hyaline membranes in Lebanon. *Pediatrics,* **29**, 332

Figure 1 is taken by permission from *British Medical Bulletin.*

CHAPTER 4

THE EFFECT OF OBSTETRICAL HAZARD ON THE LATER DEVELOPMENT OF THE CHILD

CECIL MARY DRILLIEN

OVER 100 years ago Little (1862) drew attention to possible handicapping sequelæ of obstetric complications in his classic paper, "On the influence of abnormal parturition, difficult labour, premature birth and asphyxia neonatorum on the mental and physical condition of the child." During the past ten years, as therapeutic advances have succeeded in preventing or treating many hitherto lethal or incapacitating diseases in childhood, so pædiatric practice has become increasingly concerned with handicapping and psychosomatic conditions which may be of pre- or perinatal origin. In addition, these same advances have resulted in more damaged children surviving infancy or early childhood. There has also been increasing emphasis on the importance of possible minor sequelæ of obstetric complications. Recently a pædiatrician (Smith 1962) has commented on the right of the premature infant not only to survival but to a college education, and an obstetrician (Walker 1960) has stressed that although less than 10% of babies are lost in the perinatal period or are recognisably damaged or defective, only some 10% reach university levels of educational attainment. Walker suggested that anoxia and other causative factors of prenatal damage are unlikely to be "all-or-none" insults, and questioned how many children are "damaged just a little so that they are well below their potential level but not obviously defective."

Prematurity

Early literature. The major studies published prior to 1953 have been reviewed by Wallich and Fruhinsholz (1911), Benton (1940) and Alm (1953). The data presented and conclusions drawn are widely contradictory. Many samples were highly selective with regard to social grouping. Others introduced bias by being drawn from children seen in pædiatric or psychiatric consultation. Few utilised adequate controls for comparison and conclusions were seldom based on reproducible testing techniques. Numbers were often inadequate and the proportion of children untraced rather high.

Recent studies. The more important investigations reported in the last ten years are summarised in the Table on pages 84–85.

Recent investigators have avoided some of the methodological defects of the earlier work in that most studies are based on larger numbers; the samples are drawn from all, or a predetermined selection by birth weight of all premature infants born in a specified area or maternity hospital practice; control groups of mature infants have been studied concurrently and standardised tests and examination techniques have been utilised. In some investigations adequate numbers of prematures in the lower birth weight groups have been included, allowing the distinction to be made between the larger prematures, many of whom are small babies born at or near term, and the smaller infants who appear to be those at greater risk.

There is, however, still some disagreement about prognosis for the prematurely born. This may be due in part to the rather unsatisfactory definition of prematurity, by birth weight, laid down by the World Health Organisation in 1948. It was anticipated then and subsequent experience has confirmed, that an upper limit of $5\frac{1}{2}$ lb. (2500 g.) is not applicable in many underdeveloped countries nor to a lesser extent in more advanced communities. In 1957 it was agreed that more realistic criteria might be established and a study of birth weights in 18 countries was initiated (W.H.O. 1961). The preliminary analysis based on 23,000 births showed that many of the babies included within the limits of the definition previously adopted are not born prematurely. Of particular interest was the finding that in areas with a relatively low mean birth weight this was accounted for by a small excess of babies born before 37 weeks gestation and a marked excess of low birth weight babies born at or near term.

When considering the later development of so-called premature infants it is important to take note of the various causes of low birth weight. Workers in Winnipeg (Grewar, Medovy and Wylie 1962) have proposed a re-classification of prematurity to include both birth weight and gestation time. Certainly, differentiation should be made between the small near-term baby, frequently born to a mother of poor physique (Drillien 1957); the true premature, i.e. the infant premature both by birth weight and gestation time; and prematures who are markedly under the expected weight for their gestational age.

Findings in recent surveys. The most comprehensive post-war investigation from the viewpoint of sample selection is provided by the group obtained from children born during the National Maternity Survey of 1946 (Royal College of Obstetricians and Gynæcologists and the Population Investigation Committee 1948). This survey is unique as the only investigation of later growth and development of a fully-representative sample of prematurely born children and closely matched mature controls on a national scale, and is also notable for the long period of successful follow-up. The birth weight distribution of the sample is that of the surviving prematures in the general population, with over one-half having a birth weight between 5 and $5\frac{1}{2}$ lb. (2270–2500 g.). The pre-school findings are of limited value, being based on answers to a questionnaire completed by local authority health visitors, but at 8 years over 80%, and at 11 years 71% of surviving National Survey children in primary schools completed a series of standardised tests of intelligence and educational attainment (Douglas 1956, 1960). Small but statistically significant differences were found between the prematures and the controls at 8 years, and at 11 years rather bigger differences were observed. Moreover, at this age only 9·7% of prematures gained entry to Grammar School compared with 22·0% of controls. Premature children resulting from uncomplicated pregnancies had consistently greater handicaps than those

Place	Source of		Numbers of		Dates of birth
	Premature subjects	Controls	Prematures	Controls	
STOCKHOLM (Alm 1953)	All hospital births	Matures matched for social class	1012 single and multiple births all males	1018 single births	1902–21
NATIONAL SURVEY (Douglas 1956, 1960)	All births (Great Britain) one week	Matures matched for various social indices	676 single births	676	March 1946
BALTIMORE (Knobloch et al. 1956; Harper et al. 1959)	A sample by birth weight of all births in Baltimore	Matures matched for various social indices	585 negro and white single births	585	1952
BIRMINGHAM (May 1958)	All births in Birmingham	Matures matched for living conditions	95 single births, uncomplicated obstetric history and no obvious defect noted at birth	95	July–Dec. 1948
EDINBURGH I (Drillien 1964)	A sample by birth weight of all hospital births	Random sample of hospital matures	381 single and multiple births	214	1953–55
WINNIPEG (Grewar et al. 1962)	All hospital births	Random sample of hospital matures	736 single and multiple births	100	1953–56
NEW YORK (BROOKLYN) (Freedman 1961)	A sample by birth weight of all hospital births	Random sample of hospital matures having uncomplicated obstetric history	351 single negro births	50	1956–58 (Prems.) 1959–60 (Controls)
NEW YORK (CORNELL) (Dann et al. 1958)	All hospital births	Siblings for 47% of prematures	116 white and non-white single and multiple births	34	1940–52
DENVER, COLORADO (Lubchenco et al. 1963)	All hospital births	—	94 single and multiple births	—	1947–50
PARIS (Rossier 1962)	All births from a premature unit	—	175 single and multiple births	—	1948–51
EDINBURGH II (Drillien 1964)	All hospital births	Mature controls from Edinburgh I and siblings for 71% of school-age prematures	112 single and multiple births	214	1948–60
M.R.C. (McDonald 1962)	All hospital births from 19 prematures units	—	1128 single and multiple births	—	Oct. 1951– May 1953

BLE

TURITY SURVEYS

At last examination		Birth weight composition of premature group	Special emphasis	Data obtained from
Age	% lost			
27–46 yrs.	1	79% > 2000 g.		Records from Government agencies, e.g. military, educational, census
11+ yrs.	47 exc. deaths} 29	80% > 4½ lb. (2090 g.)	Fully representative sample on National scale	At 8 and 11 + years educational tests, verbal and non-verbal intelligence tests, and teachers' reports on behaviour
3–5 yrs.	23	12% 1500 g. or less 32% 2000 g. or less	Neuropsychiatric sequelæ by race and birth weight	Neurological examination, IQ testing (Gesell and TML)
7–8 yrs.	28	5 lb. (2270 g.) or less	No known cause for prematurity	Growth, medical history, IQ testing (Wechsler and Goodenough), educational tests, social maturity (Vineland), emotional development (Raven controlled projection)
5–7 yrs.	at 5 yrs.} 12 exc. deaths} 10	43% 4½ lb. (2090 g.) or less		*Pre-school:* physical examination, medical history, developmental testing (Gesell) at 6–12 monthly intervals. *In school:* IQ testing (TML), behaviour assessment (Bristol Social Adjustment Guide)
?3–6 yrs.	24	27% > 2000 g.		Questionnaires by Public Health nurses; children suspected of abnormality further investigated
30–33 mos.	23 exc. deaths} 20	24% 1500 g. or less	Hyperbilirubinæmia	Neurological and physical examination, developmental testing (Gesell—gross motor; Cattell and Stanford-Binet)
4–11 yrs.	37 exc. deaths} 36	All 1280 g. or less	Very low birth weight	Medical, neurological, ophthalmological examination, IQ testing (TML), social maturity (Vineland)
10 yrs.	33	All 1500 g. or less	Very low birth weight	Medical, neurological, ophthalmological examinations, electroencephalography, IQ testing (WISC)
4–7 yrs.	11 exc. deaths} 9	All 1500 g. or less	Very low birth weight	20% assessed on answers to a questionnaire. 80% neurological and opthalmological examinations, IQ testing (TML)
3–15 yrs.	At 4 yrs. or earlier} 15 exc. deaths 8	All 3 lb. (1360 g.) or less	Very low birth weight	*Pre-school:* physical examination, developmental testing (Gesell) at 6–12 monthly intervals *School-age:* physical examination, IQ testing (TML), teachers' reports on educational attainment and behaviour
6–8 yrs.	5 exc. deaths} 3	All 4 lb. (1820 g.) or less	Neurologic and ophthalmic disorders in very low birth weight	Questionnaires completed by health visitors; children suspected of abnormalities further investigated

from pregnancies in which there was a history of toxæmia, antepartum hæmorrhage or induction. Douglas concluded that, apart from a small well-defined group who were heavily handicapped, other differences between prematures and matched controls were explainable on the grounds of environmental disadvantages which remained unrecognised until the children reached 11 years.

These findings agree with those of Alm (1953) who succeeded in tracing after intervals of 27–46 years all but 1% of the male infants born prematurely in Stockholm hospitals in the years 1902–21. Compared with a group of mature male infants born concurrently, prematures showed a small but significant excess of overt mental and neurological disorder. In other respects such as fitness for military service, criminality and the need for various forms of public relief, there were no statistically significant differences between prematures and controls. Four-fifths of the prematures in Alm's sample were over 2000 g. (4·4 lb.) at birth.

From Birmingham, May (1958) reported on a sample of premature children compared individually with controls of the same age, sex and living conditions at ages 7 and 8 years. On a battery of intelligence and achievement tests the only significant difference between prematures and controls was that premature boys had significantly lower scores than their control partners in arithmetic tests. The premature children selected for testing were those of 5 lb. (2270 g.) or less, legitimate, single born, free from gross mental or physical defect detectable at birth, and born after an uncomplicated pregnancy and in most cases by a spontaneous vertex delivery. May concluded that premature children whose low birth weight could not be accounted for by adverse prenatal factors would, provided they escaped disabling defect, show the same range of development as normal full term children of the same social situation.

From Baltimore, Knobloch and her associates (Knobloch *et al.* 1956) reported their findings for 500 prematurely born infants and 492 matched controls at 40 weeks, and again when the children were between 3 and 5 years (Harper, Fischer, Rider 1959). The Gesell developmental scale was applied at both examinations and the Terman Merrill "L" Form Test at the re-examination. The children were also subjected to a careful neurological examination at both ages. In this study an attempt was made to equalise more nearly the numbers in different birth weight groups. All surviving babies whose birth weight was 1500 g. (3·3 lb.) or less were included, with the remainder selected from the weight groups between 1501 and 2500 g. (3·3–5·5 lb.). Matched controls were again used but here more precise social indices were employed than in other studies and included details of educational level of mother and season of birth. The information about social background was obtained by a small team of investigators in close contact with the families and with each other, and these workers considered that their matching technique had still successfully eliminated environmental differences between premature and control groups at the time of their last examination (Pasamanick 1962).

The incidence of mental and neurological defect increased with decreasing birth weight. At 40 weeks 51% of infants with a birth weight of 1500 g. or less were considered to have some neurological or intellectual defect, compared with 13% of full term controls. The difference between small prematures and matures increased between 40 weeks and re-examination at 3–5 years. At this age little difference was found between prematures over 2000 g. (4·4 lb.) at birth and mature controls.

A sample of 351 singleton negro babies, all of whom weighed 2100 g. (4 lb. 10 oz.) or less at birth, and 50 mature controls is being studied in the Department of Psychiatry in New York Medical College (Freedman *et al.* 1960). It was stipulated that each mature infant should be the product of a normal labour and delivery and should not require resuscitation or show clinical signs of repiratory distress. When all children had reached the age of 18 months it was reported (Freedman 1961, 1962) that a significant linear relationship had been found between developmental status and degree of maturity, with males showing more impairment than females. It was thought unlikely that differences between premature and term infants were a reflection of the poorer social environment associated with prematurity, as both survey and control infants came from the same very underprivileged social strata. An excess of impairment in male prematures as compared with females has also been reported by Lezine (1958).

Grewar and his associates in Winnipeg (Grewar *et al.* 1962) agreed that overt neuropsychiatric handicap, particularly cerebral palsy and mental retardation, increased with decreasing birth weight. In a group of infants of differing birth weight the incidence of such defects was 5% when birth weight was over 2000 g. (4·4 lb.) and 17% in the group 1000–1500 g. (2·2–3·3 lb.). In Montreal, Rabinowich, Bibace and Caplan (1961) found a greater discrepancy between prematures and controls aged 11 years than in a younger group of children aged 7½ years. At both ages mean IQ of controls was 116. At 7½ years mean IQ of premature subjects was 108 and that of the 11-year-old prematures 104. Prematures and controls all came from private and semi-private confinements. Rabinowich concluded that there were real differences between prematures and matures in the areas of general intelligence, motor coordination and also in certain aspects of perceptual functioning.

In Edinburgh, groups of hospital born premature infants and mature controls selected at random were studied from birth to 7 years (Drillien 1964). In the pre-school period scores on developmental testing for singletons and twins fell steadily with decreasing birth weight, twins showing consistently lower scores than singletons of like birth weight at all ages. Developmental ability was related to socio-economic status but in all social groupings prematures of 4½ lb. (2041 g.) or less at birth were at a disadvantage as compared with mature controls from similar homes. There was little difference in mental ability between those prematures who were over 4½ lb. at birth and the controls, except for those children coming from the best homes, where more children in this birth weight group were premature by gestation as well as birth weight. Intelligence testing in school (TML scale) gave similar results to those found in the pre-school period, with a marked excess of dull, retarded and defective children when birth weight was 4½ lb. or less, more particularly if there were additional adverse factors in environment (Fig. 1).

In school prematurely born children showed an excess of behaviour disturbance and were more likely to be working below their intellectual capacity than maturely born children of like intelligence from similar homes.

Babies of very low birth weight. A number of studies have concentrated on the later development of the smaller prematurely born babies. Improved techniques in premature baby care have been particularly successful in raising the survival rate of these babies (Rider *et al.* 1957, Drillien 1958).

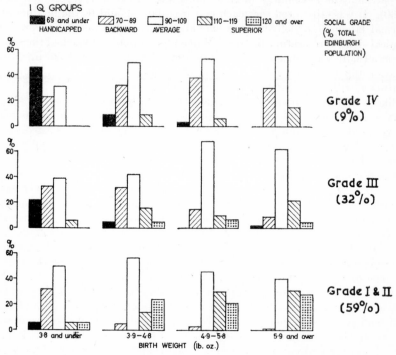

FIG. 1. Effect of birth weight, and environment on intellectual ability at age 5–7 years.

(Social Grade 1 = middle class; Grade II = superior working class; Grade III = average; Grade IV = poor)

Figs. 1–3 reproduced by courtesy of E. & S. Livingstone Ltd.

McDonald (1962) traced after an interval of 6–8 years all but 3% of surviving children who had originally been enrolled in the Medical Research Council investigation of oxygen therapy and retrolental fibroplasia. The sample comprised all infants who weighed not more than 4 lb. (1814 g.) at birth admitted to one of nineteen premature baby units between 1951 and 1953. Some neurological or ophthalmological disorder was found in 22·6% of surviving children. In addition, over one-half of the survey children who had died were known to have had a neurological disorder. The incidence of cerebral palsy amongst survivors was 6·6% and of gross mental defect (IQ 50 or less) 2·7% compared with 0·3% and 0·6% of the general population (McDonald 1961). Some of the cases of retrolental fibroplasia were certainly iatrogenic in origin and would not be found in children born in more recent years. Nevertheless, this study reveals a disturbingly high incidence of later defect in children of low birth weight.

The later development at 3 to 10 years of children discharged alive from the New York Hospital, with birth weights ranging from 600 g. (1·5 lb.) to 1280 g. (2·8 lb.) (Dann, Levine and New 1958) showed a lower incidence of severe handicap in those who were re-examined (two-thirds of the total sample). Apart from defects of vision noted in 56%, significant physical defect was found in 12% of children. Only 16% had estimated intelligence quotients below 80, although mean IQ in the premature group was 14 points below that of full term sibs. Of the children not examined 44% were known to be mentally retarded, which indicates that those presenting for examination were a selected sample with regard to mental grade.

A study of prematurely born children from Denver, Colorado (Lubchenco et al. 1963) revealed that two-thirds of a group of infants who weighed 1500 g. (3·3 lb.) or less at birth showed some visual or central nervous system defect at 10 years, although one half of the defects were not seriously crippling. Growth retardation was severe. School failures among children with normal intelligence were seen in 30% of the group. The incidence and severity of handicaps was inversely related to birth weight.

A more optimistic report comes from Paris (Rossier 1962). Rossier considered that only 12% of children weighing 1500 g. (3·3 lb.) or less at birth showed mental retardation and 7% serious motor defects when reassessed at 4 to 7 years. The children were last examined 7 years before publication of this paper and it would be informative to have more recent assessments, particularly regarding educational disposal, and also to have been given more precise details of testing procedures and the criteria of normality employed.

In Edinburgh a group of 110 children of birth weight 3 lb. (1360 g.) or less have been under study (Drillien 1964); 72 of these have passed the age of 5 years. Over one-third of the school age children are ineducable in normal school for reason of physical or mental defect, or both. Over one-third are in normal school but are educationally retarded, and less than one-third are doing class work appropriate to their age (Fig. 2). Only 30% of school age children were said to show no disturbance of behaviour. Restlessness and hyperactivity were the most commonly reported behaviour problems. Some congenital defect and/or mental retardation was found in three-quarters. Of 51 children with sibs for comparison, 76% were considered to be of poorer ability than any of their larger born sibs.

From the studies quoted above there appears to be a majority agreement that the larger prematurely born children do not show any marked impairment in mental ability compared with maturely born children from a similar environment. Below a weight of about 4½ lb. (2050 g.) there appears to be an increasing incidence of mental retardation and neurological defect as birth weight decreases, and this cannot be accounted for solely by the impoverished environment of the premature subjects. Although the reported incidence of serious handicap in the extreme prematures varies in different centres, there seems little doubt that a substantial proportion of these infants exhibit a variety of physical and mental handicaps.

4

In the three studies by Alm, Douglas, and May, it was concluded that apart from a small excess of severely defective children, the prematurely born are little different from matures with respect to intellectual ability and social adjustment. All three studies included a preponderance of prematures in the birth weight range which other authors have shown to be associated with little residual handicap. Alm's study was designed to detect only the grosser forms of disability and May's sample was highly selective. Both Douglas and May excluded children who were ineducable in normal school; 7% were excluded from the National Survey sample at 11 years for this reason. In this latter

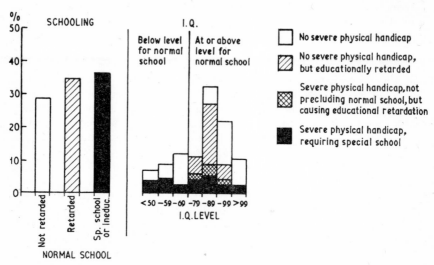

Fig. 2. Educational disposal of 72 children born 1948–56, of birth weight 3 lb. (1360 g.) or less.

investigation it seems unlikely that the rather small differences in environment between prematures and their matched controls recognised at 11 years, could account for the quite substantial difference in the proportions of definitely ·dull children found on intelligence testing (21 and 9%) and the much smaller proportion of prematures gaining entry to Grammar School. Freedman (1961) makes the suggestion that the premature may be particularly vulnerable to the effects of an impoverished and depriving environment, and that a higher correlation of socio-economic variables with test scores may be expected in the premature than in the term infant. Other authors have confirmed that the prematurely born from a poor environment appear to show increasing impairment relative to mature controls with increasing age (Harper et al. 1959, Grewar et al. 1962, Drillien 1964).

Baird (1959) and other workers in Aberdeen (Fairweather and Illsley 1960) consider that prematurity per se plays a comparatively small part in the ætiology of mental handicap, as relatively few very small infants survive, and that mental retardation in larger prematures is more often due to environmental or genetic causes. However, as Knobloch and Pasamanick (1962) have pointed out, extreme prematurity is associated with a higher incidence of damage than is found in any other prenatally affected or determined condition with the exception of mongolism.

The demonstration of a raised incidence of defect in prematurely born children raises the basic question as to what is the primary cause of such defect. Polani (1959) suggested that in some cases, possibly by reason of individual peculiarity of biological maturation, premature birth might deprive the infant of the intra-uterine environment which may be essential to final maturation of the nervous system. If the premature delivery itself is the cause of the later defect, improvements in the techniques of premature baby care, in particular those directed towards more nearly simulating the intra-uterine environment, might be expected to improve the child's chance of later normality. On the other hand, if the baby is born prematurely because of developmental defect already present (as suggested by Collier 1924), such improved techniques might lead to the survival of an increasing number of defective children. Rossier (1962) and others (e.g. Alm 1953, Hess, Mohr and Bartelme 1934, Douglas 1956) believe that severe defect in the prematurely born is usually due to intracranial hæmorrhage sustained at delivery. Others (e.g. Reid 1959, Knobloch and Pasamanick 1962, Ingram 1963) consider that "birth injury" in the premature more commonly results from intra-uterine hypoxia, following such conditions as pre-eclamptic toxæmia and ante-partum hæmorrhage, which are frequently associated with prematurity.

From the immediate postnatal condition of the infant it is impossible to differentiate between cerebral damage due to birth injury, and that due to malformation. In the Edinburgh longitudinal study it was found that the incidence of postnatal symptoms suggestive of abnormalities of the central nervous system increased with decreasing birth weight, but that at later ages there was no significant difference in mental ability between children of like birth weight who had or had not exhibited such symptoms. There was little difference in the incidence of complications of pregnancy and/or delivery in non-handicapped children of like birth weight to the handicapped, although rather more of the latter exhibited abnormal postnatal signs. Moreover, the large number of associated abnormalities, which must have arisen at an early stage of fœtal development, found in the lower birth weight babies, would support the hypothesis that in many cases both prematurity and subsequent defect were due either to an underlying developmental abnormality in the fœtus or to another factor producing both prematurity and defect.

Eastman et al. (1962) reported that a variety of congenital defects were found much more commonly in a group of cerebral palsy patients, many of whom were of very low birth weight, than in control children or in the population at large. It would appear that in these patients the primary cause of the cerebral palsy was unlikely to have been premature birth or obstetrical complications.

Neonatal nutrition. It is possible that restrictions in early feeding of small prematures may have a deleterious effect on later development (Smith 1962). Animal experiments have shown that restriction of growth in suckling rats, however much they are fed after three weeks, prevents their ever attaining normal adult size and reduces their activity and inquisitiveness during their

entire growth period (Lát, Widdowson and McCance 1960). Falkner and
Steigman (1962) reported that small premature infants offered a formula
averaging 42 cals./oz. had a greater gain in weight than those taking a
weaker formula averaging 26 cal./oz. The infants were divided into birth
weight groups of less than 3 lb. (1360 g.), 3·0–3·9 lb. (1360–1770 g.) and
4·0–4·9 lb. (1814–2223 g.). The tendency to higher weight gain with increased
caloric intake was particularly notable in the lowest birth weight group.

In the Edinburgh study of children of very low birth weight about twice
as many of those born in the years 1953 and 1954 when delayed feeding was
routine practice, show severe handicap as those born before and after this
period. Taking the group as a whole significant correlation coefficients were
obtained between scores on the Terman Merrill "L" Form Test at 5 years
or later and such factors in the postnatal history as the percentage of birth
weight lost, the days on which the lowest weight was recorded and birth
weight regained, and the days on which fluid and milk feeds were started
(Drillien 1963). It is possible, of course, that during the years 1953–54
the survival rate of defective children was improved by the regime of delayed
feeding or that dehydration resulting from fluid restriction was an added
insult in cases with a degree of prenatal brain damage.

Finberg and Harrison (1955) have suggested that hypernatremia resulting
from dehydration may result in brain damage, in a study of the clinical and
neurological state of infants with diarrhœa. It seems possible that neurological damage in small prematures may result from their tendency to dehydration and disturbances in the electrolyte and acid base balances, a
tendency which may be further aggravated by fluid restriction.

Intra-uterine growth retardation. This term should be applied only to those
infants who are markedly underweight for their gestation time, and not to the
more common group of pseudo-prematures who are born near term with a
weight of 5–5½ lb. (2270–2500 g.) often to mothers of small stature and poor
physique. Warkany, Monroe and Sutherland (1961) suggested that the term
intra-uterine growth retardation should be reserved for those having a birth
weight 40% or more below the expected weight for gestational age. It is
estimated that this group accounts for rather less than 0·2% of the surviving
new born population born at term. If premature and stillborn infants are
included the incidence rises to over 0·2%. Rumbolz and McGoogan (1953)
reviewed 20 cases including stillbirths, all of whom weighed 2000 g. (4·4 lb.)
or less at term, and workers in Cincinatti (Warkany et al. 1961) reported on
27 cases seen in consultant practice. The ætiology appears to be multiple.
Rumbolz, Edwards and McGoogan (1961) considered that "placental insufficiency" resulting in inadequate supplies of oxygen and nutriments to the
fœtus was the most important cause of the condition. Over one-half of the
placentas examined were very small and all had infarcts. In a study of perinatal mortality (Bound, Butler and Spector 1956) 18% of perinatal deaths
in a hospital practice were found on necropsy to be associated only with
maceration. It was thought that the majority of deaths in this group were
due to placental insufficiency. It was noted that a high proportion of
the mothers had complications of pregnancy such as toxæmia, hypertension, antepartum hæmorrhage and diabetes, and these complications were

associated with gross abnormalities in placental structure. Malpas (1956) has criticised the conception of placental insufficiency as a primary factor in the ætiology of intra-uterine death, and considers that demonstrable pathological abnormalities in the placenta are more often secondary to pathological conditions of the fœtus.

The cases reported by Warkany et al. (1961) showed a variety of congenital defects and 15 of 22 survivors were mentally subnormal. Genetic and familial factors were implicated in some cases and placental anomalies in others. It is, of course, possible that both placental anomaly and slow growth of the fœtus might be due to another independent factor. Pick (1954) stated that the children he studied, who were "malnourished in prenatal life," regained their birth weight rapidly if adequately fed postnatally and developed into normal children. The majority of Pick's cases were retarded in birth weight, but unlike Warkany's not much retarded in length.

Complications of Pregnancy and Delivery

That birth injury (i.e. damage sustained by the fœtus in the last trimester of pregnancy or during labour and delivery) is associated not only with a raised incidence of stillbirths and neonatal deaths, but also with the development of cerebral palsy, has been reported by many authors since the appearance of Little's paper. The literature on the causes and effects of hypoxic and traumatic damage to the infant has been reviewed by Ingram (1964).

A series of well-controlled retrospective enquiries from Baltimore has demonstrated that a variety of neuropsychiatric disorders, as well as cerebral palsy, are associated with a raised incidence of obstetric complications. These studies have been summarised by Pasamanick and Knobloch (1958). Recognising that fœtal and neonatal deaths are associated with prematurity and with complications of pregnancy and delivery, it was postulated that in the children who survived these complications, a series of neuropsychiatric disabilities would result. Depending on the degree and location of the cerebral injury, these would vary in severity from gross neuromuscular and intellectual impairment to minor disability. This hypothesis of "a continuum of reproductive casualty" was tested in studies of seven clinical entities. Five were found to be significantly associated with complications of pregnancy and/or prematurity. These were cerebral palsy; epilepsy; mental deficiency; behaviour disorders and reading difficulties. Tics were found to be significantly associated with complications of pregnancy but not with prematurity, and childhood speech disorders were not associated significantly with either pregnancy complications or with prematurity when dissociated from other neurological or intellectual defects. The influence of difficult labour and operative procedures at delivery was not thought to be of such importance as that of prolonged and probably hypoxia-producing complications of pregnancy such as toxæmia, hypertension and ante-partum bleeding. Although these studies provide firm evidence that hypoxic birth injury is an ætiologic factor of some importance in a variety of neuropsychiatric disabilities, they also demonstrate that such complications can only be of major importance in a minority of cases. The association of pregnancy complications and prematurity with later defect was most marked in the cases of cerebral palsy,

38% of whom were born to mothers with complications, as compared with 21% of normal children. This finding does not explain why the 21% of normal children escaped serious sequelæ from the same complications, nor what were the ætiological factors responsible for the 62% of cerebral palsied children born after uncomplicated pregnancies. Carstairs (1961) reviewing these and other related studies pointed out that statistically significant associations between pregnancy complications and later defect do not necessarily imply equal significance in practical terms of the number of cases thus affected.

Ingram (1964) calculated the number of possible and probable hypoxic, traumatic and toxic insults to which patients in different categories of cerebral palsy may have been subjected as a result of abnormalities of parturition. A high proportion of patients with acquired hemiplegia had no insults. A high proportion of patients suffering from dyskinesia and congenital hemiplegia suffered many insults and in other types of congenital cerebral palsy about one-fifth of cases suffered no insults and one-third many insults. Ingram concluded that in a minority of patients birth injury was of no ætiological significance in the development of cerebral palsy; in another minority birth injury was the only cause and in between there was a series of patients in whom birth injury and other ætiological factors were both important in varying degrees. In another ætiological study of congenital cerebral palsy in Edinburgh (Drillien, Ingram and Russell 1962) 65% of a group of mature diplegics were born after a complicated pregnancy and/or delivery, compared with 38% of a mature control group of hospital born infants. There was a greater excess of abnormalities of labour and delivery than of complications of pregnancy. When premature diplegic patients were compared with premature controls, no difference was found in the incidence of pregnancy complications, but there was a significant excess of disorders of labour and delivery in the diplegic group. Abnormalities of the neonatal period suggestive of cerebral abnormality were significantly increased in both mature and premature diplegic groups, particularly if there had been obstetric complications. However, 35% of the mature diplegics and 52% of the premature diplegics exhibited abnormal postnatal signs following a completely normal preganancy and delivery, compared with 1·5% and 10·5% of the control groups. These findings suggest that although perinatal injury may be the ætiological factor of major importance in some patients with congenital diplegia, in others multiple contributory ætiological factors are operating which may cause the child to be abnormal before birth or predispose him to sustain damage from hypoxia or birth trauma.

Prenatal emotional stress. The idea that emotional shock or stress during pregnancy may have an adverse effect on the developing fœtus has travelled in a full circle from being taken for granted in folk medicine, entirely discounted as unscientific and superstitious, to being once more considered as a reasonable hypothesis and worthy of experimental testing. Experimental work in animals has established that purely psychogenic stress during pregnancy has a deleterious effect on the offspring. Thompson (1957) demonstrated that pregnant rats who were exposed to anxiety by the fear of an electric shock (this fear being developed before pregnancy) were delivered of offspring who were slower to leave the open cage, took longer to discover food when hungry, and covered less ground than pups born to control mothers. Keeley (1962) subjected pregnant albino mice to stress by crowding. The subsequent litters were less active and defæcated less often than control mice. These differences were still noticeable at 100 days of age, whether the mice were raised by a crowded or an uncrowded mother and in spite of starvation. Keeley thought that abnormal endocrine activity in the crowded pregnant female might impair the development of fœtal response systems. Stott (1962a) has reviewed some epidemiological studies of animal populations which indicate that when population density reaches a certain point, before there is an actual food shortage, changes take place which have the effect of reducing the population. Signals of incipient overcrowding, in advance of food shortage, result in reduced fertility and reduced survival rate of the young; in addition those young who do survive exhibit aberrations of behaviour and poor viability.

It is well known that emotional shock or distress such as the fear of extra-marital pregnancy may result in amenorrhœa presumably due to endocrine disturbance. The German anatomist Stieve (1942) carried out necropsies of women imprisoned and subsequently executed during the Hitler regime. He found degenerative ovarian lesions which he attributed exclusively to nervous shock as the women were in a well nourished condition at the time of their death. In a later paper (Stieve 1943) he reported that the incidence of amenorrhæa in this group was 85% compared with 11% of women undergoing ordinary terms of imprisonment.

It has been suggested (Wortis and Freedman 1962) that the high incidence of premature labour among women of low socio-economic class may be related to stressful situations in their life experience. A larger number of disturbed and neurotic women were found among mothers of prematures than mothers from a similar social background giving birth to full-term infants.

Workers in Novia Scotia have also suggested that some cases of abortion and premature delivery may be due to a specific response of the pregnant woman to emotional stress (Tupper 1960). Proliferative lesions were demonstrated in the placentas and an agglutinating factor found in the maternal serum of women having abortions and premature deliveries, similar to the findings in the tissues and serum of patients with collagen disorders such as rheumatoid arthritis. Since these latter conditions are considered by some psychiatrists to be psychosomatic in nature, 22 women with a history of habitual abortion were given weekly psychotherapy. All but 2 (9%) had viable babies. Of 18 women treated in an identical manner but having no psychotherapy only 5 (28%) produced living children.

Stott (1957) carried out case studies on 102 mentally retarded children of normal physical appearance and 450 mentally normal controls; some were sibs of mentally subnormal children and others came mainly from superior type homes. The mothers reported "pregnancy stresses" (two-thirds of them being of an emotional type and one-third physical illnesses) among 66% of the retarded but only 30% of the normals. Such a retrospective finding is open to the objection that the mothers of the retarded children may have been more prone to report disturbances during pregnancy than those of the mentally normal; nevertheless, some internal corroboration was provided by the much higher incidence (76% as opposed to 29%) of non-epidemic early illness following pregnancy stress for both the retarded children and the normal controls. That pregnancy stress and infantile illness were both due to a common cause of bad home conditions seems unlikely as the association was, if anything, rather less noticeable in families regarded as inadequate than in the superior homes. When prematurely born children, twins, and those reported as having had an abnormal delivery were excluded, the association between pregnancy stress and early illness still remained about the same. There was also a significantly greater incidence (Stott 1959) of a defect of temperament termed "unforthcomingness" in children born to women having stress in pregnancy, in particular when the stress occurred or was heightened during the last trimester. This was not related to early ill-health, maternal deprivation or cultural inadequacy of the home. The types of behaviour observed after pregnancy stress bore a striking resemblance to the behavioural aberrations seen in the offspring of experimental animals subjected to anxiety during pregnancy. In a further study (Stott 1961) he reported a marked preponderance of psychogenic shock in the first trimester of pregnancies resulting in the birth of mongol children. In a control group of non-mongoloid mental defectives fewer shocks were reported and the highest incidence was in the second trimester. Stott suggested that this finding could be reconciled with the known facts of chromosomal abnormalities, if the pregnancy stresses which tended to be prolonged anxiety rather than sudden accidents, operated by interference with the regular, presumably hormonal mechanisms, by which abnormal embryos are destroyed. A retrospective study of mentally defective children in Edinburgh (Drillien and Wilkinson 1964) confirmed Stott's findings of a significantly increased incidence of severe emotional stress in the pregnancies of mothers giving birth to mongol infants, compared with those having non-mongoloid defectives. This was particularly marked in the case of mothers of 40 years and older. In most cases stress was pre-conceptional in origin. It was suggested that endocrine disturbance resulting from emotional stress might be causatively associated with the chromosomal anomalies found in mongolism. That factors of maternal physiology must have some ætiological significance in mongolism is evidenced by the marked excess of cases born to elderly mothers.

Retrospective studies of this nature are open to criticism and Stott's findings were not confirmed by McDonald (1958). In a prospective study she could not demonstrate any significant relationship between anxiety or emotional shock reported at about the twelfth week of pregnancy and later incidence of abortion, stillbirth, neonatal death or major congenital defect. Nevertheless, this seems to be an area which merits further investigation, preferably using prospective methods of enquiry and paying due regard to time and place of interview. It is unlikely that an accurate history of early stresses and anxieties can be obtained in a routine antenatal clinic, as attempted by McDonald.

Neonatal Apnœa, Asphyxia and Anoxia

A number of recent prospective studies have been designed to study the residual effects of neonatal apnœa and asphyxia. An initial difficulty arises in terminology; *apnœa, asphyxia* and *anoxia* often being used interchangeably. The term *apnœa* means only failure to breathe, whilst the terms *asphyxia* and *anoxia* indicate a reduced oxygen content of the blood. This is present in apnœa but can occur without failure to breathe. In some studies the diagnosis of asphyxia has been based on the clinical condition of the child, particularly as regards his muscle tone and colour, although it has been shown that in the immediate postnatal period cyanosis does not necessarily parallel oxygen saturation as measured (Apgar *et al.* 1955). It is estimated that between 5 and 10% of newborns have difficulty in establishing respiration after birth (Graham *et al.* 1957) and it seems likely that the later development of children exhibiting neonatal apnœa as compared with children having no respiratory difficulty will depend on the primary cause of the failure to breathe rather than the presence or absence of this particular sign. The infant who has suffered hypoxia in the last trimester is more likely to suffer damage from a short period of postnatal apnoea than the mature infant not previously hypoxic (ten Berge 1961), whose apnœa may result from prolonged labour, difficult delivery or maternal sedation.

Efforts to assess the degree of asphyxia by measurements of arterial oxygen saturation in the first few hours of life and to relate different degrees of asphyxia to later development have indicated that immediate postnatal oxygen content may not adequately reflect early asphyxia. Pennoyer and her co-workers (Pennoyer *et al.* 1956) found that reduced oxygen saturation was most commonly associated with complications of delivery and to a lesser extent with the type of anæsthesia or analgesia given to the mother. On the other hand, the immediate clinical condition of the infant seemed to be influenced chiefly by intra-uterine hypoxia associated with complications of pregnancy. Although these intra-uterine complications were not reflected in lower cord values at the time of delivery, such infants were less likely to have achieved normal oxygenation (saturation of 90% or over) by one hour after delivery and their clinical condition was more likely to be unsatisfactory. A similar finding was reported by Apgar and her colleagues (Apgar *et al.* 1955). No significant correlation was found between levels of capillary blood oxygen content measured in the first three hours after birth and intelligence levels (Stanford-Binet test) at $2\frac{1}{2}$–$4\frac{1}{2}$ years. In a later study by these same workers early asphyxia was assessed on a history of perinatal complications as well as by level of oxygen content in neonatal blood (Shachter and Apgar 1959). Statistically significant relationships were demonstrated between multiple clinical criteria of perinatal asphyxia and several psychologic signs of brain damage, but no relationships were shown with oxygen content measurements. Perinatal events considered likely to indicate the presence of asphyxia included complications of pregnancy, premature delivery and the need for neonatal resuscitation. There is no further breakdown to indicate whether infants requiring resuscitation but being of normal birth weight and having no evidence of fœtal hypoxia, differed in the incidence of later defect from those where such defect might have been primarily related to the prematurity or prenatal complications; thus this study gives no indication as to the possible effect of purely postnatal apnœa.

A positive relation between umbilical vein oxygen levels at birth and neurological abnormality was reported by Minkowski (1959). Using the techniques developed by André-Thomas and St.-Anne Dargassies (1960) evidence of neurological damage was demonstrated in 29% of 71 neonates in whom saturation was below 50%, compared with less than 3% of 98 infants having a saturation of more than 60%. 74 of the 206 infants originally examined were followed up for three years. Of these 6 were found to have persistent significant neurological abnormalities, all of them coming from the group with less than 50% saturation at birth. These abnormal children constituted 14% of the total infants followed up in this group.

A follow-up study of infants subjected to prolonged labour, and others considered to be asphyxiated (described as having asphyxia livida or pallida, or delayed respiration for longer than one minute) is being carried out from the Mayo Clinic (Keith, Norval and Hunt 1953, Keith and Gage 1960). Control groups of infants born after relatively short uncomplicated labours and those who did not have asphyxia or delayed respiration are also being studied. At both the first examination (at ages 1 to 7 years) and the second (at 8 to 14 years) there was no evidence of any difference in the incidence of neurological abnormality in children surviving the early months of life, between survey and control subjects. Information regarding the development and progress of survey children was gathered mainly from answers to questionnaires, presumably completed by the parents. Only 11% of the survey children traced at the second re-examination were personally examined and given an intelligence test. 59% of the controls were available for re-examination. This marked difference in the proportion of survey and control children returning for re-examination throws some doubt on the validity of the criteria of normality accepted for the former group.

An attempt to differentiate between different types of neonatal apnœa was made by Ernhart, Graham and Thurston (1960). Here the term *apnœa* was applied only to infants who were observed to be "not breathing," and *anoxia* was used to cover both the apnœic cases and those with various clinical signs of intra-uterine difficulty or evidence of possible interference with the oxygen supply to the fœtus. The cases were subdivided into those with postnatal apnœa only, those with possible prenatal anoxia, and those considered to exhibit both prenatal and postnatal anoxia. All survey subjects and control infants were full-term. At re-examination at 3 years neurological and psychological testing was carried out. Significant differences were found between survey and control children, the group who had both pre- and post-natal anoxia showing the biggest differences, and those with post-natal apnœa only the smallest. The distribution curves for scores on the Stanford-Binet test showed that the entire curve for survey subjects was displaced downwards. These curves suggested that anoxia is associated with a slight reduction in intelligence amongst all subjects so traumatised, rather than being a major source of severe damage in a small group of children. Impairment was more marked on tests of conceptual ability than in vocabulary skill. No differences were found in perceptual-motor functioning, though this was possibly due to insensitive measures of testing. A quite different conclusion was reached by workers in Chicago (Benaron *et al.* 1960) who re-examined, at ages 3 to 19 years, 41 of 43 children originally selected from a group of over 40,000 new born infants as being the most profoundly anoxic, together with an equal number of normal control infants. The anoxic children were also compared with their sibs. There was no significant difference in mean IQ between anoxic and control children, although the former group had a greater incidence of obvious mental retardation, 20% of anoxic children and 2·5% of controls having an IQ less than 70. Electroencephalographic abnormalities were found in 36% of the anoxic children and in none of the controls. The authors concluded that anoxia does not produce a generalised lowering of function but rather overt abnormality in isolated instances. All children studied came from an underprivileged section of the community. It is difficult to reconcile the quite opposite conclusions reached in these last two investigations.

A high incidence of pathological conditions, attributed to hypoxic brain damage, was found in a series of 125 full term children, who comprised all who could be traced of a total of 201 infants showing asphyxia at birth, born in Dusseldorf between 1956 and 1959 (Hüter 1962). Only 43% of the children were considered normal after neurological examination and mental testing (Bühler Hetzer tests) at 2 to 6 years. The incidence of disability increased with the severity of the immediate postnatal condition of the child. 65% of children with Grade I asphyxia survived and were considered to be normal at re-examination, compared with 15% of those with Grade III asphyxia (following the classification of Flagg and Wulf). Delayed mental development was taken to be IQ less than 85, and it was stated that the majority of neurological defects noted and diagnosed as infantile cerebral palsy were of a minor degree. Over three-quarters of the mothers had clinical evidence of pre-eclampsia at the time of confinement and delivery was complicated in over one-half. In addition, many had received analgesics for alleviation of pain or required anæsthetics for operative termination of pregnancy, and it was thought that these medications may have increased fœtal hypoxia in some cases.

A study from Aberdeen (Fraser and Wilks 1959, Atkinson et al. 1962) probably gives the best indication of the residual effects to be expected after postnatal apnœa. Infants studied were all mature legitimate singletons born between 1947 and 1951 in a hospital with high standards of obstetric care. In one-half of the older children the failure to breathe was attributed to mechanically difficult birth. Among the 1950–51 births the proportion of asphyxia due to physical trauma appeared to have declined. Moderate asphyxia was defined as regular breathing not established for three to five minutes. In severe cases regular respiration and cry began usually in 15–30 minutes. The children were re-examined between $7\frac{1}{2}$ and $11\frac{1}{2}$ years. As well as neurological examination they were subjected to testing of intelligence (WISC), educational attainments, motor ability, manual dexterity, perceptual ability and personality rating. Few of the asphyxiated children showed any obvious intellectual or neurological defects and some of the defects found were thought to be unrelated to incidents at birth. Minor differences were found in motor ability, manual dexterity and perceptual ability. The later report on electroencephalogram findings of 32 severely asphyxiated children and their matched controls showed no difference in the two groups, when submitted to an assessor knowing nothing of the history or clinical findings. At this date 145 infants who had been severely asphyxiated at birth were available for examination. Disorders which might have been related to condition at birth such as cerebral palsy, epilepsy or overt nerve deafness were found in 15 cases (10%).

In general, hypoxia is likely to be suspected only if there are pre-, para- or post-natal complications. Heyns (1961) however, considers that some degree of hypoxia occurs in all labours. He maintains that improved oxygenation *in utero* by means of pregnancy decompression prevents loss or impairment of neurones resulting from the normal processes of labour and delivery. Results are given of developmental testing (on the Gesell scale) of white and Bantu infants whose mothers had or had not received decompression during pregnancy. It was found that the decompression babies were superior in mental and physical development to those not having decompression. At the time of the last examination (Heyns 1962) all the decompression babies were still under 24 months. It seems possible that improved oxygenation of the fœtus could result in accelerated neuronal maturation with early acceleration of development. It will be interesting to note whether these infants maintain their superiority in later ages.

From these various reports it would appear most likely that in the absence of fœtal hypoxia few maturely born infants who fail to breathe for 15 minutes or longer suffer gross damage, although minor impairment may be relatively common. Postnatal apnœa associated with fœtal hypoxia and prematurity is more likely to be associated with subsequent neurological or intellectual defect.

The contradictory reports from different centres may be a reflection of differing standards of obstetric care, and also of the quality of the re-examinations.

Minimal Brain Damage

The term *minimal brain damage* appears to have fallen into disrepute because of the rather indiscriminate application of this label to children exhibiting minor motor dysfunction, certain forms of abnormal behaviour or having specific educational difficulties, whether or not there is reasonable evidence of such damage having occurred. Recently this concept was examined by members of different disciplines at an International Study Group (Bax and MacKeith 1962). The suggestion was put forward that, as this diagnosis is made on symptoms, it would be preferable to use the term "minimal brain dysfunction" rather than the anatomical one of brain damage. However, there are certain cases showing minor neurological abnormalities in the new born period, and/or evidence of some impairment in motor function or intellectual ability or disturbances of behaviour in later childhood, where there is also strong presumptive evidence of brain damage having occurred during pregnancy or at the birth. To these conditions the term *minimal brain damage* might legitimately be applied. Some of the cases referred to in the last section (e.g. Fraser and Wilks 1959, Shachter and Apgar 1959) come into this category.

Prechtl (1960) has demonstrated a highly significant excess of minor neurological abnormality in maturely born neonates following complications during pregnancy or at birth. At 1½ to 4 years the incidence of behaviour problems was 70% of those who had had obstetric complications and abnormal postnatal findings, 38% of those with complications but normal neonatal test results and 12% of the control group. There was no difference in developmental ability up to the age of 2 years (assessed on the Griffiths test) between those who had exhibited postnatal signs and those who had not. On the Bühler test (given after the age of 2) the neonatally normal group had a developmental quotient above 100 significantly more often than children from the abnormal group, indicating a slight but definite impairment in intellectual functioning in the latter.

Prechtl described two distinct syndromes which he attributed to minimal brain damage, (1) the hypokinetic baby who is often hypotonic, drowsy and apathetic, and (2) babies exhibiting the hyperexcitability syndrome. These babies are hyperkinetic, often hypertonic, and show sudden changes of state from being drowsy to being wide awake and difficult to pacify. A striking symptom exhibited by many is a shuddering movement, particularly well seen in the arms, when the baby is disturbed. Of 32 children who had exhibited hyperexcitability in the new born period, 70% showed the choreiform syndrome when re-examined between 1½ and 4 years. This syndrome is characterised by frequent small chorea-like twitches in all muscles, hyperactivity, short concentration span, fluctuations of attention and instability of mood. These children have learning difficulties when they are at school (Prechtl 1962; Prechtl and Stemmer 1962). Elsewhere Prechtl (1961) questioned whether some of the later behaviour disturbance might have been due to anxious or rejecting attitudes of the mother resultant on the abnormal behaviour of their infants, in that "neurologically abnormal babies do not make adequate partners in the child-mother interaction."

Ingram (1963) proposed a clinical classification of the various syndromes which have been included under the heading of *minimal brain damage*, which term he defined as "a condition of the brain which may be responsible in whole or in part for abnormalities of a child's motor, linguistic, adaptive or social behaviour and which cannot be classified easily into the existing major categories of chronic neurological or mental disease in childhood." The three clinical groups proposed were, (1) those disorders in which there is strong evidence of a fairly constant association between abnormalities of brain structure and particular symptoms and signs, such as the choreiform syndrome (which Ingram considers to be a mild dyskinesia or choreoathetosis), minor degrees of cerebral palsy and the hyperkinetic behaviour syndrome associated with temporal lobe damage; (2) disorders such as developmental dysphasia, dyslexia, and dysgraphia and some cases of "clumsiness," in which there is evidence of an associated detectable brain injury or abnormality in some patients but not in all; and (3) various symptoms of behaviour disturbance in which brain abnormality may be an inconstant contributory cause. Ingram pointed out that identical syndromes and symptoms to those in the last two categories may be due to familial or environmental factors. However, in some cases there is a history highly suggestive of birth injury and in others minor focal neurological findings, of little importance in themselves, but which indicate that the brain is probably abnormal.

Windle (1960) demonstrated neurohistological defects in the brains of monkeys which had been resuscitated after being deliberately asphyxiated at birth. Only transient signs of neurological abnormality were detected postnatally, but later psychological testing elicited statistically significant behaviour differences between asphyxiated and control groups.

The experience of the two groups of Edinburgh prematurely born children (Drillien 1964) indicated that most cases of mental retardation or gross neurological abnormality were unlikely to result from the effect of perinatal damage to a potentially normal central nervous system, there being no

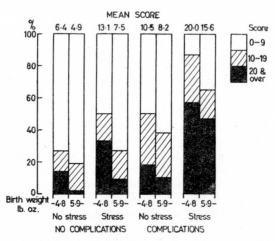

FIG. 3. Effect of birth weight, environmental stress, and obstetric complications on assessment of behaviour disorders at 6½ to 7½ years.

evidence of an excess of obstetric complications in the handicapped group as compared with those of like birth weight without major handicap, although there was an excess of all types of congenital defect. However, in the field of behaviour quite marked differences were found between children who had or had not been subjected to certain obstetric complications.

An assessment of behaviour as observed in school was made by class teachers towards the end of the second year, using the Bristol Social Adjustment Guide (Stott and Sykes 1956, Stott 1962b). The children were divided by *birth weight*, by presence or absence of early familial *stress* likely to result in disturbed behaviour, and by presence or absence of severe *complications* of pregnancy and/or delivery. Little difference was found between the larger prematurely born children of over 4½ lb. (2040 g.) and maturely born children having the same environmental background and parturition experiences, but mean adverse score for behaviour and the proportion of children considered unsettled or maladjusted was significantly higher in small prematures of 4½ lb. or less than in mature controls. Children of all birth weights subjected to severe familial stress showed an increase in adverse behaviour. This was more marked when birth weight had been 4½ lb. or less. Where there had been severe complications of pregnancy and/or delivery, a striking excess of disturbed behaviour was found in all birth weight groups, whether or not the child had been subjected to stress in the pre-school years (Fig. 3). An arbitrary grading was applied to obstetric complications to give some indication of their severity, and disturbed behaviour was found to increase significantly with the severity of the complications. A comparison of twin pairs gave an opportunity of studying the effect of birth weight and the birth process on later behaviour, in children whose hereditary endowment and postnatal environment would be roughly similar. In 21 of 73 pairs there was a marked difference in behaviour as observed in school and in all but 3 of these 21 pairs the more disturbed twin was either second born or subjected to a more traumatic delivery. When all twin pairs were considered the smaller members in pairs of like sex showed significantly more disturbance of behaviour, particularly if they were also second born. Males showed more disturbance than females if second born. In this study low birth weight, prenatal conditions likely to cause fœtal hypoxia, and potentially traumatic methods of delivery were all quite significantly associated with disturbed behaviour seven years later. Obstetric complications appeared to have the effect of lowering the resistance level to stressful situations encountered in early childhood.

Reproductive History of Mother

From the various studies already discussed two important points emerge. (1) There seems little doubt that a variety of obstetrical complications are causatively associated with degrees of later impairment ranging from gross mental and neurological defect to minor impairment of motor and intellectual function and disorders of behaviour, and (2) while a minority of children apparently sustain damage from obstetric complications, the majority escape without serious sequelæ. Even in the case of extreme prematurity where the incidence of obvious defect may be as high as 50%, there are some children who are of superior intelligence, have no congenital or other physical defect and are emotionally stable. One must suppose that in certain cases the fœtus or neonate is particularly susceptible to sustain damage from a variety of pre- or perinatal stresses, which other infants not so predisposed survive unscathed. Ernhart et al. (1960) suggested that characteristics inherent in the subject such as genetic factors may be associated with both perinatal complications and later inferiority. Steer and Binney (1962) postulated that in some cases of cerebral palsy there might be a congenital or developmental defect of fœtus or placenta which caused the neurological defect, and this in turn was responsible for anoxia and other obstetric abnormalities. Benda (1957) considered that premature delivery was not infrequently due to abnormal development of the fœtus, being "an attempt of Nature to interrupt an unsuccessful pregnancy."

There are indications that the primary cause of prematurity and later defect may be some disturbance of maternal physiology, possibly an endocrine imbalance. McDonald (1959) has demonstrated a familial predisposition to prematurity, and observed that mothers with this tendency also have frequent abortions. Eastman et al. (1962) found that a highly significant excess of previous conceptions of mothers of cerebral palsy patients had resulted in abortion or stillbirth as compared with controls.

Studies of the reproductive histories of mothers of diplegic patients in Edinburgh (Ingram and Russell 1961, Drillien *et al.* 1962) showed a similar excess of other conceptions having an abnormal outcome in the maternal histories of premature diplegic patients, and a significant excess of subfertility amongst the mothers of mature diplegic patients, subfertility being defined as difficulty in conceiving after marriage and long, unwanted gaps between pregnancies. Subfertility was more evident immediately before the birth of the diplegic patient than at other times in the mother's reproductive history.

In both the Edinburgh premature studies (Drillien 1964) mothers of low birth weight babies were found to be less successful in their other conceptions than were mothers of normal full-term infants. In addition, mothers of premature children with mental or neurological defect appeared to be less successful than those having children of like birth weight without handicap. The conception immediately preceding the birth of a small premature was the most likely to be abnormal in outcome.

A number of other authors have also reported an excess of abnormalities in the conceptions immediately preceding or succeeding a child with a congenital defect. Murphy (1947) studied the reproductive histories of all mothers of children with a congenital malformation who died during a five year period in Philadelphia. He found that abortions, stillbirths and premature births occurred more often than would be expected by chance in the pregnancies immediately preceding and following the pregnancy which resulted in the birth of the congenitally defective child. In addition, he noted that the birth of the defective child was preceded by a period of relative sterility significantly more often than were the births of its normally developed siblings. Record and McKeown (1950) studying congenital malformations of the central nervous system, found that the highest incidence of a recurrent malformation was in the pregnancy prior to or subsequent to that of another affected subject, They thought this indicated that some adverse environmental factor was tending to operate for a certain period of time in the mother's life.

The hypothesis that in certain cases the developing fœtus is unduly susceptible to intra-uterine disturbances, and that this predisposition may be genetic in origin, has been tested in an ætiological study of clefts of lip and palate (Drillien 1963). These defects were selected for study because they appear to be hereditary in origin in some cases and due to environmental causes in others. Quite significant differences were demonstrated between those cases having a positive family history of cleft and those where no family history was obtainable. Mothers giving birth to children with clefts of lip and/or palate, *in the absence of a family history*, were found to be more likely to have lost the products of other conceptions by abortion, stillbirth or infant death; they were more likely to have difficulty in conceiving with long, unwanted gaps between conceptions; and they were more likely to have other children with apparantely unrelated congenital defects. The mothers' reproductive histories showed similarities to those of mothers having defective children associated with prematurity or obstetrical complications in the third trimester. In addition, children having clefts showed a highly significant excess of other congenital defects when there was no family history of cleft. Mothers giving birth to children with clefts where there was a positive family history were little different in their reproductive capacity to mothers of unaffected control children.

The incidence of congenital defects other than clefts in the five nearest groups of relatives to the affected children was examined. No difference was found in incidence of other defects between the group of children with clefts and a positive family history and the control group. There was, however, a highly significant excess of families recording one or more defective relatives, and an excess in the total number of defective relatives, when the survey child was the only known member of the family with a cleft. Thus in the family history-negative group the tendency to produce an abnormal child was not confined to the particular mating which produced the child with a cleft, but was also apparent in other members of the family. It might seem unlikely that different malformations including cleft lip and palate should alternate freely within one family; nevertheless this possibility was strengthened by the observation that defects found in relatives were of the same type as those not uncommonly found in the cleft children themselves with a negative family history.

An unexpected finding in this study was a highly significant excess of severe menstrual disorders reported by mothers of cleft children, more especially when there was no family history of cleft and when the cleft infant was stillborn or died in the neonatal period. It was thought that an endocrine disturbance might act as the precipitating environmental insult in certain cases.

Conclusions

In this field of research it is unlikely that much more can be gained by repeated follow-up studies using the methodology of most of the investigations reviewed here, in which children judged to be at special risk because of premature birth or perinatal complications are compared at later ages with control children who have not been subjected to these obstetric hazards. With additional refinements in techniques of neurological and psychological testing it may be possible to determine more precisely those areas of intellectual or behavioural functioning most likely to be affected by minor degrees of damage. This would be useful. It would also be useful to possess more accurate methods of measuring fœtal hypoxia and placental function; more precise definitions of what obstetricians mean by such terms as "prolonged labour," and "fœtal distress," and criteria for measuring the severity of such complications as pre-eclamptic toxæmia and ante-partum bleeding. Even with standardised criteria and the use of similar testing techniques in later childhood, findings from different centres are still likely to be at variance, since the samples of mothers and children studied will differ in respect to other ætiological factors whether of maternal physiology, intra-uterine environment, genetic constitution of the fœtus, or circumstances affecting the child at later ages, all of which probably determine the outcome in infants subjected to various adverse influences during pregnancy or at birth. What seems to be needed now is a series of enquiries designed to define the nature of the additional factors which predispose some babies to malformation or to permanent damage as a result of prematurity or birth injury.

REFERENCES

ALM, I. (1953) The long term prognosis for prematurely born children. *Acta pædiat.* **42**, Suppl. 94

ANDRÉ-THOMAS, CHESNI, Y., ST.-ANNE DARGASSIES, S. (1960) The neurological examination of the infant. *Little Club Clinics in Developmental Medicine.* No. 1, National Spastics Society, London

APGAR, V., GIRDANY, B. R., MACKINTOSH, R., TAYLOR, H. C. (1955) Neonatal anoxia; a study of the relation of oxygenation at birth to intellectual development. *Pediatrics*, **15**, 653

ATKINSON, C., FRASER, M., LOWIT, I., PAMPIGLIONE, G. (1962) EEG and clinical follow-up studies of children who suffered from neonatal asphyxia and of a matched control group. *Electroenceph. clin. Neurophysiol.* **14**, 282

BAIRD, D. (1959) The contribution of obstetrical factors to serious physical and mental handicap in children. *J. Obstet. Gynœc. Brit. Emp.* **66**, 743

BAX, M., MACKEITH, R. (1962) ed. Minimal Cerebral Dysfunction. Papers from the International Study Group. *Little Club Clinics in Developmental Medicine, No. 10*, National Spastics Society. Heinemann, London

BENARON, H. B. W., TUCKER, B. E., ANDREWS, J. T., BOSHES, B., CURRAN, J., FROMM, E., YACRZYMSKI, G. K. (1960) Effect of anoxia during labour and immediately after birth on the subsequent development of the child. *Amer. J. Obstet. Gynec.* **80**, 1129

BENDA, C. E. (1957) Neuropsychiatric and neuropathological aspects of prematurity. *Ann. Pædiat. Fenn.* **3**, 109

BENTON, A. L. (1940) Mental development of prematurely born children. A critical review of the literature. *Amer. J. Orthopsychiat.* **10**, 719

BOUND, J. P., BUTLER, N. R., SPECTOR, W. G. (1956) Classification and causes of perinatal mortality. *Brit. med. J.* **2**, 5003

CARSTAIRS, G. M. (1961) Apropos de l'étiologie des troubles psychiatriques chez les enfants. Quelques études longitudinales de cohorte. In *La Psychiatrie de l'Enfant.* Vol. IV. Fasc. 1, Presses Universitaires de France, Vendôme.

COLLIER, J. (1924) The pathogenesis of cerebral diplegia. *Brain*, **47**, 1

DANN, M., LEVINE, S. Z., NEW, E. V. (1958) The development of prematurely born children with birth weights or minimal postnatal weights of 1000 g. or less. *Pediatrics*, **22**, 1037

DOUGLAS, J. W. B. (1956) Mental ability and school achievement of premature children at 8 years of age. *Brit. med. J.* **1**, 1210

DOUGLAS, J. W. B. (1960) "Premature" children at primary school. *Brit. med. J.* **1**, 1008

DRILLIEN, C. M. (1957) The social and economic factors affecting the incidence of premature birth. *J. Obstet. Gynœc. Brit. Emp.* **64**, 161

DRILLIEN, C. M. (1958) Growth and development of children of very low birth weight. *Arch. Dis. Childh.* **33**, 10

DRILLIEN, C. M. (1963) Aetiological studies of clefts of lip and palate. *Brit. Ass. Plastic Surgeons (Research Group) Meeting*

DRILLIEN, C. M. (1964) *The Growth and Development of the Prematurely Born Infant.* Livingstone, Edinburgh

DRILLIEN, C. M., INGRAM, T. T. S., RUSSELL, E. M. (1962) Comparative ætiological studies of congenital diplegia in Scotland. *Arch. Dis. Childh.* **37**, 282

DRILLIEN, C. M., WILKINSON, E. M. (1964) Emotional stress and mongoloid births. *Develop. Med. Child Neurol.* **6**, 140

EASTMAN, N. J., KOHL, S. G., MARSEL, J. E., KAVALER, F. (1962) The obstetrical background of 753 cases of cerebral palsy. *Obstet. Gynec. Survey*, **17**, 459

ERNHART, C. B., GRAHAM, F. K., THURSTON, D. (1960) Relationship of neonatal apnœa to development at three years. *Arch. Neurol.* **2**, 504

FAIRWEATHER, D. V. I., ILLSLEY, R. (1960) Obstetric and social origins of mentally handicapped children. *Brit. J. prev. soc. Med.* **14**, 149

FALKNER, F., STEIGMAN, A. J. (1962) The physical development of the premature infant. I. Some standards and certain relationships to caloric intake. *J. Pediat.* **60**, 895

FINBERG, L., HARRISON, H. E. (1955) Hypernatremia in infants. An evaluation of the clinical and biochemical findings accompanying this state. *Pediatrics*, **16**, 1

FRASER, M. S., WILKS, J. (1959) The residual effects of neonatal asphyxia. *J. Obstet. Gynœc. Brit. Emp.* **66,** 748

FREEDMAN, A. M. (1961) The effect of hyperbilirubinemia on premature infants. Progress Report. New York Medical College Department of Psychiatry.

FREEDMAN, A. M. (1962) Long-term anterospective study of premature infants. *Wld. ment. Hlth.* **14,** 9

FREEDMAN, A. M., BRAINE, M., HEIMER, C., KNOWLESSAR, M., O'CONNOR, W. J., WORTIS, H., GOODMAN, B. (1960) The influence of hyperbilirubinemia on the early development of the premature. *Psychiat. Res. Rep. Amer. psychiat. Ass.* 13

GRAHAM, F. K., CALDWELL, B. M., ERNHART, C. B., PENNOYER, M. M., HARTMANN, A. F. (1957) Anoxia as a significant perinatal experience. A critique. *J. Pediat.* **50,** 556

GREWAR, D. A. I., MEDOVY, H., WYLIE, K. Q. (1962) The fate of the expremature; prognosis of prematurity. *Canad. med. Ass. J.* **86,** 1008

HARPER, P. A., FISCHER, L. K., RIDER, R. V. (1959) Neurological and intellectual status of prematures at three to five years of age. *J. Pediat.* **55,** 679

HESS, J. H., MOHR, G. J., BARTELME, P. F. (1934) *The Physical and Mental Growth of Prematurely Born Children.* Univ. Press, Chicago

HEYNS, O. S. (1961) A device to improve fœtal oxygenation. *Trans. Coll. Physns. S. Afr.* **5,** 1

HEYNS, O. S. (1962) Use of abdominal decompression in pregnancy and labour to improve fœtal oxygenation. *Develop. Med. Child Neurol.* **4,** 473

HÜTER, VON K. A. (1962) Über Beziehungen zwischen intra- und postpartaler Hypoxie sowie zerebralen Spätschäden beim Kind. *Geburtsh. u. Frauenheilk.* **22,** 846

INGRAM, T. T. S. (1963) Chronic brain syndromes in childhood, other than cerebral palsy, epilepsy and mental defect. In *Little Club Clinics in Developmental Medicine,* No. 10, ed. Bax, M., MacKeith, R.

INGRAM, T. T. S. (1964) *Pœdiatric Aspects of Cerebral Palsy,* Livingstone, Edinburgh

INGRAM, T. T. S., RUSSELL, E. M. (1961) The reproductive histories of mothers of patients suffering from congenital diplegia. *Arch. Dis. Childh.* **36,** 34

KEELEY, K. (1962) Prenatal influence on behaviour of offspring of crowded mice. *Science,* **135,** 44

KEITH, H. M., GAGE, R. P. (1960) Neurologic lesions in relation to asphyxia of the newborn and factors of pregnancy. A long term follow-up. *Pediatrics,* **26,** 616

KEITH, H. M., NORVAL, M. A., HUNT, A. B. (1953) Neurologic lesions in relation to the sequelae of birth injury. *Neurology,* **3,** 139

KNOBLOCH, H., PASAMANICK, B. (1962) Mental subnormality. (An etiological review.) *New Engl. J. Med.* **266,** 1045, 1092, 1155

KNOBLOCH, H., RIDER, R. V., HARPER, P., PASAMANICK, B. (1956) Neuropsychiatric sequelae of prematurity. *J. Amer. med. Ass.* **161,** 581

LÁT, J., WIDDOWSON, E. M., McCANCE, R. A. (1960) Some effects of accelerating growth. Pt. III. Behaviour and nervous activity. *Proc. Roy. Soc.* **B.153,** 347

LEZINE, I. (1958) Le development psychomoteur de femmes prématurés. *Études neo-natal.* **7,** 1

LITTLE, W. J. (1862) On the influence of abnormal parturition, difficult labour, premature birth and asphyxia neonatorum on the mental and physical condition of the child especially in relation to deformities. *Trans. Obst. Soc. London,* **111,** 293. Reprinted 1958. *Cerebr. Palsy Bull.* **1,** 5

LUBCHENCO, L. O., HORNER, F. A., REED, L. H., HIX, I. E. JR., METCALF, D., COHIG, R., ELLIOT, H. C., BOURG, M. (1963) Sequelæ of premature birth. Evaluation of premature infants of low birth weights at ten years of age. *Amer. J. Dis. Child.* **106,** 101

MALPAS, P. (1956) Criticism of hypothesis of placental insufficiency. *J. Obstet. Gynœc. Brit. Emp.* **63,** 199

MAY, E. S. (1958) The later development of prematurely born children. Ph.D. Thesis, Univ. Birmingham. Quoted in Crosse, V. M. (1961) *The Premature Baby,* 5th Ed., Churchill, London

MINKOWSKI, A. (1959) The relation between umbilical vein oxygen levels at birth and neonatal and infant neurological symptoms and signs. In *Oxygen Supply to the Human Fœtus,* ed. Walker, J., Turnbull, A. C., Blackwell, Oxford

MURPHY, D. P. (1947) *Congenital Malformations. A Study of Parental Characteristics with Special Reference to the Reproductive Process,* 2nd Ed., Lippincott, Philadelphia.

McDONALD, A. D. (1958) Maternal health and congenital defect. A prospective investigation. *New Engl. J. Med.* **258,** 767

McDONALD, A. D. (1961) Maternal health in early pregnancy and congenital defect. Final report on a prospective inquiry. *Brit. J. prev. soc. Med.* **15,** 154

McDONALD, A. D. (1962) Neurological and ophthalmic disorders in children of very low birth weight. A survey with the Society of Medical Officers of Health. *Brit. med. J.* **1**, 895

McDONALD, I. S. (1959) Familial predisposition to prematurity. *Scot. med. J.* **4**, 190

PASAMANICK, B. (1962) Brain damaged children. *Brit. med. J.* **1**, 558, 1625

PASAMANICK, B., KNOBLOCH, H. (1958) Race, complications of pregnancy and neuropsychiatric disorder. *Social Problems*, **5**, 268

PENNOYER, M. M., GRAHAM, F. K., HARTMANN, A. F. with JONES, D., McCOY, E. L., SWARM, P. A., MEYER, R. J., ENDRES, R. K. J. (1956) The relationship of paranatal experience to oxygen saturation in newborn infants. *J. Pediat.* **49**, 685

PICK, W. (1954) Malnutrition of the newborn secondary to placental abnormalities. *New Engl. J. Med.* **250**, 905

POLANI, P. E. (1959) Effects of abnormal brain development on function. *Cerebr. Palsy Bull.* **1**, No. 7, 27

PRECHTL, H. F. R. (1960) The long term value of the neurologic examination of the newborn infant. In *Little Club Clinics in Developmental Medicine, No. 2*, ed. Bax, M., MacKeith, R. National Spastics Society, Heinemann, London

PRECHTL, H. F. R. (1961) The mother-child interaction in babies with minimal brain damage. A follow-up study. Tavistock Study Group on Child-Mother Interaction

PRECHTL, H. F. R. (1962) Reading difficulties as a neurological problem in childhood. A.A.C.C. Conference on Dyslexia. Baltimore. *Develop. Med. Child Neurol.* **4**, 206

PRECHTL, H. F. R., STEMMER, C. J. (1962) A choreiform syndrome in children. *Develop. Med. Child Neurol.* **4**, 119

RABINOWICH, M. S., BIBACE, R., CAPLAN, H. (1961) Sequelæ of prematurity. Psychological test findings. *Canad. med. Ass. J.* **84**, 822

RECORD, R. G., McKEOWN, T. (1950) Congenital malformations of the central nervous system. II. Maternal reproductive history and familial incidence. *Brit. J. soc. Med.* **4**, 26

REID, D. E. (1959) Remote effects of obstetrical hazards on the development of the child. *J. Obstet. Gynæc. Brit. Emp.* **66**, 709

RIDER, R. V., HARPER, P. A., KNOBLOCH, H., FETTER, S. E. (1957) An evaluation of standards for the hospital care of premature infants. *J. Amer. med. Ass.* **165**, 1233

ROSSIER, A. (1962) The future of the premature infant. *Develop. Med. Child Neurol.* **4**, 483

ROYAL COLLEGE OF OBSTETRICIANS AND GYNÆCOLOGISTS AND THE POPULATION INVESTIGATION COMMITTEE (1948) *Maternity in Great Britain*, Oxford Univ. Press, London

RUMBOLZ, W. L., EDWARDS, M. C., McGOOGAN, L. S. (1961) The small full term infant and placental insufficiency. *West. J. Surg.* **69**, 53

RUMBOLZ, W. L., McGOOGAN, L. S. (1953) Placental insufficiency in the small undernourished full term infant. *Obstet. Gynec.* **1**, 294

SHACHTER, F. F., APGAR, V. (1959) Perinatal asphyxia and psychologic signs of brain damage in childhood. *Pediatrics*, **24**, 1016

SMITH, C. A. (1962) Prenatal and neonatal nutrition. *Pediatrics*, **30**, 145

STEER, C. M., BINNEY, W. (1962) Obstetric factors in cerebral palsy. *Amer. J. Obstet. Gynec.* **82**, 526

STIEVE, H. (1942) Der Einfluss von Angst und psychischer Erregung auf Bau und Funktion der weiblichen Geschlechtsorgane. *Zbl. Gynäk.* **66**, 1698

STIEVE, H. (1943) Schreckblutungen aus der Gebärmutterschleimhaut. *Zbl. Gynäk.* **67**, 866

STOTT, D. H. (1957) Physical and mental handicaps following a disturbed pregnancy. *Lancet*, **1**, 1006

STOTT, D. H. (1959) Evidence for prenatal impairment of temperament in mentally retarded children. *Vita hum.* **2**, 125

STOTT, D. H. (1961) Mongolism related to emotional shock in early pregnancy. *Vita hum.* **4**, 57

STOTT, D. H. (1962a) Cultural and natural checks on population growth. In *Culture and Evolution of Man*, ed. Montagu, M. F. A. Univ. Oxford Press, New York

STOTT, D. H. (1962b) *The Social Adjustment of Children*, 2nd Ed., Univ. London Press, London

STOTT, D. H., SYKES, E. G. (1956) *The Bristol Social Adjustment Guides*, Univ. London Press, London

TEN BERGE, B. S. (1961) The influence of the placenta on cerebral injuries. *Cerebr. Palsy Bull.* **3**, 323

THOMPSON, W. R. (1957) Influence of prenatal maternal anxiety on emotionality in young rats. *Science*, **125**, 698

TUPPER, C. (1960) The problem of prematurity. *Canad. med. Ass. J.* **83,** 51

WALKER, J. (1960) Obstetric viewpoint on cerebral palsy. *Cerebr. Palsy Bull.* **2,** 61

WALLICH, V., FRUHINSHOLZ, A. (1911) Avenir eloginé du prématuré. *Ann. Gynécl. Obstét.* **8,** 625

WARKANY, J., MONROE, B. B., SUTHERLAND, B. S. (1961) Intra-uterine growth retardation. *Amer. J. Dis. Child.* **102,** 127

WINDLE, W. F. (1960) Effects of asphyxiation of the fetus and the new born infant. *Pediatrics,* **26,** 565

WORLD HEALTH ORGANISATION (1961) Public health aspects of low birth weight. 3rd Report of Expert Committee on Maternal and Child Health. W.H.O. Technical Report Series No. 217

WORTIS, H., FREEDMAN, A. M. (1962) Maternal stress and premature delivery. *Bull. Wld. Hlth. Org.* **26,** 285

CHAPTER 5

IDIOPATHIC HYPOGLYCÆMIA IN THE NEWBORN

GERALD NELIGAN

". . . the frequent occurrence in the normal newborn infants of cyanosis, irritability, listlessness, and muscular disorders, such as hypotonicity, hypertonicity and twitchings, might very well be due sometimes to hypoglycemia which is almost a 'normal' occurrence during the first few days of life." (Hartmann and Jaudon 1937)

THE possibility suggested in the first part of the above quotation has received ample confirmation, but only in isolated cases until the past few years, during which a number of small series of cases of symptomatic hypoglycæmia have been described by Cornblath, Odell and Levin (1959), Cornblath, Baens and Lundeen (1961), Haworth, Coodin, Finkel and Weidman (1963), Brown and Wallis (1963), and Neligan, Robson and Watson (1963). The delay has largely been due to the fact, mentioned in the last part of the quotation, that blood sugar levels which would be expected to produce symptoms of hypoglycæmia in older children are regularly found during the first few days of life in babies who are perfectly well. Systematic use of a therapeutic test has been largely responsible for the recent clarification of the position. The idea which had to be accepted, and used as a tool in studying the problem, was that if abnormal neurological signs can be promptly and completely abolished by intravenous glucose in an adequate dose, this constitutes good evidence that the abnormality was due to hypoglycæmia, even in a newborn baby. There is now general agreement that this is so, with the difference that in the newborn the blood sugar level has to fall below about 20 mg./100 ml. before any clinically detectable abnormality occurs. There is also admittedly greater difficulty in excluding other diagnoses during the first few days, when the brain has recently been exposed to the risk of damage by trauma and anoxia, and may currently be exposed to other possible biochemical disturbances such as a questionably low blood level of calcium. But the dramatic response to intravenous glucose of a true and uncomplicated case (repeated after an interval of hours or days if treatment is inadvertently stopped too soon) provides the most convincing possible evidence that symptomatic hypoglycæmia does occur even in the newborn.

Within the past year some progress has also been made towards the possibility of understanding the conditions under which symptoms arise. There certainly need be no fall in the blood glucose level, which may have been very low indeed for as long as 48 hours previously. It has seemed tempting to postulate that the brain may be using an alternative metabolic fuel during this period, and that symptoms do not arise until this too is exhausted. Edwards (1964) has reported that in newborn calves rendered hypoglycæmic by intravenous insulin there is a compensatory rise in blood lactate levels (provided the splanchnic nerves are intact) which appears to prevent the development of symptoms. It seems possible that a similar mechanism exists in the human newborn.

Normal Blood Sugar Level

Some of the difficulties in establishing a normal range of values for the neonatal period have been due to differences between the analytical methods which have been used. The glucose oxidase method of Huggett and Nixon (1957) is specific for glucose. The chemical methods which come nearest to it, and which have been used for most of the published observations, are based on those described by Nelson (1944) and Somogyi (1945). They are adequate for this purpose, so long as there is no pathologically raised level of galactose or fructose. Similar results are being obtained by the method used in automatic analysers in which the non-sugar reducing substances are eliminated by dialysis. The chemical methods have the advantage that fluoride can be used to eliminate any risk of glycolysis after the blood is collected, which may otherwise be troublesome (Baens, Oh, Lundeen and Cornblath 1961).

All observers are agreed in recording a more or less abrupt fall in the blood sugar level of the normal baby after birth, to reach its lowest after some hours or at latest on the second or third day, often at a level which would be expected to cause hypoglycæmic symptoms in an older child. The earlier work defining this tendency to hypoglycæmia was fully reviewed by Smith (1959), who also discussed the mechanisms which could be involved but did not consider any single explanation adequate. None has been provided by the reports published subsequently, that there is a well-marked rise in the blood sugar level following intravenous injection of glucagon (Cornblath, Levin and Marquetti 1958); that there is a well-marked rise in adrenalin output when hypoglycæmia is deliberately produced with insulin (Greenberg, Lind and von Euler 1960); and that there is little rise in the already very low level of the plasma insulin-like activity in response to a large intravenous dose of glucose (Baird and Farquhar 1962). In view of the results of their own investigations, Cornblath, Wybregt and Baens (1963) have suggested that the tendency to hypoglycæmia at this age is due to the metabolic demands of the disproportionately large brain of the newborn exceeding the liver's capacity to supply sufficient carbohydrate to maintain a "normal" blood sugar level by adult standards, during the initial period of relative starvation.

A further difficulty about trying to establish a normal range of values at this age lies in knowing how to define a normal baby for this purpose. The infants of diabetic mothers are obvious candidates for separate consideration, and are discussed in the following chapter of this book. Premature infants have also usually been reported separately, and Cornblath, Baens and Lundeen (1961) recorded a mean blood glucose level of 35 mg./100 ml. on the third day in a group of babies who weighed less than 2 kg. at birth. They also noted lower levels in the babies who developed a variety of symptoms not attributable to hypoglycæmia, but specifically including the respiratory distress syndrome, than in those who remained well. There is some doubt whether the baby's blood glucose level may vary with changes in body temperature under normal conditions, but none about the tendency for severe accidental chilling to cause hypoglycæmia (Mann and Elliott 1957). The extent to which the possible effects of a variety of factors may have to be taken into account is illustrated in the paper by Cornblath, Ganzon *et al.* (1961). They concluded that the mother's blood sugar level at the time of delivery affects the baby's cord blood level but not his subsequent response to glucagon, and that this response is less good in the premature than the mature, less good in the mature within the first 3 hours than after the first 6 hours, and less good in the baby delivered by cæsarean section without being exposed to labour than in the baby exposed to labour and then delivered either vaginally or by section—but that all these differences are abolished if ten times the standard test dose of 30 μg./kg. is used.

Symptomatic Hypoglycæmia

Against this background of uncertainty there was no acceptable basis for attributing any newborn baby's neurological disturbance to his "hypoglycæmic" blood sugar level (since it was known that the well-looking baby in the next cot might be just as "hypoglycæmic"), until the therapeutic test with intravenous glucose was systematically applied. The test is based on the observation that in the uncomplicated case the clinical abnormality can be promptly and completely abolished by raising the blood sugar level to more than 20 mg./100 ml., and keeping it there till the baby demonstrates his ability to maintain it on his ordinary diet without special help. The first report of a series of cases of "symptomatic neonatal hypoglycæmia" in which the diagnosis was based on this test was published by Cornblath *et al.* (1959). This and subsequent reports are agreed in finding that in such cases the "true" blood sugar level is less than 20 mg./100 ml. Cornblath, Baens *et al.* (1961) went further, saying that "persistent levels below 20 mg./100 ml. are abnormal." Such levels were associated with abnormal behaviour in 7 of the 8 babies in whom they occurred.

But the diagnosis is far from straightforward in many cases, as was well shown by the correspondence in the *Lancet* which followed publication of the papers by Brown and Wallis (1963) and Neligan *et al.* (1963). Blood sugar levels below 20 mg./100 ml. are even more likely to be found, transiently, in a variety of abnormal states than in normal babies. When such hypoglycæmia is associated with accidental chilling, with respiratory distress or with cerebral damage due to trauma, anoxia or infection, or to the hypoglycæmia itself, treatment with intravenous glucose cannot be expected to produce a complete cure. But it may theoretically (and in practice) produce partial clearing of the abnormal signs, either by eliminating any which are being directly caused by the (secondary) hypoglycæmia, or by some quite unrelated effect such as reduction of cerebral œdema by osmosis. Correction of the hypoglycæmia in such cases can do no harm, and may do some good, provided a watch is kept upon the blood sugar levels, since these may easily be raised above acceptable limits by the large doses of glucose which are characteristically required in the true "idiopathic" case. It may also be reassuring later, if signs of permanent brain damage develop, to know that this cannot have been caused by such an easily treatable cause as hypoglycæmia. But incomplete relief of the symptoms by an adequate test dose of glucose implies that those which persist must have another cause, which requires investigation in the hope that it too may be treatable.

The clinical course of a typical mild uncomplicated case is summarised in Fig. 1. Baby W. weighed 4 lb. 9 oz. (2070 g.) when delivered by forceps on account of signs of slight fœtal distress, after an uncomplicated pregnancy lasting 277 days from the first day of the last menstrual period. At the age of 17 hours he had a series of mild apnœic attacks, responding quickly to toe-flipping. When examined at 19 hours he appeared semi-conscious and no Moro response could be elicited, though he was rather irritable when handled.

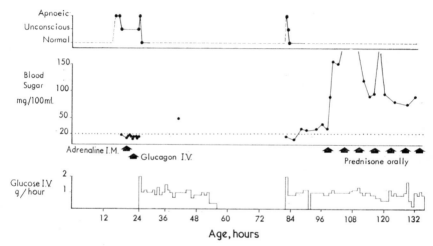

FIG. 1. Baby W., weight 2,070 g. at 39 weeks, course over first 5½ days (see text). In the upper *clinical* section the unbroken line represents continuous, and the broken line intermittent, observation. *Blood sugar* shown in the middle section; *treatment* by intravenous glucose, intramuscular adrenaline, intravenous glucagon, and oral prednisone shown in the bottom section.

His "true" blood sugar level was later reported as 16 mg./100 ml. Since his symptoms were mild it was considered justifiable to delay intravenous treatment with glucose long enough to investigate his response to adrenalin (0·03 ml./kg. of a 1:1000 solution intramuscularly), followed after two hours by glucagon (30 µg./kg. intravenously). There was no change in his clinical state or his blood sugar levels. At the age of 26 hours he had another apnœic attack, and further delay was considered unjustifiable: the fluid in the scalp vein drip (which had been kept open with 0·9% sodium chloride solution) was changed to 10% glucose solution. After 6 ml. had been run in rapidly he became pink, appeared normal in his behaviour, and within a few minutes had a normal Moro response. He remained well, with his drip running at about 9 ml. hourly. When it slowed and then stopped at the age of 56 hours he was taking 30 ml. of milk 3-hourly by bottle and so was left to see if he could manage without extra help. At 82 hours, however, he had another apnœic attack just when a feed was due. He was again found to be semi-conscious with increased tone but no Moro response. A new drip was immediately set up and after 10 ml. of 10% glucose solution had been run in rapidly his behaviour became normal again. At the age of 98 hours his response to adrenal glucocorticoids was assessed by starting treatment with oral prednisone, while maintaining his glucose infusion at as nearly constant a rate as possible. The blood sugar level responded dramatically, reaching a peak of 235 mg./100 ml. after 10 hours and then returning to more normal levels. Intravenous treatment was stopped on the sixth day of life, his blood sugar level was well maintained after the prednisone was stopped, and he appeared well at the time of discharge from hospital.

Various important aspects of the syndrome can be illustrated by reference to his case-history.

Clinical picture. The onset is usually a little later than this, during the second or third day of life, and often in relation to the time of the first feed in our experience. This picture of mild apnœic attacks with a semi-conscious or dazed appearance and irritable, "jittery" movements when roused, but no satisfactory Moro response, is typical of the milder cases: in the more severe cases the picture is dominated by alarming apnœic attacks or convulsions and a state of deep coma. There does not appear to be any characteristic difference from the picture that may be produced by other causes of mild or severe disturbances of cerebral function (traumatic, chemical or infective) except in so far as the latter may give rise to localising signs such as raised fontanelle tension and cranial nerve palsies.

Diagnosis depends upon the result of the therapeutic test in a baby who shows a suggestive neurological disturbance. In the case of Baby W. the full routine diagnostic procedure was not carried out, and it was considered justifiable to delay the start of treatment by some hours for the reasons stated. Our usual routine, when confronted with a baby in whom the diagnosis has to be considered, is first to take blood (and cerebro-spinal fluid, as a rule) for the appropriate analyses, and then straight away and without waiting for the results to test the response to adequate doses first of calcium then of glucose. The intravenous route is optimal, because it can ensure that the blood level of the substance administered is raised rapidly by a predictable amount. In the case of glucose, rapid administration of 10–20 ml. of a 10% solution can be expected to raise the blood sugar level by 50–100 mg/100 ml., at least transiently, depending upon the size of the baby and his blood volume. This will temporarily correct any degree of hypoglycæmia, without danger of producing harmful hyperglycæmia if the initial level turns out to have been normal. If the injection of either substance produces prompt and complete correction of the neurological abnormality, this can be accepted as *prima facie* evidence that its cause was a pathologically low level of that substance. In the case of glucose, the infusion of 10% glucose can be continued at a rate of about 90–110 ml./kg./24 hr. while awaiting confirmation of the diagnosis by a report that the initial blood sugar level was less than 20 mg./100 ml. Other ways of raising the blood glucose level initially have been described, but they appear more appropriate to the phase of treatment, under which heading they are discussed. For the purpose of the initial therapeutic test, if there is any technical difficulty about making the injections into a scalp vein, the umbilical route can be used instead.

The possibility that symptomatic hypoglycæmia may be due to one of the rare but well-defined causes, such as glycogen storage disease or a pancreatic islet cell tumour, cannot easily be excluded at this stage. Such causes need to be considered seriously if the spontaneous recovery which is characteristic of the "idiopathic" case does not occur within the first week or so of life. No case of leucine-sensitive hypoglycæmia appears to have been described at this age, and the onset of symptoms is often either before the baby has had any milk or clearly unrelated to feed-times. But if there is any doubt, the appropriate test can be performed in due course (Cochrane, Payne, Simpkiss and Woolf 1956).

Clinical background. This aspect is relevant both to the clinical diagnosis and the prevention and treatment. The factors predisposing to hypoglycæmia which have already been mentioned are environmental chilling, respiratory distress and cerebral damage. They are mentioned again here because of the practical importance of thinking about the possibility that any associated neurological disturbance may be wholly or partly due to this complication, which can be treated.

But the factor which is illustrated by the case of Baby W. and which at present appears to be much the commonest factor in the background of the "idiopathic" cases, is the poor nutritional state at the time of birth, evidenced by a weight of 4 lb. 9 oz. (2070 g.) after a pregnancy lasting 277 days. The association was described by Usher (1961) and Zetterström (1961), who stressed that the toxæmia of pregnancy which had been present in each of the 8 cases of symptomatic neonatal hypoglycæmia described by Cornblath et al. (1959) would have tended to cause malnutrition of the fœtus, and described a disturbed relationship between birth weight and maturity in their personal cases. This way of defining intra-uterine malnutrition is convenient and relatively objective, though subject to the limitation that there may be varying degrees of uncertainty about the mother's "dates." If the physique and nutritional state of the mother are normal, lowering of the birth weight relative to a reliable estimated duration of pregnancy presumably indicates some degree of impairment of utero-placental function. Fig. 2 is a composite chart illustrating this relationship in 30 cases where the diagnosis was made by the therapeutic test of intravenous glucose. The mother's pregnancy was complicated by pre-eclamptic toxæmia in 22 of the cases. That there is a relationship between intra-uterine malnutrition and relatively low blood sugar levels has been confirmed in asymptomatic babies by Neligan et al. (1963). Their findings are summarised in Fig. 3. No light has yet been shed on the reason why only a small proportion of the babies whose blood sugar level falls below 20 mg./100 ml. show any signs of a neurological disturbance.

The connecting link between malnutrition and hypoglycæmia could be supplied by the state of the glycogen stores in the liver at the time of birth. Normally these form the main source of the glucose required to maintain an adequate blood level during the period after the newborn mammal has been abruptly deprived of the continuous "assisted transfusion" of carbohydrate from the placenta, and before he has begun to absorb adequate quantities from any other source. That the situation may easily become critical was dramatically illustrated by Shelley (1961) who used published data from 7 animal species to demonstrate the steep build-up of the glycogen concentration in the liver of the fœtus towards the end of pregnancy, and the even steeper fall after birth to reach lower levels before the end of the second day than at any later stage. She also summarised a number of animal experiments in which the concentration present at the time of birth was shown to have

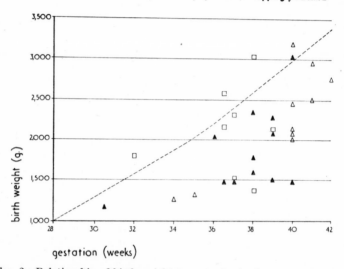

FIG. 2. Relationship of birth weight to maturity in three series of cases of symptomatic hypoglycæmia. □ cases of Cornblath *et al.* (1959); △ cases of Brown and Wallis (1963); ▲ cases of Neligan *et al.* (1963). Broken line gives mean growth curve of fœtus, based on figures of Scammon and Calkins (1924–25).

been markedly reduced in offspring whose mothers had been subjected to insulin-induced hypoglycæmia or acute starvation. No data were available at that time for the human fœtus beyond the first half of pregnancy. The difficulty is that liver tissue for analysis can only be obtained from dead babies, which has delayed the attempt to build up a series of values which could be described as "normal." More recently these difficulties have been partly overcome, largely as a result of the finding that tissues from babies who have been refrigerated within a few minutes of death are suitable for this form of analysis (Shelley 1964). The rise towards the end of pregnancy and the rapid fall after birth have been confirmed in material from 130 autopsies. The fall is even greater in cases of hyaline membrane disease (p. 64), and particularly low values were also found in cases of intra-uterine malnutrition, as defined above.

There is indirect support for the idea that neonatal hypoglycæmia in the human baby may be due to depletion of the stores of glycogen available to him. The rapid fall in the respiratory quotient, which has long been known, from near unity at the time of birth to reach its lowest level of about 0·75 on the second and third days of life (Smith 1959) indicates a change in the main source of energy from carbohydrate to fat. Failure to show the appropriate response to parenteral adrenalin and glucagon, as in the case of Baby W. and the few other babies suffering from hypoglycæmia who have been tested before treatment with glucose was begun, may indicate that there is a deficiency of the necessary substrate (liver glycogen). Also the first two

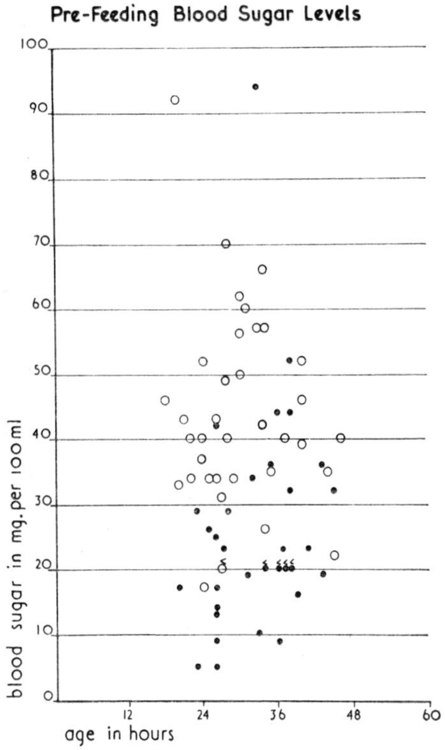

FIG. 3. "True" blood sugar level in asymptomatic babies before the first feed. ○ 36 well-nourished babies (mean birth weight 3,180 g. at 37·9 weeks); ● 33 poorly-nourished babies (2,040 g. at 38·1 weeks). In 5 of the cases the blood sugar was recorded as "< 20 mg./100 ml."

predisposing factors for hypoglycæmia, mentioned at the beginning of this section, are both conditions in which the rate of consumption of carbohydrate is likely to be increased at certain stages owing to increased energy requirements. Widdowson (1961) has shown the effect of exposure to cold and of simulated respiratory distress upon the liver glycogen content of fasting piglets during the first 24 hours of life.

In the light of these findings, the question of alimentary intake of carbohydrate assumes great interest. Haworth and Ford (1963) studied the effect of early administration of glucose by mouth upon the blood sugar levels of "premature" babies (without apparently taking into account the question of intra-uterine malnutrition) and were unable to satisfy themselves of any benefit. This question seems ripe for further study.

But poor development of enzyme systems or hormonal responses could explain the malnourished baby's proneness to neonatal hypoglycæmia, quite apart from any reduction in the liver's glycogen stores. The only direct information about such babies has been provided by Broberger and Zetter-ström (1961) and Zetterström (1961), whe found an absence of the rise in adrenalin output which normally occurs in response to hypoglycæmia induced with intravenous insulin. There is no explanation of this association between malnutrition and reduced activity of a hormone, nor of the relation-ship to the control of blood sugar levels in these babies. The whole problem is made all the more perplexing by the fact that a background of intra-uterine malnutrition is characteristic of the rare cases of congenital temporary diabetes mellitus which have been described, most recently by Hutchison, Keay and Kerr (1962).

Treatment has the aim of keeping the blood sugar at a level where the particular baby's behaviour appears normal. In general terms it seems reasonable to keep it securely above the level of 20 mg./100 ml. below which any baby is liable to show a neurological disturbance. It is one of the striking characteristics of these "idiopathic" cases that this aim may be surprisingly difficult to achieve. There is general agreement that glucose cannot be given by mouth in sufficient quantities to achieve it (Cornblath et al. 1959, Brown and Wallis 1963, Neligan et al. 1963). But Creery (1963) reported that simultaneous administration of adrenal glucocorticoids can produce a satisfactory result, and the effect of steroid therapy during continuous intravenous infusion of glucose is illustrated in Fig. 1. The intravenous route is more certain and corrects the abnormality more rapidly, which seems a matter of some urgency in any but the mildest cases. It makes rapid changes in the rate of administration possible, which is sometimes convenient. A 10% solution of glucose given at a rate of about 40–50 ml./lb. (90–110 ml./kg.) per 24 hours is usually sufficient, but it is wise to check the blood levels at intervals. If they are not satisfactory a suitable steroid can be used as an adjuvant. Treatment usually has to be continued for several days, and there are objections to using the umbilical route for this purpose, especially if the catheter has to be passed through a potentially infected umbilical vein stump. If a scalp vein infusion is impracticable, the treatment of choice would seem to be to administer equivalent volumes of 10% glucose solution by tube into the stomach, and to reinforce this with an appropriate adrenal steroid parenterally. It has been suggested that fructose may have advantages both for intravenous and intragastric use, because when in solution it is far less irritant than equivalent concentrations of glucose. But before accepting that this form of treatment is satisfactory for the individual case of sympto-matic hypoglycæmia it would be necessary to show that conversion of the fructose is being carried out satisfactorily after absorption, by demonstrating an adequate rise in the blood level of glucose, as measured by the glucose oxidase method. In any case where milk administration is long delayed, the risk of electrolyte depletion arises.

The possibility of an early clinical and biochemical relapse after a day or two of effective treatment, is also illustrated in Fig. 1. It might have been anticipated by carrying out serial blood sugar estimations after the first drip was taken down.

Prognosis. Most of the adequately treated cases reported so far have recovered spontaneously within the first week of life, and had no further trouble. But it has long been recognised that the first manifestations of idiopathic hypoglycæmia of infancy may occur during the first few days of life (McQuarrie 1954). When the diagnosis is made in the first few days, therefore, the possibility of further episodes should be taken as an indication for adequate follow-up, since these recurrences may take the form of convulsions without any of the usual accompanying signs of hypoglycæmia. So far, 2 of the 12 cases of symptomatic hypoglycæmia diagnosed among the 6,000 or so babies born in our hospital during the three years beginning September 1959, including Baby W., have had hypoglycæmic convulsions in later infancy. When this happens it seems wise to take steps to exclude one of the rare clear-cut causes, such as glycogen storage disease, islet cell tumour and leucine sensitivity, before instituting a regime of palliative treatment. This may take the form of simple modification of the diet if the history suggests that this may be effective, or a maintenance dose of glucocorticoids, continued until the expected ultimate recovery is confirmed by serial blood sugar values after withdrawal of treatment.

The magnitude of the risk that serious brain damage will be produced by persistent or recurrent hypoglycæmia is difficult to assess, for the reason which makes the assessment of any such problem in the neonatal period peculiarly difficult, namely the wide range of other factors, whether measured or not, which may be operating at the same time. But there seems to have been no adequate alternative explanation for the majority of the deaths occurring during the original episode, and the cases of permanent brain damage, reported so far (Cornblath *et al.*, 1959, Howarth *et al.* 1963, Brown and Wallis 1963). Certainly the risk of such complications forms a cogent incentive to all concerned to make the diagnosis as early as possible in every case, since the abnormality is so much more amenable to treatment than most others which involve this sort of risk at this age. Among the questions which remain to be answered is whether the babies whose blood sugar levels fall below an arbitrary figure, say 20 mg./100 ml., but who show no symptoms, are also exposed to an increased risk of brain damage and should therefore be treated. The answer to this and other questions will only come from long-term follow-up studies.

REFERENCES

BAENS, G. S., OH, W., LUNDEEN, E., CORNBLATH, M. (1961) Determination of blood sugar in newborn infants. *Pediatrics*, **28**, 850

BAIRD, J. D., FARQUHAR, J. W. (1962) Insulin-secreting capacity in newborn infants of normal and diabetic women. *Lancet*, **1**, 71

BROBERGER, O., ZETTERSTRÖM, R. (1961) Hypoglycemia with an inability to increase the epinephrine secretion in insulin-induced hypoglycemia. *J. Pediat.* **59**, 215

BROWN, R. J. K., WALLIS, P. G. (1963) Hypoglycæmia in the newborn infant. *Lancet*, **1**, 1278

COCHRANE, W. A., PAYNE, W. W., SIMPKISS, M. J., WOOLF, L. I. (1956) Familial hypoglycæmia precipitated by amino-acids. *J. clin. Invest.* **35**, 411

CORNBLATH, M., LEVIN, E. Y., MARQUETTI, E. (1958) The effect of glucagon on the concentration of sugar in the capillary blood of the newborn infant. *Pediatrics*, **21**, 885

CORNBLATH, M., ODELL, G. B., LEVIN, E. Y. (1959) Symptomatic neonatal hypoglycemia associated with toxemia of pregnancy. *J. Pediat.* **55**, 545

CORNBLATH, M., BAENS, G. S., LUNDEEN, E. (1961) Hypoglycemia in premature infants. *Amer. J. Dis. Child.* **102**, 729

CORNBLATH, M., GANZON, A. F., NICOLOPOUCOS, D., BAENS, G. S., HOLLANDER, R. J., GORDON, M. H., GORDON, H. H. (1961) Some factors influencing the capillary blood sugar and the response to glucagon during the first hours of life. *Pediatrics*, **27**, 378

CORNBLATH, M., WYBREGT, S. H., BAENS, G. S. (1963) Tests of carbohydrate tolerance in premature infants. *Pediatrics*, **32**, 1007

CREERY, R. D. G. (1963) Hypoglycæmia in the newborn. *Lancet*, **1**, 1423

EDWARDS, A. V. (1964) Resistance to hypoglycæmia in the newborn calf. *J. Physiol.* (in press)

GREENBERG, R. E., LIND, J., EULER, U. S. VON (1960) Effect of posture and insulin hypoglycemia on catecholamine excretion in the newborn. *Acta pædiat.* **49**, 780

HARTMANN, A. F., JAUDON, J. C. (1937) Hypoglycemia. *J. Pediat.* **11**, 1

HAWORTH, J. C., COODIN, F. J., FINKEL, K. C., WEIDMAN, M. L. (1963) Hypoglycemia associated with symptoms in the newborn period. *Canad. med. Ass. J.* **88**, 23

HAWORTH, J. C., FORD, J. D. (1963) The effect of early and late feeding and glucagon upon blood sugar and serum bilirubin levels of premature babies. *Arch. Dis. Childh.* **38**, 328

HUGGETT, A. ST. G., NIXON, D. A. (1957) Use of glucose oxidase, peroxidase, and O-dianisidine in determination of blood and urinary glucose. *Lancet*, **2**, 368

HUTCHISON, J. H., KEAY, A. J., KERR, M. M. (1962) Congenital temporary diabetes mellitus. *Brit. med. J.* **2**, 436

MANN, T. P., ELLIOTT, R. I. K. (1957) Neonatal cold injury due to accidental exposure to cold. *Lancet*, **1**, 229

MCQUARRIE, I. (1954) Idiopathic spontaneously occurring hypoglycemia of infants. *Amer. J. Dis. Child.* **87**, 399

NELIGAN, G. A., ROBSON, E., WATSON, J. (1963) Hypoglycæmia in the newborn: a sequel of intrauterine malnutrition. *Lancet*, **1**, 1282

NELSON, N. (1944) A photometric adaptation of the Somogyi method for the determination of glucose. *J. biol. Chem.* **153**, 375

SCAMMON, R. E., CALKINS, L. A. (1924/5) The relation between the body weight and age of the human fetus. *Proc. Soc. exp. Biol. (N.Y.)* **22**, 157

SHELLEY, H. J. (1961) Glycogen reserves and their changes at birth. *Brit. med. Bull.* **17**, 137

SHELLEY, H. J. (1964) Carbohydrate reserves in the newborn infant. *Brit. med. J.* **1**, 273

SMITH, C. A. (1959) *The Physiology of the Newborn Infant.* 3rd ed., Thomas, Illinois, U.S.A., Ch. 9, p. 12

SOMOGYI, M. (1945) Determination of blood sugar. *J. biol. Chem.* **160**, 69

USHER, R. H. (1961) In Ciba Foundation Symposium on *Somatic Stability in the Newly Born.* Churchill, London, p. 10

WIDDOWSON, E. M. (1961) Metabolic effects of fasting and food. In Ciba Foundation Symposium on *Somatic Stability in the Newly Born.* Churchill, London, p. 39

ZETTERSTRÖM, R. (1961) Carbohydrate metabolism and the rôle of the liver. In Ciba Foundation Symposium on *Somatic Stability in the Newly Born.* Churchill, London, p. 59

CHAPTER 6

THE INFLUENCE OF MATERNAL DIABETES ON FŒTUS AND CHILD

JAMES W. FARQUHAR

BABIES born to diabetic women form only a small percentage of all births, but they are the subject of disproportionate interest not to the physician, obstetrician, pædiatrician and nurse alone, but to others in the field of anatomy, physiology, pathology, chemistry, nutrition, teratology and genetics. They represent, as it were, an experiment of Nature in which growth and survival are attempted within an environment possessing growth-disturbing and lethal effects, and they suggest answers to questions on fœtal growth and development, on the cause of malformations, on placental function, on adaptation to extra-uterine life, on the action of insulin and on the function of both maternal and fœtal endocrine glands, on the ætiology of diabetes mellitus and on some of the vascular troubles which afflict both the diabetic adult and newborn child. And they also present a challenging perinatal mortality, pleasure at reducing which is tempered just a little by doubts concerning the long-term prognosis both for surviving children and for their offspring.

The subject is reviewed in the following order: external characteristics and neonatal behaviour; body structure (gross, microscopic and chemical); possible causes of altered structure and disturbed function; prenatal factors in perinatal mortality; management of the newborn; the progress of survivors.

External Characteristics and Neonatal Behaviour

External characteristics. Most newborn infants of diabetic mothers conform to the same external morphological features. They bear a striking resemblance to each other, are plump, sleek, liberally coated with vernix, full-faced and plethoric. Their gigantism is shared by the umbilical cord and the placenta. With the hairiness and the œdema which may exist, these features have been described as cushingoid. But the œdema can seldom be demonstrated at birth, and recent studies have shown that the fullness of these Pickwickian poppets is due very largely to fat. This type of baby comes in various sizes ranging from 2·5 to about 5·5 kg. depending upon the gestational age and the standard of diabetic control, but another and rarer variety exists. These ill-favoured, runted fœtuses with their thin umbilical cords, diminished vernix and dry skin suggest the dysmaturity syndrome and, having remained much the same size for several weeks *in utero* present at birth as "post-mature" at a gestational age of perhaps 36 weeks. They are to be distinguished from the very prematurely born infant of the diabetic woman which at 30 or 32 weeks looks very much like any other infant of that maturity.

Normal behaviour. During the first few days of life most of these babies conform to a slightly unusual but unalarming pattern of behaviour. Immediately after birth, if delivered by cæsarean section and then held head-down, they pour amniotic fluid from the mouth. The practice of holding them in this position for a few moments may explain why the volume of gastric contents is so small at birth in the Edinburgh series (Farquhar 1959) when compared with the previous experience of Gellis, White and Pfeffer (1949) in Boston. Respiration is established without difficulty in from 60 to 75% of cases and, as in other immature babies, breathing may be a little irregular for the first few days. The rate may be 60 or 70 per minute at one hour, but decreases steadily into the normal range during the next few hours. Such a baby lies comfortably on his back, bloated and flushed, sucking his tongue at times, legs flexed and abducted, abdominal and skeletal muscles relaxed, and lightly closed hands resting by each side of his head. "He conveys the impression of having had such a surfeit of food and fluid pressed upon him by an insistent hostess that he desires only peace so that he may recover from his excesses." But he is always and increasingly easy to disturb so that he may spontaneously or in response to very little noise or vibration engage in quick little movements which have been described variously as jittering, juddering, trembling, tremoring, twitching, or even as fits. Whatever their cause may be, they involve all the limbs as in the Moro reflex, although the arm movements are the more striking.

Toward the end of the first day and certainly on the second he will complain vigorously if he is not fed, and the longer that fluids are withheld from him, the more deeply jaundiced he is likely to become (Rudolph, Hubbell, Drorbaugh, Cherry, Auld and Smith 1959) until by the third or fourth day his complaints are silenced by weakness and he lies dry, bronzed and quiet.

Weight loss. During these first few days he was thought to lose much more weight than normal babies by shedding congenital œdema (White 1952), an opinion which was reflected in the well-known text-books of obstetrics and pædiatrics during the next few years. A statistical study disproving this view has been published (Farquhar and Sklaroff 1958). In short, the previous claims for abnormal weight loss were based on an uncontrolled evaluation of absolute weight loss from birth, but a very large baby is likely to lose more grammes than a smaller one, even although he may lose no greater a percentage of his birth weight. The percentage loss was found not to differ between early-fed babies born by cæsarean section to diabetic and non-diabetic mothers (Fig. 1). Delayed feeding and the route of delivery rather than maternal diabetes are the factors which govern it.

Oedema and diuresis. The public image of these babies is created out of such facts as the frequency of hydramnios in diabetic pregnancy, the spewing of amniotic fluid from their mouths at birth, their possibly increased urine volume, their greater weight and glossy fullness, their imagined excessive weight loss, their cyanotic attacks, respiratory distress, pulmonary adventitious sounds and cardiac failure. All of these suggest the œdema to which reference is still made (Peel 1962). But to this indirect evidence must be added the fact that some do have demonstrable œdema although observers dispute its nature. It is seldom demonstrable at birth but may develop during the first few hours of life and, as in the immature infant, can be found over the limbs and trunk. It may be more marked in babies with respiratory distress (Sutherland, Oppé, Lucey and Smith 1959) in whom increasing limb volume is demonstrable at a time when body weight is decreasing, and it may persist for a little in the presence of dehydration. They seem to pass rather

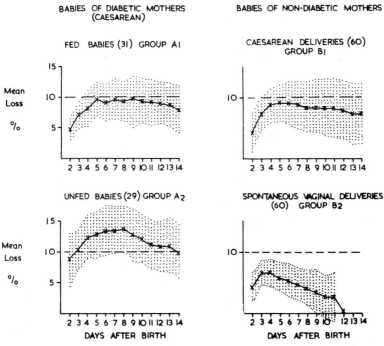

FIG. 1. Postnatal weight loss of babies as a percentage of birth weight. The shading indicates ± one S.D. about the mean.

more urine than normal controls (Fig. 2) but not in the amounts which are to be expected from patients with demonstrable pitting (Farquhar 1959, Osler 1960d). The volume seems to vary in different parts of the world and may relate to the induced state of maternal hydration just before and during delivery.

Abnormal behaviour. Even the healthiest looking baby of a diabetic mother may suffer one or more sudden episodes of deep cyanosis during which he may look quite lifeless. He is limp, commonly has respiratory arrest, and his heart rate may be reduced to infrequent beats. These attacks last for one or two minutes, and the baby then gasps and returns slowly to normal respiration, heart rate, tone and colour.

Respiratory distress of varying degree is a feature of these babies (Moore, Kay, Desmond and Dutton 1960); the subject is considered in Chapter 3, pp. 57, 69.

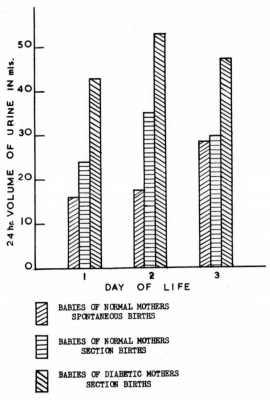

FIG. 2. Daily volume of urine passed by babies of normal and diabetic
women.

Fœtal Structure

Weight. The heaviness of most of these babies for gestational age is their
most striking abnormality. Their gigantism is generalised, although the
cranial vault, sharing less in the obesity, may look disproportionately small.
Skull measurements, however, have been reported as normal by Fischer and
Moloshok (1960). The previous descriptions by Warren and Le Compte (1952)
and by Cardell (1953a) said little or nothing about fat, and Cardell very seldom
found œdema, while Driscoll, Benirschke and Curtis (1960), working largely
from the pathological archives of the Boston Lying-in Hospital, were unimpressed by gigantism, visceromegaly or œdema. But gigantism is due in part
to fat, fat and œdema may be reduced or lost before death, and both may be
prevented to some degree by strict dietary control of the pregnant diabetic,
so that the classical features may be less obvious in some medical centres
than in others, although such babies in Boston and Edinburgh bear a striking
resemblance. The pathologist's population is not a fair sample of that seen
at birth by the clinician, and their respective findings cannot be strictly
compared. Live comparison by means of skin-fold thickness and radiological
measurements of the subcutaneous fat layer of such babies with that of

normal full-term infants and of others of the same maturity born to non-
diabetic women has shown that it is increased by from 38 to 46% over the
normal newborn and by 50% over normal infants of the same gestational age
(Osler 1960b).

Length.   The above-average length has been the subject of previous
comment by Warren and Le Compte (1952) and by Cardell (1953a) and of a
clinical study by Pedersen (1954a).   But a later investigation by Osler and
Pedersen (1960) was widely interpreted as meaning that the small difference
in length from normal infants of the same gestational age could be accounted

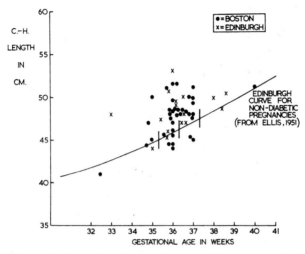

FIG. 3.   Crown-heel lengths of babies born to diabetic women in Boston
(U.S.A.) and in Edinburgh.

for by increased thickness of subcutaneous fat (Driscoll *et al.* 1960).   The
matter has received further attention from Osler (1961).   Working retrospectively from case records, he has compared the lengths of infants of diabetic
mothers, not with those of normals of the same gestation, but with the lengths
of normals in the same 200 g. weight groups.   If anything, the diabetic groups
were just a little, but not significantly, shorter.   He also provides mean
radiological measurements of the femoral and tibial diaphyses of four infants
of diabetic women and of four control babies matched for weight instead of
for maturity.   The bone length of the diabetic group is shorter by approximately 0·5 cm.   Thus babies of diabetic women maintain a normal birth
weight–length ratio.   But this is not in dispute for no one has claimed that
such babies are disproportionate.   If, however, they have maintained a
normal weight–length ratio, then weight and length are both abnormal for
gestation.   Nothing much is known of comparable girths, but if babies of
diabetics are fatter, then, when matched with babies of the same length and
weight, the different density of their tissue should involve their occupying a
greater volume.   The real controversy, however, concerns the cause of their
increased, if proportionate, length.   A recent small prospective study of accurately measured crown-heel lengths in both Boston and Edinburgh (Fig. 3)

again suggests that these babies are longer than controls of the same gestational age (Farquhar 1962b). This difference is unchanged by some days of no or low caloric intake, and this makes it less easy to explain in terms of soft-tissue layers.

Radiological measurements, other than of the dead, are generally avoided now unless indicated for clinical reasons, and the dead cannot provide normal values. Changes in linear measurements are usually less impressive than are those in volume or weight, but they are important to an understanding of fœtal growth in diabetic pregnancy. A need persists for an accurate prospective survey with accurate equipment and standardised technique, which includes simultaneous controls from non-diabetic women matched for all those factors which can influence fœtal size. The cause of premature birth so often influences fœtal growth *per se* that the collection of such a series is difficult.

Ossification. The development of ossification centres in such babies does not correspond to their length or weight but to their gestational age or less. Thus growth outstrips maturation (Osler and Pedersen 1960).

Other structures. Both brain and heart may be of abnormal size (Driscoll *et al.* 1960, Miller 1944, Cardell 1953a), the lungs may be the site of hyaline membrane formation (see p. 57), and an interesting and important predisposition to renal thrombosis may exist (Takeuchi and Benirschke 1961).

Congenital malformations. Reports are at their most controversial and intriguing when they deal with the incidence of congenital malformations. As in all studies of the frequency of malformation, the answer obtained depends upon the accepted definition of congenital malformation, upon the size and nature of the population, upon the inclusion or otherwise of stillbirths (which may escape physicians and pædiatricians), upon the thoroughness and the repetition of examination, and upon the autopsy of all cadavers. Furthermore, comparison of incidence in various communities also depends completely on the homogeneous nature of the study throughout the community.

Comparisons of the incidence of very serious or lethal malformations in some of the larger series is possible. Peel and Oakley (1950) found 6·3% compared with an incidence of 0·94% in the same hospital for non-diabetic pregnancy; Pedersen and Brandstrup (1956) found 3%, and Gellis and Hsia (1959) reported an incidence of 2·9% of lethal malformations which they compared with 0·75% in non-diabetic pregnancy reported from the same hospital by Reid (1956). In the best known autopsy series (in which, of course, there is likely to be a much higher incidence of malformation than in the general population) Driscoll *et al.* (1960) found, from autopsy records, 24·1% of gross malformations, most of which were classed as major and two thirds (16·8%) of which were lethal. Only Cardell (1953a) has published figures for personally-conducted and simultaneous autopsies on infants of diabetic and non-diabetic women. In reaching a malformation incidence of 25 and 20·2% respectively, he dismisses the difference as insignificant.

The range of malformations is wide and shows no tendency to specific combinations. Thus they involve the cardiovascular, central nervous, genitourinary and alimentary systems as well as the skeleton of which the vertebral column seems either to be more susceptible or better suited to the recognition of deformity.

Experience of malformations in the Edinburgh series has already been published (Farquhar 1959) but has been extended (Farquhar 1961). Still-births and neonatal deaths have been submitted to autopsy in 95% of cases and only two badly macerated stillbirths have been omitted. Abnormalities have been compared with those selected at random from the archives of the pædiatric pathology service at the same hospital over the same period (Table I) and no significant difference was found.

TABLE I

ABNORMALITIES PRESENT FROM BIRTH IN CHILDREN OF
DIABETIC MOTHERS AND IN CONTROLS
(EDINBURGH 1948–1959: 182 babies, including 3 sets of twins)

Diabetic Pregnancies	*Non-diabetic Pregnancies*
STILL-BIRTHS	
Total 23. *Autopsy Performed on* 21	Total 21. *Selected at Random*
1. Anencephaly.	1. Phocomelia; Meckel's diverticulum; patent urachus.
2. Hypoplastic thymus.	2. Severe talipes.
	3. Encephalocele; adrenal hypoplasia.
NEONATAL DEATHS	
Total 15. *Autopsy Performed on All*	Total 15. *Selected at Random*
1. Unilateral renal agenesis.	1. Arnold-Chiari; hydrocephalus; unilateral renal agenesis.
2. Widely patent ductus arteriosus	2. Renal agenesis; hypoplastic lungs; lacunar skull.
(7 had pulmonary hyaline membrane)	3. Renal hypoplasia.
	(4 had pulmonary hyaline membrane)

The surviving children were examined several times during the newborn period but have since been examined on from one to three further occasions up to the age of 12 years. Almost all have been examined by the same person but a few exceptions living in other parts of the U.K., the Republic of Ireland, or overseas have been examined by the kindness of local pædiatricians who have followed instructions governing the examination of children in Edinburgh. A small number has been lost from the series for a variety of reasons (Table II). Of the two deaths, one healthy child was killed in a road accident, but the other, in whom no abnormality was detected in hospital, died suddenly at home aged four weeks, and on the basis of a cardiac murmur heard just before death the family doctor diagnosed congenital heart disease. No autopsy was obtained. Each child has been matched as closely as possible with another, conceived in the same month of the same year and born in the same hospital to a non-diabetic woman of the same age and parity. These controls were examined with the same care by the same person along with the children of diabetic mothers. A medical history has been taken on each occasion and evaluation of general growth and development has been followed by systematic clinical examination. Such diagnostic aids as radiography and electrocardiography have been employed only where clinical suspicion was aroused, and routine radiological examination of the skeleton

TABLE II

144 CHILDREN SURVIVING THE NEWBORN PERIOD

LOST FROM THE SERIES—2 by death, 3 by emigration, 1 lost trace, 1 by adoption, and 2 by intention (a mongol and a post-meningitic amentia)
TOTAL 9

135 SURVIVING CHILDREN OF DIABETIC MOTHERS COMPARED WITH THE SAME NUMBER OF CONTROLS

Diabetic Pregnancies	*Non-diabetic Pregnancies*
1. Patent ductus arteriosus.	1. Coarctation of the aorta.
2. Cardiac murmurs, probably organic, 3. but without disability or other sign.	2. Pulmonary stenosis.
	3. Aberrent left coronary artery (died at 10 years).
4. Cardiac murmurs, possibly organic, 5. but without disability or other sign.	4. Cardiac murmurs, probably organic, 5. but without disability or other 6. signs. 7.
6. Sacral agenesis.	8. Cerebral palsy.
7. Ataxic diplegia with deafness.	9. Idiopathic epilepsy.
8. Mental defect (neonatal period normal).	10. Severe rotatory nystagmus.
9. Cleft vertebræ; hemivertebræ; scoliosis (little disability).	11. Congenital ptosis.
10. Bilateral cataract.	12. Facial hemiatrophy and ptosis.
11. Large abdominal lymphangioma.	13. Congenital stenosis naso-lacrimal duct.
12. Unilateral hydronephrosis (no obstruction found and not progressive).	14. Epidermolysis bullosa.
13. Fused bifid thumb.	15. Icthyosis.
14. Tight tendo-calcaneus (no physical or intellectual disability).	16. Hypertrophic pyloric stenosis; bilateral club feet.
15. Fused upper central incisors.	17. Oesophageal hiatus hernia?
16. Inguinal hernia.	18. Oesophageal hiatus hernia.
17. Squints—10.	19. Inguinal herniæ. 20.
18. Benign heart murmurs—11.	21. Absent finger nail.
	22. Squints—7.
	23. Benign heart murmurs—9.

has been avoided. These abnormalities have been listed which were judged by the same examiner to be of sufficient functional or cosmetic importance (Table II). The presence of some organic cardiac murmurs in non-diabetic cases was not disclosed to their parents because the children were without complaint, but they will be recalled for further study. There is little difference in the incidence of malformations in the two groups, but some are clearly inherited disorders while others may result from factors operating in early pregnancy. A much larger study than this may be required to settle the argument, but two things are clear: (a) even should there be a statistically significant difference between the groups, the individual diabetic mother in Edinburgh need have no greater fear of fœtal malformation than the non-diabetic woman, and (b) large numbers of cases are no substitute for careful planning, examination and recording. With regard to the mongol child, no record has been found of an increased incidence of this abnormality among babies of diabetic women, but Farquhar (1962c) has commented upon the high incidence of mongolism among the diabetic child population of Scotland, and there is a little evidence that some mongols have minor disturbances of carbohydrate metabolism (Bixby and Benda 1942, Dutton 1961).

Placenta. White (1945) stated that the placenta usually deviates from the normal in size, that it is notably large, that the cord is abnormally thick and that infarcts may be present. It may be very small in some cases. According to Farquhar (1959) the placental-to-fœtal weight ratio does not differ from that in non-diabetic pregnancy, and this accords with the pathological experience of Driscoll et al. (1960).

Histological Findings in Fœtus

Pancreas. Unusual size of the pancreatic islets, for which many references are given by Pedersen (1952) and by Farquhar (1958), has been the subject of both excitement and scepticism among pathologists because of the variations which may occur in size and in site of islets, not only in the pancreas of such babies but in those of infants of non-diabetic women. The observations of Tejning (1947) make their hypertrophy almost certain, and their area in such babies and in controls has been measured both by Cardell (1953b) and by Woolf and Jackson (1957). Expressing their figures in terms of percentage of total pancreatic area, the workers in both investigations found the "diabetic group" to have on average about 4 times the normal area of islet tissue. A direct relationship between the degree of islet hypertrophy and fœtal weight has been claimed both by Cardell (1953b) and by Driscoll et al. (1960). The latter found appreciable islet hypertrophy in four-fifths of the babies studied. Much must yet be learned about the histology of the fœtal islets (Ferner 1952, Robb 1961) but infants of diabetic mothers appear to have more β-cells than the usual 50% present in the newborn, and islet hypertrophy represents the result of β-cell hyperplasia (Hultquist, Lindgren and Dalgaard 1946, Cardell 1953b, Woolf and Jackson 1957, Driscoll et al. 1960). This suggests either an increased capacity or a block in the secretion of insulin (Farquhar 1959).

Other structures. Increased myocardial glycogen was thought to account for part of the cardiomegaly observed in earlier studies, but this experience was unshared by Warren and Le Compte (1952) or by Cardell (1953b). Similar findings have been reported in relation to the liver but no descriptions of muscle or subcutaneous tissue glycogen content are available, and the observations of Klein, Marks, Roldan, Sherman and Fetterman (1962) on the initial insulin treatment of juvenile diabetes suggest that the latter may be rewarding.

Increased extramedullary erythropoiesis has been reported (Cardell 1953a,

Driscoll *et al.* 1960), and increased normoblastæmia was described by Berglund and Zetterström (1954).

Follicle development in female infants has been noted previously, but hyperplasia of testicular interstitial cells has received less attention (Bayer 1942) although it was noted by Driscoll *et al.* in 38%. Similar findings are reported by Geoghegan and Drury (1962) and by Scott (1962) who has found that they are more readily recognised than pancreatic islet hypertrophy and that the pattern remains clear for some considerable time even in the macerated fœtus. The specificity of these changes is rejected by Rewell (1962).

The small blood vessels of established diabetics have become the object of much attention in recent years, with particular emphasis on their involvement in the degenerative complications of the disease. The conjunctival vessels are accessible to the bio-microscope and for skilled photography using such equipment as that described by Edgerton (1962). The recent literature on this subject has been briefly reviewed (Farquhar 1962a, 1962b).

Placenta. The calcification of the maternal uterine vessels found by White (1952) in pregnant diabetics is rare in Edinburgh. According to Burstein, Soule and Blumenthal (1957) the placentas of diabetic mothers differ from those of normal, toxæmic or hypertensive women in that about one-third show marked endarteritis, and the affected vessels progress to vascular obliteration or thrombosis and true infarct formation. The placenta has been examined by the electron microscope (Wislocki and Dempsey 1955) but it is difficult tissue to get and handle in the undamaged fresh state.

Chemical Changes

Body composition. The œdema which a proportion of these babies may develop during the first few hours was once thought to exist at birth, to be the cause of their excessive weight, and to be followed (as it was shed) by remarkable weight loss. But their weight loss does not differ significantly from that of infants of non-diabetic women (Farquhar and Sklaroff 1958). Careful studies on living immediately-newborn babies by Osler (1960a, 1961) have shown that those of diabetics have significantly less total body and extracellular water than is normal, and these findings have been confirmed by Cheek, Maddison, Malinek and Coldbeck (1961) and by Clapp, Butterfield and O'Brien (1962). They are interpreted as implying the presence of increased body fat, and this is in keeping with Osler's fat thickness measurements. Direct analysis of one cadaver by Fee and Weil (1960) showed that fat was moderately increased for an infant of comparable size and markedly increased for gestational age when compared with those figures given by Widdowson and Spray (1951). The body-water/protein ratio corresponded more with gestational age than with body size, and the inter-relationship of electrolyte values suggested a slight increase in intracellular but none in extracellular fluid. A further 8 bodies have since been analysed, and first calculations suggest confirmation of increased body fat from the 34th week of gestation (Fee and Weil 1962).

Varying degrees of uncompensated acidosis at birth have been described by Lowrey, Graham and Tsao (1954), Reardon, Field, Vega, Carrington, Arey and Baumann (1957), Segal, Sutherland, Lucey, Drorbaugh, Cherry and Hsia

(1957), and Reardon (1959), and this may be independent of acid-base balance in the mother (Kaiser and Goodlin 1958). Similar findings are described for infants of prediabetic women (Carrington, Shuman and Reardon 1957).

The diminished O_2-saturation of cord blood in these babies, together with their vigorous erythropoiesis and normoblastæmia, led Berglund and Zetterström to the conclusion that they were exposed to prolonged prenatal hypoxia, and this received some support from the observations of Walker (1954), MacKay (1957) and Prystowski (1957). As a result of many further studies, however, Prystowski, Hellegers and Bruns (1960) warned that, "it is tempting to associate the reduced gradients in clinically abnormal pregnancies with a diminution in oxygen transfer to the fœtus, but until other aspects of placental oxygen transfer are evaluated, it would seem wise to hold such feelings in abeyance."

Apparently inconsistent changes in serum potassium have been reported. According to Björklund (1953) they may be sufficiently low to produce changes in the electrocardiogram, and a possible need to give potassium to such babies was mentioned by Peel (1955). Normal levels have been reported by Lowrey et al. (1954), Zetterström and Aberg (1955), Clayton (1956), and Gellis and Hsia (1959).

Serum calcium levels were found by Gittleman, Pincus, Schmerzer and Saito (1956) to be low in babies born after complicated non-diabetic pregnancy and/or delivery. Zetterström and Arnhold (1958) found a mean of 8·5 mg./100 ml. during the first two days of life in babies of diabetic women, while Craig (1958) and Craig and Buchanan (1958) described levels of from 8 to 6 mg. or less with an ultrafilterable component of 4·9 mg. or less. This has also been the experience of Gittleman, Pincus, Schmerzer and Annecchiarico (1959) and of Rose (1960). The serum phosphorus level was reported to be raised by Zetterström and Arnhold (1958), Gittleman et al. (1959) and Rose (1960).

Much has been written about the significance of the hypoglycæmia which can be found in most of these babies, and, for a time, in a high proportion of normal newborn infants of normal women. The relevant literature of the previous fifty years or so was extensively reviewed by Pedersen (1952) and by Farquhar (1956a, 1958). The subject is dealt with briefly on p. 139 and in greater detail in Chapter 5.

Increased amounts of corticosteroids have been reported in the amniotic fluid, the blood or the urine of babies of diabetic women by Hoet and Lukens (1954), Björklund and Jensen (1955), Farquhar (1956b), Klein and Taylor (1960) and Lloyd (1961), but not in the careful and authoritative study made by Migeon, Nicolopoulos and Cornblath (1960), nor in the amniotic fluid investigation by Baird and Bush (1960). The urinary corticoid excretion during the first few days of life in a small number of infants of diabetic and prediabetic mothers has been compared with that of healthy infants who had suffered neonatal stress and for details of this the writer is indebted to Dr. Constance Forsyth and her colleagues. Using the method previously described by Birchall, Cathro, Forsyth and Mitchell (1961), Forsyth and Cathro (1962) found that infants of diabetic mothers tended to show high levels of corticoid excretion (Fig. 4) reflected in all areas of the chromatogram. They also

showed high levels of steroids giving sodium-fluorescence. The baby who
showed an extremely high level had an exchange transfusion at birth, but
the others had a normal course, and a proportion continued to show high
corticoid output, while babies of prediabetic women showed normal excretion
on each day. Most of the stressed infants of non-diabetic women suffered

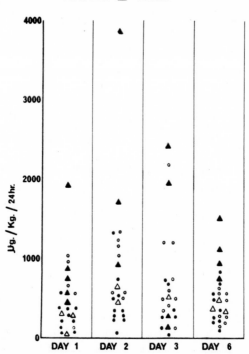

BLUE—TETRAZOLIUM—REDUCING   STEROIDS

FRACTION Ⅲ TOTALS

FIG. 4. Total blue-tetrazolium-reducing steroid excretion in micrograms
per kilogram of body weight per 24 hours. (By courtesy of Dr Constance
C. Forsyth.)

▲ Infants of diabetic mothers.
△ Infants of prediabetic mothers.
● Healthy full-term and premature infants.
○ Sick full-term and premature infants (e.g. with respiratory distress).

from respiratory distress and their raised corticoid excretion was less sustained than in the diabetic group. As only one of the babies born to diabetic
mothers suffered stress, Forsyth and Cathro suggest that their high corticoid
excretion was directly related to maternal diabetes.

Of the plasma protein fractions, Ditzel and Moinat (1957) found that some
pregnant diabetics had significant increases in β-lipoprotein and in α_2-
glycoprotein during the last trimester. The abnormal pre-β-lipid fraction was
found by Vernet and Smith (1961) to increase in successful diabetic pregnancy
from the 25th week and to fall rapidly after delivery, whereas in unsuccessful

cases it rose earlier, reached higher levels and persisted for some time after the infant's birth. The cholesterol, phospholipid, α-, β- and γ-lipoprotein levels of infants of diabetic women in Edinburgh (Lloyd 1961) were compared with normal values as determined by Rafstedt and Swahn (1954). Little difference is apparent in cord levels, but the mean values for the two groups vary during the first week of life (Fig. 5). Unfortunately for this short investigation, the eleven babies available to it pursued normal courses. Lastly,

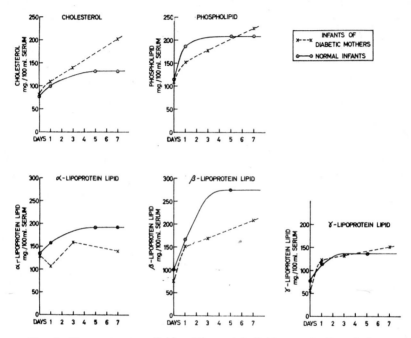

FIG. 5. Changes in serum lipid and lipoprotein lipid concentrations during the first week of life in infants of normal and diabetic mothers.

Sirek, Sirek and Leibel (1961) found that the hexose, hexosamine and sialic acid contents of the carbohydrate moiety conjugated with plasma proteins (the glycoproteins) were significantly raised in babies whose mothers were without recognisable clinical or biochemical disturbance other than their diabetes. Later (1962) they showed that the electrophoretic pattern of serum proteins differed distinctly and consistently from that of normal controls of the same gestational age. The pattern of the diabetic group has a larger number of distinct arcs of which that in continuation of the orosomucoid and that in the siderophilin region are the most striking.

Possible Causes of Gigantism

Genetic. Although there is such a thing as familial fœtal gigantism unassociated with diabetes, the development of fœtal overgrowth in diabetic pregnancy largely depends upon the maternal environment, and if some unrecognised inherited characteristic of fœtal tissue plays any part, it ceases obvious operation from birth for at least some years. The possibility of fœtal outsize among babies fathered by diabetic men is not so clear. They were found to be somewhat heavier than those of non-diabetic fathers by Jackson (1954, 1960) and this experience is shared by Pirart (1955) and by Kellock (1961), but not by Babbott, Rubin and Ginsburg (1958) nor by FitzGerald, Malins, O'Sullivan and Wall (1961). Pyke (1960) found the evidence inconclusive. Thus one author failed to provide the data on which his statement was based, while others employed an unsatisfactory questionnaire technique.

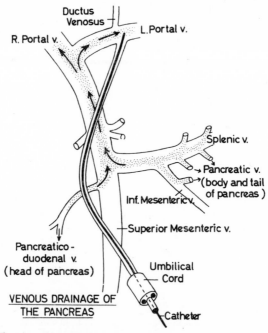

Fig. 6. Showing the sampling catheter positioned proximal to the veins which drain the pancreas.

How many men between 16 and 92 years of age can provide from memory details of their reproductive history without either forgetfulness or exaggeration? A properly controlled prospective study should be undertaken in an obstetric unit where details of paternal health are also indexed, or from a diabetic clinic with good obstetric-pædiatric liaison.

Hyperinsulinism. A high carbohydrate diet favours obesity, and the "sugar babies" described by Trowell and Jelliffe (1958) resemble those of diabetic women. Present opinion holds that increased secretion of insulin by the fœtal pancreas is responsible in whole or in large part for the baby's size, in particular for his obesity, and it may promote skeletal growth in experimental animals (Salter and Best 1953, Salter, Davidson and Best 1957). Advanced ossification need not occur, as linear growth and maturation of bone seem to be controlled by different factors (Leeming 1962). The pancreatic islet hypertrophy, β-cell hyperplasia, postnatal hypoglycæmia, obesity and possible increase in tissue glycogen all favour such a possibility, and Osler (1960b) suggests that the release of water by glycogenolysis causes the increased urinary volume and possibly the postnatal œdema. The intravenous glucose tolerance of newborn infants of diabetic and normal women has been studied by Baird and Farquhar (1962). While the most surprising feature of this investigation, later confirmed by Schwartz, Bowie and Mulligan (1962), Mulligan and Schwartz (1962), Larsson (1963) and Cornblath (1963), is the poor tolerance of normal mature newborn babies, it also demonstrates that infants of diabetic women have a tolerance akin to that of normal adults. Baird and Farquhar also measured the insulin-secreting capacity of the newborn. By catheterising the umbilical vein for the appropriate distance (Fig. 6) they were able to obtain blood near to its discharge from the pancreas.

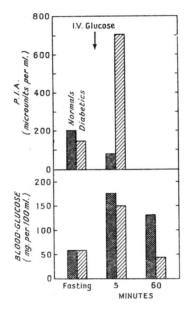

Fig. 7. Plasma insulin activity in response to an intravenous glucose load.

After a fasting-sample for insulin-assay had been taken from the babies, they were given a glucose load by rapid intravenous injection and a second sample was taken exactly five minutes later. The resulting mean values for plasma insulin-like activity are shown in Fig. 7. The experiment may be criticised on grounds of the rat-diaphragm method of assay used, the differing maturity of the babies studied, and the time at which the second sample was taken, but the difference between the groups seems to be clear. It has been confirmed by Stimmler, Brazie and O'Brien (1964), who used the immunochemical method of insulin assay described by Morgan and Lazarow (1963).

The poor tolerance of normal newborns can be improved by injecting insulin along with the glucose load. The average tolerance of babies of diabetic and normal women in Baird and Farquhar's series, plotted on a semi-logarithmic scale, are shown in Fig. 8. To these are added the tolerances of two normal babies who received the same amount of glucose and also soluble insulin 0·13 unit/kg. (one baby was given the insulin subcutaneously 5 minutes before the glucose load and the other received both glucose and insulin in the same intravenous injection). The resultant change in gradient does not mean that the poor tolerance of normal newborns necessarily results from limited ability to secrete insulin, but it is in keeping with the belief that the better tolerance of infants of diabetic women results from their greater secretion or better release of the hormone.

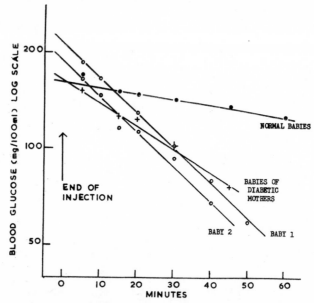

Fig. 8. The mean tolerance to an intravenous load of glucose of babies born to diabetic and normal women. Babies 1 and 2 are infants of normal women, but the rate at which they remove from circulation an injected load of glucose has been influenced by exogenous insulin. The arrow indicates the point at which the intravenous injection of glucose ended.

The popular explanation for the β-cell hyperplasia and enhanced insulin production of these babies is maternal hyperglycæmia, but such other diabetogenic factors as pituitary growth hormone, adrenal corticosteroids and an insulin-antagonist have been considered. The hyperglycæmia hypothesis has been persuasively advanced by Pedersen (1952), Osler and Pedersen (1960), Osler (1960a, 1960b, 1960c, 1960d), Pedersen and Osler (1961) and Osler (1961), although it did of course pre-date them (Skipper 1933). In essence it states that the fœtal blood glucose closely follows the maternal one, and that maternal-fœtal hyperglycæmia stimulates the developing fœtal β-cells to increased size and function. It is the converse of the belief expressed by Gerrard and Chin (1962) that the syndrome of poor fœtal nutrition and transient neonatal diabetes mellitus results from inadequate prenatal stimulation of the fœtal β-cells. The simplicity of the concept recommends it but it suffered a temporary set-back with the recognised existence of prediabetes because many authorities then, and some such as Peel now (1962), felt that β-cell hyperplasia and gigantism of a fœtus whose mother had no recognisable sign of established diabetes mellitus, could not be attributed to maternal hyperglycæmia.   But a maternal blood glucose just short of the renal threshold and unaccompanied by ketosis or diabetic degenerative disease may stimulate the baby's pancreas and favour fœtal over-nutrition with greater success than one which is very high.

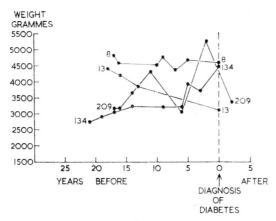

Fig. 9. Patterns of family birth weights in prediabetic and diabetic pregnancy.

Pancreatic islet hypertrophy can certainly be produced either in animals assured of continuous raised blood glucose levels, or in the fœtuses of others subjected to pancreatectomy (Farquhar 1962b).   In human pregnancy the hyperglycæmia hypothesis is lent some support by the experience of Pedersen (1954b), Pedersen and Brandstrup (1956) and of Oakley (1961a, 1961b) who have shown that birth weight may be reduced to the normal range by prolonged and very strict control of the maternal blood glucose throughout each 24 hours for much of the pregnancy.   Reference has already been made to the positive correlations between body weight and the degree of pancreatic islet hypertrophy, and between body weight and maternal blood glucose figures. Furthermore the newborn of non-diabetic women with Addison's disease are smaller than normal even when post-mature (Osler 1962).   But if hyperglyc-æmia alone explains fœtal overgrowth, then the progressive impairment of carbohydrate tolerance implicit in the concept of prediabetes should be accompanied by rising fœtal birth weight in successive pregnancies.   This can happen but clear exceptions exist (Farquhar 1962a, 1962b).   Thus in Fig. 9 various patterns of family birth weight can be seen during the pre-diabetic years.   Birth weight can be consistently high in each pregnancy (e.g. family 8 in Fig. 9), or may tend to increase (family 134), or sometimes may decrease (family 13).   Such patterns (further examples are given by Farquhar 1962a) suggest the existence of another factor, possibly a genetic one, and a prospective study is needed to examine the relationship between fœtal weight and carbohydrate tolerance and the body build of both parents and their relatives.

The experiments of Young (1953, 1961) and of others suggest that pituitary growth hormone (PGH) may play a part in causing diabetes mellitus. The injection of purified PGH raises the blood sugar of pancreatectomised and hypophysectomised baboons and the animals become ketotic (Gillman, Gilbert, Epstein and Allan 1958). Similarly it promotes pronounced hyper-glycæmia and ketosis when given to hypophysectomised human diabetics (Luft, Ikkos, Gemzell and Olivecrona 1958, Raben 1959, Hernberg 1960), and the recent symposium on the effects of human hypophysectomy and adrenalectomy suggests a pituitary rôle in the diabetic disorder (Diabetes 1962, Sprague 1962). Many reviews of the subject published in the 1950's favour PGH as the cause of fœtal overgrowth in diabetic pregnancy. Great difficulties have been experienced in measuring PGH but Ehrlich and Randle (1961) believe that increased activity can be demonstrated in some diabetic subjects and favour the rôle of the hormone in causing fœtal gigantism. Variations in PGH activity, or in the susceptibility of fœtal tissue to it, would be necessary explanations of the wide differences in birth weight which can occur in successive pregnancies. Such a possibility was dismissed by Pedersen and Osler in their publications of 1960–61 for it fails to fit with their observations on fœtal body composition, but Ehrlich and Randle counter this by pointing out that fat mobilization by PGH can be suppressed in both animals and humans by providing the subject with free access to glucose or food (Salter and Best 1953, Raben and Hollenberg 1960). The recent demonstration by Roth et al. (1963) that hypoglycæmia strongly stimulates PGH production is interesting, but unequivocal pancreatic islet hypertrophy was reported by Driscoll et al. (1960) and Driscoll (1963) in at least 3 such babies who were born with absent or destroyed hypothalamo-hypophyseal axes, and this would seem to exclude fœtal pituitary-adrenal hormones in the production of their unique morphology. The report of enlarged pituitary acidophil cells in babies of diabetic mothers (Gaunt, Bahn and Hayles 1962) must still be treated with caution. In any case the maternal pituitary is the likelier source of PGH and its excessive activity should suppress the fœtal acidophil cells rather than stimulate them, and other objections exist to a simple pituitary explanation of fœtal gigantism (Farquhar 1962b).

Pancreatic islet hypertrophy may result from the diabetogenic effects of hyperadrenocorticism, but even though the newly-born babies of diabetic mothers may excrete rather more corticosteroids in the urine than do those of normal women, the concept (Farquhar 1956b) of their being tiny cases of congenital Cushing's syndrome now seems to have been wrong. In the late 1940's a combination of obesity, plethora, hirsutes, œdema, weight loss, diuresis, enlargement of the adrenal cortex, stress, and inexplicable postnatal deterioration and death could not fail to excite interest. And when increased urinary steroid excretion was suspected in the mother (Hoet and Lukens 1954) and then claimed for the baby, the case for hyperadrenocorticism looked good. But the babies of women with Cushing's syndrome are believed to be of normal birth weight (Jackson 1955) and those of diabetic women with

Addison's disease still grow large (Osler and Pedersen 1962).   One by one the imagined stigmata of hyperadrenocorticism have been disproved or otherwise explained, and only some controversy over urinary steroid excretion remains.

The possible rôle of a maternal insulin-antagonist (Vallance-Owen, Hurlock and Please 1955) is of consuming interest and has been reviewed recently (Farquhar 1962b).   The probable permeability of human placenta in diabetic pregnancy to maternal acquired insulin-antibodies has been claimed by Spellacy and Gœtz (1963).   They suggest that this may be relevant to the fœtal morphology in diabetes, but acquired insulin-antibody and intrinsic insulin-antagonist cannot be assumed to have identical effects on the baby. By blocking the effectiveness of insulin the antagonist causes increased insulin secretion, but the hormone's action on lipogenesis is less suppressed so that obesity may develop and the young acute diabetic may retain insulin-like activity (Taylor 1963), findings which match the histological observations of Maclean and Ogilvie (1959).   The low molecular weight of the antagonist may make possible its crossing of the placental barrier with similar effects on the fœtus, including β-cell hyperplasia, obesity and, possibly, accelerated growth.

Possible Causes of Disturbed Function*
Gigantism and mortality are separable.   As a group these babies are fat, as a group they have a high morbidity, and in the past death during obstructed labour claimed many who survived to term.   Thus fœtal gigantism, disturbance of function, and even death are often regarded as having a common ætiology.   This need not be true.   While the possible cause of their unique morphology has been partly unravelled, the causes of morbidity and mortality remain matters for speculation.   When considering them it is fundamental to remember that the stillbirth rate is normal for normal women mated with diabetic men (Rubin 1958, Jackson 1960) and that stillbirths exceed neonatal deaths in most reported series of diabetic pregnancies.   Thus the root trouble is not directly genetic, operates before the start of extra-uterine existence, and concerns the diabetic environment.

Hypoglycæmia.   Neonatal hypoglycæmia receives specific attention in Chapter 5, but some remarks relevant to infants of diabetic mothers are necessary.   The association of hypogylcæmia and clinical disturbance in such babies was carefully examined by Pedersen (1952), Komrower (1954) and Farquhar (1956a) and each concluded that while hypoglycæmia occurs, it is commonly asymptomatic and that clinical disturbance is usually due to other factors.   Recent personal studies (unpublished) using a glucose oxidase method have not altered this view.

In the period 0–4 hours the blood sugar tends on average to fall to lower levels in the babies of diabetic women than in controls, but thereafter the difference is not great.   In particular, the babies of diabetic mothers rarely contribute to that small group of babies who develop prolonged hypoglycæmia with symptoms, generally after the first 24 hours, and who form the subject of Chapter 5.

For these reasons great caution should be exercised before attributing to

* Respiratory distress syndrome is treated in Chapter 3, pp. 57, 69.

hypoglycæmia symptoms which are far more likely to be the result of other causes, such as anoxia, respiratory distress syndrome, intracranial bleeding, congenital malformation or sepsis.

Hypocalcæmia. The "jitteriness" so often seen in these babies has been explained on a basis of hypocalcæmia (Craig 1958, Zetterström and Arnhold 1958, Gittleman *et al.* 1959), but there are some facts which raise doubts about this explanation. For instance, hypocalcæmia is a frequent concomit-ant of exchange transfusion when citrated blood is used, but does not necessar-ily produce any symptoms (Farquhar and Smith 1958). Even when symp-toms in the neonatal period are associated with hypocalcæmia, calcium given by injection often does not affect the symptoms.

Potassium levels. Changes in serum potassium are just as difficult to correlate with clinical behaviour as are calcium levels, and the two may need to be considered together (Farquhar and Smith 1958). ECG evidence of hypo-kalæmia was described by Björklund (1953b), but the ECG was normal in the experience of Gellis and Hsia (1959) and of Page *et al.* (1960). Keith *et al.* (1961) in a study of babies with respiratory distress whose mothers were diabetic, concluded that alteration in serum potassium was unlikely to be the only explanation for ECG changes.

One recent death at age 36 hours was associated with a serum potassium of 12 mEq./l. The baby's progress had been normal, with no respiratory symptoms, until the acute onset of grey cyanosis and tachycardia. His blood glucose exceeded 60 mg./100 ml. He had received no chloramphenicol. The ECG record was quite disorganised and provided no clear evidence of hyperkalæmia. He died before treatment could be effected, and autopsy was entirely negative. The case is unique in the Edinburgh series.

Hypoadrenocorticism. Adrenal failure as a cause of disturbance and death has been reviewed (Farquhar 1956b) and although suppression of fœtal adrenocortical function by maternal steroids does seem possible, almost every death occurs either when fœtal needs are being met *in utero*, or during the first postnatal hours when circulating maternal corticosteroids are adequate. Acute neonatal hypoadrenocorticism now seems an unlikely cause of death.

Respiratory arrest. Those cyanotic attacks which are not superimposed upon respiratory distress have shown in the past a close association either with the giving of oral fluids or with the presence of mucus in the pharynx (Farquhar 1959). But they can occur without such causes and have the quality of the temporary respiratory arrest sometimes seen in premature infants.

Vascular accidents. Vascular accidents are common in the brain and elsewhere (Driscoll *et al.* 1960) and may be fatal or productive of physical and mental handicap. They may result from hypoxic or traumatic delivery (Farquhar 1959), and so their incidence may vary according to obstetrical and anæsthetic technique.

Prenatal Factors in Perinatal Mortality

The high incidence of intra-uterine death, and the speed with which neonatal disturbance follows vaginal or abdominal birth, imply that the perinatal mortality is largely decided by prenatal conditions in the fœtus or in his environment, and not by such secondary abnormalities as hypoglycæmia, hypocalcæmia, hypo- or hyperkalæmia, hypo- or hyperadrenocorticism, hypotension, pulmonary hyaline membrane, vascular accidents, fluid shifts or hyperbilirubinæmia.

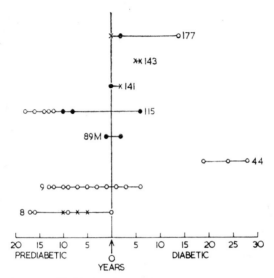

FIG. 10. Viable fœtal mortality in diabetic women.

○ survivor
× neonatal death
● stillbirth

Maternal. The relationships between birth weight and mortality and the obstetric history of individual diabetic women have been studied (Farquhar 1959, 1962a, 1962b). The fate of each infant born to diabetic mothers in the Simpson Memorial Maternity Pavilion between 1948 and 1961 has been plotted on a chart like that of Fig. 10, where each birth is shown against the appropriate year of the mother's diabetic life. The perinatal mortality during the *prediabetic* and *diabetic* years was found to be 135 and 250 per 1000 viable fœtuses respectively. In those pregnancies in which diabetes was first diagnosed it was 370, and among primiparous diabetic pregnancies it was 230 per 1000. But of greater interest is the fact that of the 108 families in the series 57 of them (with 185 babies) had not a single death, while the remaining 51 families (with 203 babies) had a perinatal mortality of 380 per 1000. Thus over half of the women in the series bore families of at least 2 children without loss and the others shared all the perinatal deaths. Half of those families which are unmarred by fœtal loss were born entirely within the mother's diabetic years and, as in family 44 (Fig. 10), long after establishment of the diagnosis. This freedom from fœtal loss fails to correlate with the quality of diabetic control.

Birth weight. The perinatal state of each child is related to birth weight and gestational age in Fig. 11. The curve represents birth weight at various gestational ages for non-diabetic pregnancy at the same hospital (Ellis 1951). The incidence of respiratory distress, of stillbirth and of neonatal death is much greater among the 118 infants of 3000 g. or less than among the 87 who exceeded this weight, and this holds true even if only those babies

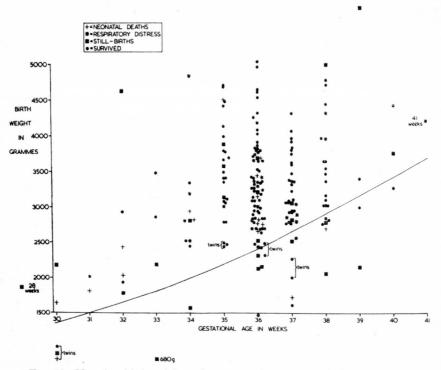

Fig. 11. Maturity, birth weight and outcome of 205 babies of diabetic women.

of 36 weeks gestation or more are considered (Farquhar 1962a). Examples of co-existing high birth weight and survival rate are shown in Fig. 12.

Control and severity of maternal diabetes. In the light of these observations consideration may now be given to those prenatal factors which influence survival. Strict control of the maternal blood glucose level throughout the second half or more of pregnancy, and all the extra care that goes with it, clearly improves survival (Pedersen 1954b, Pedersen and Brandstrup 1956, Osler 1961, Oakley 1961a, 1961b, Peel 1961) but it has not reduced it below a figure several times greater than that for non-diabetic pregnancy. Even women who are free from complicating nephropathy and who have enjoyed optimal care may have a dismal record of foetal loss, while others can be consistently successful without exercising particular caution. Women with nephropathy have, as a group, a higher foetal mortality rate and smaller babies (Oppé, Hsia and Gellis 1957), and the Edinburgh series suggests that, irrespective of the existence of maternal nephropathy, babies of 3000 g. or less are likelier to have serious trouble. This experience is shared by Malins (1962) and by Brandstrup, Osler and Pedersen (1961) who are also unhappy about very big babies. In Edinburgh, given freedom from the dangers of prolonged labour and hypoxia, large babies are safer than small ones, and while this conflicts with the notion advanced by others that simple fœtal hyperglycæmia is the harmful factor, it is in keeping with the principle enunciated by McCance (1959) and by McCance and Widdowson (1961) that growth has protective properties.

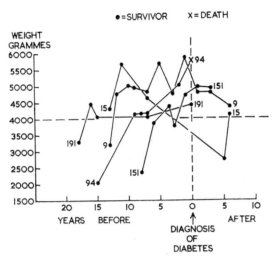

FIG. 12. Examples of high fœtal survival rate at high birth weight in the prediabetic and diabetic pregnancies of 5 women.

Placental failure. This evidence, with that already reviewed, supports the belief that perinatal disturbance and mortality result from prenatal under-nutrition, hypoxia and impaired elimination of carbon dioxide and other metabolites. The distress or death of large babies may be due to difficult delivery or to late failure of the placenta on which their very size makes them unusually dependent. Apart from such clinical and biochemical observations, however, direct proof of placental insufficiency is very difficult to obtain. Myometrial blood flow was judged normal by Brudenell, Miles and Coleman (1961), and in a further report Peel (1962) stated that it was actually increased where pregnancy ended in perinatal death or in respiratory distress. The significance of these results is obscure, but blood flow in the uterine wall cannot be a measure of the complex functions of the placenta. Simple histological examination of the placenta has revealed little, but electron microscopy and other techniques have shown remarkable changes in blood capillaries and other structures throughout the body in persons suffering from diabetes mellitus (Colwell 1960, Bloodworth 1963, Newell 1963). Hereditary basement membrane disease is an attractive hypothesis, but similar small vessel changes have been described in pure pancreatic diabetes (Burton, Kearns and Rynearson 1957, Duncan, MacFarlane and Robson 1958), and they occur in animals with induced diabetes. Thus both normal cells and those with a possible inherited metabolic fault respond to the diabetic milieu. The cells of the delicate placental microvilli and the fine related blood vessels are exposed to a fast flow of diabetic blood. As part of an organ which often ages prematurely even in normal pregnancy, these delicate structures may be expected to change in some subtle way which could interfere with fœtal nutrition, excretion and even with survival. Should prenatal disturbance of the fœtus be explicable in this way, then its partial prevention by meticulous control of maternal hyperglycæmia, together with the activity of another harmful factor, more serious in some women than in others and perhaps connected with a hormone of the pituitary-adrenal cells, must be assumed.

On these grounds placental insufficiency may be suspected where there exists a history of previous intra-uterine death or of frail and perhaps distressed babies and/or poor or arrested growth of the fœtus late in the current pregnancy. Under such circumstances premature delivery is probably wise. Conversely, a history of trouble-free birth of robust infants favours delivery nearer to term. Untried diabetic primipara, having received optimum medical and obstetric care, are best delivered by section at about the 37th week.

Management of the Newborn

The baby may require skilled resuscitation and after occlusion of the cord with double ligatures and the giving of vitamin K, he is transferred to an incubator with humidified environmental temperature of 30–32°C where he is carefully examined for malformations and early signs of respiratory distress. The thick cord is religatured at 12 hours, or alternatively a plastic self-adjusting cord-clamp may be used from birth.

The treatment of respiratory distress is dealt with in Chapter 3, p. 72.

Routine determinations of the blood glucose are unnecessary, but when suggestive physical signs and a blood glucose of less than 30 mg./100 ml. co-exist beyond the age of 8 hours, then safe measures should be taken to establish normoglycæmia (Farquhar 1964). Glucagon is simple and effective, the dose of 30 μg./kg. being given by intramuscular injection to spontaneous births, and ten times this amount to section deliveries. Proven, prolonged hypoglycæmia may be treated in the manner described in Chapter 5. Early feeding has been advocated by Reardon (1959), this probably has little effect on mortality, but may reduce the severity of neonatal jaundice (Rudolph et al. 1959, Hubbell and Drorbaugh 1962). Oral glucose water feeds may be given with great care toward the end of the first day and may be replaced with a milk formula after 24 hours. Effective suction should be available for clearing the airway in the event of inhalation. Injections of calcium have little effect but the rare danger of co-existing hypocalæmia and hyperkalæmia should be remembered. The latter may be treated effectively with glucose and insulin and the addition of an exchange resin where necessary. Removal from incubator-care and continuous observation should be possible by the fourth or fifth day of life.

Maternal lactation has been variable in most reports of diabetic pregnancy but in a society where enthusiastic breast-feeding may be the exception, the factor responsible for poor lactation in individual women is hard to find (Farquhar 1959).

Progress of Survivors

Most survivors of the first week of life who are free from deformity or mental handicap enjoy normal health during the first decade and concern thereafter relates only to their possible development of diabetes mellitus. The incidence of congenital malformations has yet to be discovered (p. 126) but the more disabling ones may prove to be a little commoner than in the normal population but less common than has been predicted from poorly conducted studies. Future research in the field will require means of knowing with certainty of hypoglycæmia in very early pregnancy, more exact measurement of diabetic severity, detailed histories of malformations among relatives (including perinatal deaths) and knowledge of parental consanguinity and of the increasing range of drugs, including the more toxic urinary antimicrobials, to which the diabetic woman may be exposed near the time she conceives. Visual and auditory disabilities (Dekaban 1959a, 1959b, Dekaban and Magee 1958, Hiekkala and Koskenoja 1961a, 1961b, Jorgensen 1961, Kelemen 1955, 1960) require further study for they may escape routine examination. Intellectual assessment is desirable in view of the report by Hiekkala and Koskenoja but, as with malformations, comparison with controls is essential and disability will require interpretation in the light of such facts as inheritance (obstetric history), perinatal metabolic disturbance, and birth injury.

Growth. Few people have reported long-term growth studies of children born to diabetic women. According to White, Koshy and Duckers (1953) these boys and girls are commonly above average height and weight up to and including adolescence, but Fredrikson, Hagbard, Olow and Reinand (1957), Hagbard, Olow and Reinand (1959) and Hagbard (1961) in a series of reports found that whereas the children of prediabetic mothers are probably of normal height and weight, those of diabetic mothers are as a group shorter and heavier than normal. Growth was judged normal in the series reported by Hiekkala and Koskenoja. The standing heights and naked weights of surviving children in the Edinburgh series are presented in Fig. 13a–d. The same measurements are plotted for the control children who were used in the malformation study. The degree of control could not extend to such factors as birth weight, parental physique and social status. Lines which represent the mean ± 3 standard deviations (S.D.) for Edinburgh boys and girls are drawn on each graph and were calculated from data published by Thomson (1956) and Provis and Ellis (1955). Almost all the children lie within ± 2 S.D. of the mean for height at any age, and children of both diabetic and non-diabetic mothers form the few exceptions. This largely holds also for weight, but among the exceptions the older children of diabetic mothers certainly predominate. This may be significant and further observations will be made. Only those who engage in a long-term, periodic follow-up involving not only normal control children but rather sick mothers can appreciate the task of keeping the groups complete. In an earlier study (Farquhar 1959) no clear relationship emerged between birth weight and later weight or height.

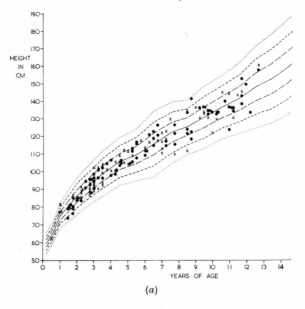

(a)

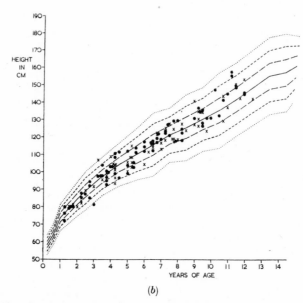

(b)

FIG. 13 (a, b). Standing heights of (a) male (b) female children of diabetic mothers and controls compared with the crown-heel length of normal Edinburgh boys and girls.

×   child of diabetic woman
●   child of non-diabetic woman

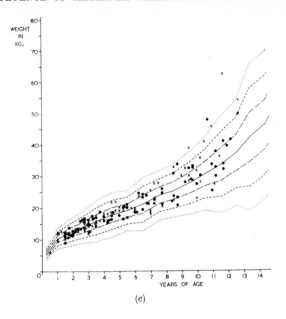

(c)

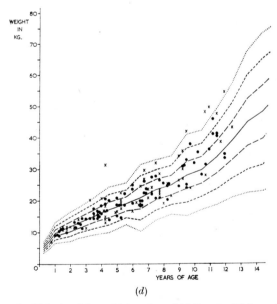

(d)

FIG. 13 (c, d). Naked weights of (c) male and (d) female children of diabetic mothers and of normal controls compared with the naked weights of normal Edinburgh boys and girls.

× child of diabetic woman
● child of non-diabetic woman

Diabetes mellitus. The likelihood of diabetes in surviving children of diabetic women has been stressed by Peel and Oakley (1950) and estimated as a 1 in 4 chance by Reis, De Costa and Allweiss (1950), while Harris (1950–51) calculated that 1·4% might be diabetic by 40 years of age. Ditzel, White and Duckers (1954) found from oral glucose tolerance tests on such children that over 9% gave diabetic curves, that the test was borderline in a further 17%, and that these children showed precocious growth and changes in the small vessels of the conjunctiva. The incidence of diabetes mellitus was 1·2% in the series reported by Hiekkala and Koskenoja (1961) and only 0·19% in that of Hagbard (1961). No case has yet appeared in the Edinburgh series.

REFERENCES

BABBOT, D., RUBIN, A., GINSBURG, S. J. (1958) The reproductive characteristics of diabetic men. *Diabetes*, **7**, 33

BAIRD, C. W., BUSH, I. E. (1960) Cortisol and cortisone content of amniotic fluid from diabetic and non-diabetic women. *Acta endocr. (Kbh.)*, **34**, 97

BAIRD, J. D., FARQUHAR, J. W. (1962) Insulin-secreting capacity in newborn infants of normal and diabetic women. *Lancet*, **1**, 71

BAYER, J. (1942) Die Hypertrophie der Pankreasinseln bei Neugeborenen diabetischer Mütter in ihren Beziehungen zu den anderen Regulatoren des Zuckerstoffwechsels. *Virchow's Archives*, **308**, 659

BERGLUND, G., ZETTERSTRÖM, R. (1954) Infants of diabetic mothers: I—Fœtal hypoxia in maternal diabetes. *Acta pœdiat.* **43**, 368

BIRCHALL, K., CATHRO, D. M., FORSYTH, C. C., MITCHELL, F. L. (1961) Separation and estimation of adrenal steroids in the urine of newborn infants. *Lancet*, **1**, 26

BIXBY, E. M., BENDA, S. E. (1942) Glucose tolerance and insulin tolerance in mongolism. *Amer. J. ment. Defic.*, **47**, 158

BJÖRKLUND, S. I. (1953a) Children of diabetic mothers. *Nord. Med.*, **49**, 582

BJÖRKLUND, S. I. (1953b) Children of diabetic mothers: electrocardiographic studies in the newborn. *Acta pœdiat.* **42**, 526

BJÖRKLUND, S. I., JENSEN, C. C. (1955) Infants of diabetic mothers, with special reference to neonatal adrenocortical function as assessed by urinary excretion of 17-ketosteroids. *Acta endocr. (Kbh.)*, **18**, 133

BLOODWORTH, J. M. B. (1963) Diabetic microangiopathy. *Diabetes*, **12**, 99

BRANDSTRUP, E., OSLER, M., PEDERSEN, J. (1961) Perinatal mortality in diabetic preganancy: the relationship to management during pregnancy and to fœtal age and weight. *Acta endocr. (Kbh.)*, **37**, 434

BRUDENELL, J. M., MILES, J. M., COLEMAN, A. (1961) The clearance of radioactive sodium from the myometrium of the pregnant diabetic. *J. Obstet. Gynœc. Brit. Comm.*, **68**, 238

BURSTEIN, R., SOULE, S. D., BLUMENTHAL, H. T. (1957) Histogenesis of pathological processes in placentas of metabolic disease in pregnancy. II. The diabetic state. *Amer. J. Obstet. Gynec.*, **74**, 96

BURTON, T. Y., KEARNS, T. P., RYNEARSON, E. (1957) Diabetic retinopathy following total pancreatectomy. *Proc. Mayo Clin.* **32**, 735

CARDELL, B. S. (1953a) The infants of diabetic mothers: a morphological study. *J. Obstet. Gynœc. Brit. Emp.* **60**, 834

CARDELL, B. S. (1953b) Hypertrophy and hyperplasia of the pancreatic islets in newborn infants. *J. Path. Bact.* **66**, 335

CARRINGTON, E. R., SHUMAN, C. R., REARDON, H. S. (1957) Evaluation of the prediabetic state during pregnancy. *Obstet. Gynec. N.Y.* **9**, 664

CHEEK, D. B., MADDISON, T. G., MALINEK, M., COLDBECK, J. H. (1961) Further observations on the corrected bromide space of the neonate and investigation of water and electrolyte status in infants born of diabetic mothers. *Pediatrics*, **28**, 861

CLAPP, W. M., BUTTERFIELD, J., O'BRIEN, D. (1962) Body water compartments in the premature infant, with special reference to the effects of the respiratory distress syndrome and of maternal diabetes and toxemia. *Pediatrics*, **29**, 883

CLAYTON, S. G. (1956) The pregnant diabetic. *J. Obstet. Gynœc., Brit. Emp.* **63**, 532

COLWELL, A. R. (1960) Histology of small blood vessel disease in diabetes. *Diabetes*, **9**, 503

CORNBLATH, M., WYBREGT, S. H., BAENS, G. S. (1963) Studies of carbohydrate metabolism in the newborn infant, VII. *Pediatrics*, **32**, 1007

CRAIG, W. S. (1958) Clinical signs of neonatal tetany: with especial reference to their occurrence in newborn babies of diabetic mothers. *Pediatrics*, **22**, 297

CRAIG, W. S., BUCHANAN, M. F. G. (1958) Hypocalcæmic tetany developing within 36 hours of birth. *Arch. Dis. Childh.*, **33**, 505

DEKABAN, A. (1959a) Arhinencephaly in an infant born to a diabetic mother. *J. Neuropath, exp. Neurol.*, **18**, 620

DEKABAN, A. S. (1959b) The outcome of pregnancy in diabetic women. II—analysis of clinical abnormalities and pathologic lesions in offspring of diabetic mothers. *J. Pediat.*, **55**, 767

DEKABAN, A. S., MAGEE, K. R. (1958) Occurrence of neurological abnormalities in infants of diabetic mothers. *Neurology*, **8**, 193

DIABETES (1962) A symposium on the influence of hypophysectomy and of adrenalectomy on diabetic retinopathy. **11**, 461

DITZEL, J., MOINAT, P. (1957) The responses of the smaller blood vessels and serum proteins in pregnant diabetic subjects. *Diabetes*, **6**, 307

DITZEL, J., WHITE, P., DUCKERS, J. (1954) Changes in the pattern of the smaller blood vessels in the bulbar conjunctiva in children of diabetic mothers. *Diabetes*, **3**, 99

DRISCOLL, S. G. (1963) Personal communication

DRISCOLL, S. G., BENIRSCHKE, K., CURTIS, G. W. (1960) Neonatal deaths among infants of diabetic mothers. *Amer. J. Dis. Child.*, **100**, 818

DUNCAN, L. J. P., MACFARLANE, A., ROBSON, J. S. (1958) Diabetic retinopathy and nephropathy in pancreatic diabetes. *Lancet*, **1**, 822

DUTTON, G. (1961) The fasting blood sugar of mongols. *J. ment. Defic. Res.*, **5**, 10

EDGERTON, H. E. (1962) Concentrated strobe lamp. *J. Biol. Photograph. Assoc.*, May, p. 45

EHRLICH, R. M., RANDLE, P. J. (1961) Serum growth hormone concentrations in diabetes mellitus. *Lancet*, **2**, 233

ELLIS, R. W. B. (1951) Assessment of prematurity by birth weight, crown-rump length, and head circumference. *Arch. Dis. Childh.*, **26**, 411

FARQUHAR, J. W. (1956a) The significance of hypoglycæmia in the newborn infant of the diabetic woman. *Arch. Dis. Childh.*, **31**, 203

FARQUHAR, J. W. (1956b) The possible influence of hyperadrenocorticism on the fœtus of the diabetic woman. *Arch. Dis. Childh.* **31**, 483

FARQUHAR, J. W. (1958) The child of the diabetic woman. *M.D. Thesis*, University of Edinburgh

FARQUHAR, J. W. (1959) The child of the diabetic woman. *Arch. Dis. Child.* **34**, 76

FARQUHAR, J. W. (1961) Round table conference on diabetic pregnancy. IVth Congress of the International Diabetes Federation, Geneva

FARQUHAR, J. W. (1962a) Birth weight and survival of babies of diabetic women. *Arch. Dis. Childh.* **37**, 321

FARQUHAR, J. W. (1962b) Maternal hyperglycæmia and fœtal hyperinsulinism in diabetic pregnancy. *Postgrad. med. J.*, **38**, 612

FARQUHAR, J. W. (1962c) Diabetic children in Scotland and the need for care. *Scot. med. J.* **7**, 119

FARQUHAR, J. W. (1964) in *Current Pediatric Therapy*, ed. by Gellis, S. S. and Kagan, B. M. W. B. Saunders Co., Philadelphia.

FARQUHAR, J. W., SKLAROFF, S. A. (1958) The post-natal weight loss of babies born to diabetic and non-diabetic women. *Arch. Dis. Childh.* **33**, 323

FARQUHAR, J. W., SMITH, H. (1958) Clinical and biochemical changes during exchange transfusion. *Arch. Dis. Childh.* **33**, 142

FEE, B., WEIL, W. B. (1960) Body composition of a diabetic offspring by direct analysis. *Amer. J. Dis. Child.*, **100**, 718

FEE, B., WEIL, W. B. (1962) Personal communication

FERNER, H. (1952) *Das Inselsystem des Pankreas*. Georg Thieme, Stuttgart.

FISCHER, A. E., MOLOSHOK, R. E. (1960) Diabetic and prediabetic pregnancies with special reference to the newborn. *J. Pediat.* **57**, 704

FITZGERALD, M. G., MALINS, J. M., O'SULLIVAN, D. J., WALL, M. (1961) IVth Congress of the International Diabetes Federation, Geneva

FORSYTH, C. C., CATHRO, D. M. (1962) Xth International Congress of Paediatrics, Lisbon

FREDRIKSON, H., HAGBARD, L., OLOW, I., REINAND, R. (1957) Follow-up investigation of children of diabetic mothers. *Nord. Med.* **57**, 669

GAUNT, W. D., BAHN, R. C., HAYLES, A. B. (1962) A quantitative cytologic study of the anterior hypophysis of infants of diabetic mothers. *Proc. Mayo Clinic*, **37**, 345

GELLIS, S. S., HSIA, D. Y-Y. (1959) The infant of the diabetic mother. *Amer. J. Dis. Child.* **97,** 1

GELLIS, S. S., WHITE, P., PFEFFER, W. (1949) Gastric suction: a proposed additional technic for the prevention of asphyxia in infants delivered by cesarean section. *New Engl. J. Med.,* **240,** 533

GEOGHEGAN, F., DRURY, M. I. (1962) Testicular changes in infant of diabetic mother. *Lancet,* **1,** 1243

GERRARD, J. W., CHIN, W. (1962) The syndrome of transient diabetes. *J. Pediat.* **61,** 89

GILLMAN, J., GILBERT, C., EPSTEIN, E., ALLAN, J. C. (1958) Endocrine control of blood sugar, lipæmia and ketonæmia in diabetic baboons. *Brit. med. J.,* **2,** 1260

GITTLEMAN, I. F., PINCUS, J. B., SCHMERZER, B. S., SAITO, M. (1956) Hypocalcemia occurring on the first day of life in mature and premature infants. *Pediatrics,* **18,** 721

GITTLEMAN, I. F., PINCUS, J. B., SCHMERZER, B. S., ANNECCHIARICO, F. (1959) Diabetes mellitus or the prediabetic state in the mother and the neonate. *Amer. J. Dis. Child.* **98,** 342

HAGBARD, L. (1961) *Pregnancy and Diabetes Mellitus.* Charles C. Thomas, Springfield

HAGBARD, L., OLOW, I., REINAND, T. (1959) A follow-up study of 514 children of diabetic mothers. *Acta pædiat.* **48,** 184

HARRIS, H. (1950–51) Familial distribution of diabetes mellitus: study of relatives of 1241 diabetic propositi. *Ann. Eugen. (Lond.),* **15,** 95

HERNBERG, C. A. (1960) The effect of human growth hormone on severe juvenile diabetes after hypophysectomy. *Acta endocr. (Kbh.),* **33,** 559

HIEKKALA, H., KOSKENOJA, M. (1961a) A follow-up study of children of diabetic mothers. Part I. General findings. *Ann. pædiat. Fenn.* **7,** 17

HIEKKALA, H., KOSKENOJA, M. (1961b) A follow-up study of children of diabetic mothers. Part II. Defective children. *Ann. pædiat. Fenn.,* **7,** 32

HOET, J. P., LUKENS, F. D. W. (1954) Carbohydrate metabolism during pregnancy. *Diabetes,* **3,** 1

HUBBELL, J. P., DRORBAUGH, J. E. (1962) Xth International Congress of Pædiatrics, Lisbon

HULTQUIST, G. T., LINDGREN, I., DALGAARD, J. B. (1946) Congenital hyperplasia of islands of Langerhans with increase in beta cells in fœtuses of diabetic mothers. *Nord. Med.,* **31,** 1841

JACKSON, W. P. U. (1954) Large babies and (pre)diabetic fathers. *J. clin. Endocr.,* **14,** 177

JACKSON, W. P. U. (1955) A concept of diabetes. *Lancet,* **2,** 625

JACKSON, W. P. U. (1960) Diabetic embryopathy. *S. Afr. med. J.,* **34,** 151

JORGENSEN, M. B. (1961) The influence of maternal diabetes on the inner ear of the fœtus. *Acta otolaryng. (Stockh.)* **53,** 49

KAISER, I. H., GOODLIN, R. C. (1958) Alterations of pH, gases and hemoglobin in blood and electrolytes in plasma of fœtuses of diabetic mothers. *Pediatrics,* **22,** 1097

KEITH, J. D., ROSE, V., BRAUDO, M., ROWE, R. D. (1961) The electrocardiogram in the respiratory distress syndrome and related cardiovascular dynamics. *J. Pediat.* **59,** 167

KELEMEN, G. (1955) Aural changes in embryo of diabetic mother. *Arch. Otolaryng. (Chic.)* **62,** 357

KELEMEN, G. (1960) Maternal diabetes. Changes in the hearing organ of the embryo: additional observation. *Arch. Otolaryng. (Chic.)* **71,** 921

KELLOCK, T. D. (1961) Birth weight of children of diabetic fathers. *Lancet,* **1,** 1252

KLEIN, R., MARKS, J. F., ROLDAN, E., SHERMAN, F. E., FETTERMAN, G. H. (1962) The occurrence of peripheral edema and subcutaneous glycogen deposition following the initial treatment of diabetes mellitus in children. *J. Pediat.* **60,** 807

KLEIN, R., TAYLOR, P. (1960) 17-hydroxycorticosteroids in blood of diabetic mothers and their offspring. *Pediatrics,* **26,** 333

KOMROWER, G. (1954) Blood sugar levels in babies born of diabetic mothers. *Arch. Dis. Childh.* **29,** 28

LARSSON, I. (1963) Personal communication

LEEMING, B. W. A. (1962) Endocrine control of skeletal development in man. *Brit. med. J.* **2,** 358

LLOYD, A. V. (1963) Observations on the composition of the blood in the neonatal period. *Ph.D. Thesis.* University of Edinburgh.

LOWREY, G. H., GRAHAM, B. D., TSAO, M. U. (1954) Chemical homeostasis in the newborn infants of diabetic mothers. *Pediatrics,* **13,** 527

LUFT, R., IKKOS, D., GEMZELL, C. A., OLIVECRONA, H. (1958) Effect of human growth hormone in hypophysectomised diabetic subjects. *Lancet,* **1,** 721

McCANCE, R. A. (1959) The maintenance of stability in the newly born: I—Chemical exchange. *Arch. Dis. Childh.* **34**, 361

McCANCE, R. A., WIDDOWSON, E. M. (1961) Mineral metabolism of the fœtus and newborn. *Brit. med. Bull.* **17**, 132

MacKAY, R. B. (1957) Observations on the oxygenation of the fœtus in normal and abnormal pregnancy. *J. Obstet. Gynœc., Brit. Emp.* **64**, 185

MACLEAN, N., OGILVIE, R. F. (1959) Observations on the pancreatic islet tissue of young diabetic subjects. *Diabetes,* **8**, 83

MALINS, J. M. (1962) Conference on disorders of carbohydrate metabolism, Royal College of Physicians. *Lancet,* **1**, 794

MIGEON, C. J., NICOLOPOULOS, D., CORNBLATH, M. (1960) Concentration of 17-hydroxy-corticosteroids in the blood of diabetic mothers and in blood from the umbilical cords of their offspring at the time of delivery. *Pediatrics,* **25**, 605

MILLER, H. C. (1944) Cardiac hypertrophy in newborn infants. *Yale J. Biol. Med.,* **16**, 509

MOORE, C. E., KAY, J. L., DESMOND, M. M., DUTTON, R. V. (1960) Transitional distress in infants of diabetic mothers. *J. Pediat.* **57**, 824

MORGAN, C. R., LAZAROW, A. (1963) Immunoassay of insulin two antibody system. Plasma insulin levels of normal, subdiabetic and diabetic rats. *Diabetes,* **12**, 115

MULLIGAN, P. B., SCHWARTZ, R. (1962) Hepatic carbohydrate metabolism in the genesis of neonatal hypoglycemia. *Pediatrics,* **30**, 125

NEWELL, F. W. (1963) Conference on microcirculation and diabetic retinopathy. *Diabetes,* **12**, 179

OAKLEY, W. G. (1961a) Panel discussion on diabetes during gestation and its influence on fœtal pathology and neonatal behaviour. IVth Congress of the International Diabetes Federation, Geneva

OAKLEY, W. G. (1961b) Pregnancy and diabetes. *Proc. roy. Soc. Med.,* **54**, 744

OPPÉ, T. E., HSIA, D. Y-Y., GELLIS, S. S. (1957) Pregnancy in the diabetic mother with nephritis. *Lancet,* **1**, 353

OSLER, M. (1960a) Body water of newborn infants of diabetic mothers. *Acta endocr. (Kbh.)* **34**, 261

OSLER, M. (1960b) Body fat of newborn infants of diabetic mothers. *Acta endocr. (Kbh.)* **34**, 277

OSLER, M. (1960c) Neonatal changes in body composition of infants born to diabetic mothers. *Acta endocr. (Kbh.)* **34**, 299

OSLER, M. (1960d) Renal function in newborn infants of diabetic mothers. *Acta endocr. (Kbh.),* **34**, 287

OSLER, M. (1961) *Body Composition of Newborn Infants of Diabetic Mothers.* Copenhagen

OSLER, M. (1962) Addison's disease and pregnancy. *Acta endocr. (Kbh.)* **41**, 67

OSLER, M., PEDERSEN, J. (1960) The body composition of newborn infants of diabetic mothers. *Pediatrics,* **26**, 985

OSLER, M., PEDERSEN, J. (1962) Pregnancy in a patient with Addison's disease and diabetes mellitus. *Acta endocr. (Kbh.)* **41**, 79

PAGE, O. C., GARLAND, J., STEPHENS, J. W., HARE, R. L. (1960) The electrocardiogram in infants of diabetic mothers. *J. Pediat.* **56**, 66

PEDERSEN, J. (1952) Diabetes and Pregnancy. *Blood Sugar of Newborn Infants.* Danish Science Press, Copenhagen

PEDERSEN, J. (1954a) Weight and length at birth of infants of diabetic mothers. *Acta endocr. (Kbh.)* **16**, 340

PEDERSEN, J. (1954b) Fetal mortality in diabetic pregnancy. *Diabetes,* **3**, 199

PEDERSEN, J., BRANDSTRUP, E. (1956) Fœtal mortality in pregnant diabetics. *Lancet,* **1**, 606

PEDERSEN, J., OSLER, M. (1961) Hyperglycæmia as the cause of characteristic features of the fœtus and newborn of diabetic mothers. *Danish med. Bull.* **8**, 78

PEEL, J. H. (1955) Management of the pregnant diabetic. *Brit. med. J.* **2**, 870

PEEL, J. H. (1961) Management of the pregnant diabetic. *Proc. roy. Soc. Med.* **54**, 745

PEEL, J. H. (1962) Progress in the knowledge and management of the pregnant diabetic patient. *Amer. J. Obstet. Gynec.* **83**, 847

PEEL, J. H., OAKLEY, W. G. (1950) The management of pregnancy in diabetics. *Trans. 12th Brit. Congr. Obstet. Gynœc.,* p. 161

PIRART, J. (1955) The so-called pre-diabetic syndrome of pregnancy. *Acta endocr. (Kbh.),* **20**, 192

PROVIS, H., ELLIS, R. W. B. (1955) An anthropometric study of Edinburgh school-children. *Arch. Dis. Childh.* **30**, 328

PRYSTOWSKI, H. (1957) Fetal blood studies. VII—The oxygen pressure gradient between the maternal and fetal bloods of the human in normal and abnormal pregnancy. *Bull. Johns Hopk. Hosp.,* **101**, 48

PRYSTOWSKI, H., HELLEGERS, A., BRUNS, P. D. (1960) Fetal blood studies. *Surg. Gynec. Obstet.* **110**, 495

PYKE, D. A. (1960) The genetics of heavy babies. Meeting of the Medical and Scientific Section of the British Diabetic Association, Glasgow

RABEN, M. S. (1959) Human growth hormone. *Diabetes*, **8**, 232

RABEN, M. S., HOLLENBERG, C. H. (1960) Growth hormone and the mobilization of fatty acids. *Ciba Found. Coll. Endocr.* **13**, 89

RAFSTEDT, S., SWAHN, B. (1954) Studies on lipids, proteins and lipoproteins in serum from newborn infants. *Acta pædiat.* **43**, 221

REARDON, H. S. (1959) Infants of diabetic mothers. Report of 31st Ross Conference on Pediatric Research, Columbus

REARDON, H. S., FIELD, S., VEGA, L., CARRINGTON, E., AREY, J., BAUMANN, M. L. (1957) Treatment of acute respiratory distress in newborn infants of diabetic and "prediabetic" mothers. *Amer. J. Dis. Child.* **94**, 558

REID, D. (1956) Personal communication quoted by Miller, H. C. in Advances in Pediatrics, **8**, Chicago

REIS, R. A., DE COSTA, E. J., ALLWEISS, M. D. (1950) The management of the pregnant diabetic woman and her newborn infant. *Amer. J. Obstet. Gynec.* **60**, 1023

REWELL, R. E. (1962) Testicular changes in infant of diabetic mother. *Lancet*, **2**, 153

ROBB, P. (1961) The development of the islets of Langerhans in the human fœtus. *Quart. J. exp. Physiol.* **46**, 335

ROSE, V. (1960) Infants of diabetic mothers: clinical and pathological features in a series of 25 cases. *Canad. med. Ass. J.*, **82**, 306

ROTH, J., GLICK, S. M., YALOW, R. S., BERSON, S. A. (1963) Hypoglycemia a potent stimulus to secretion of growth hormone. *Science*, **140**, 987

RUBIN, A. (1958) Studies in human reproduction: II—The influence of diabetes mellitus in men upon reproduction. *Amer. J. Obstet. Gynec.* **76**, 25

RUDOLPH, A. J., HUBBELL, J. P., DRORBAUGH, J. E., CHERRY, R. B., AULD, P. A. M., SMITH, C. A. (1959) Early versus late feeding of infants of diabetic mothers: a controlled study. *Amer. J. Dis. Child.* **98**, 496

SALTER, J., BEST, C. H. (1953) Insulin as a growth hormone. *Brit. med. J.* **2**, 353

SALTER, J., DAVIDSON, I. W. F., BEST, C. H. (1957) The effects of insulin and somato-trophin on the growth of hypophysectomised rats. *Canad. J. Biochem. Physiol.* **35**, 913

SCHWARTZ, R., BOWIE, M. D., MULLIGAN, P. B. (1962) Insulin-secreting capacity in newborn infants of normal and diabetic women. *Lancet*, **1**, 641

SCOTT, J. M. (1962) Testicular changes in infant of diabetic mother. *Lancet*, **2**, 100

SEGAL, S., SUTHERLAND, J. M., LUCEY, J. F., DRORBAUGH, J. E., CHERRY, R. B., HSIA, D. Y-Y. (1957) Determination of pH, CO_2 content, O_2 saturation, and lactate in the blood of newborn infants of diabetic mothers. *Amer. J. Dis. Child.* **94**, 562

SIREK, O. V., SIREK, A., LEIBEL, B. S. (1961) Serum glycoproteins in newborn infants of diabetic mothers. *Diabetes*, **10**, 375

SIREK, O. V., SIREK, A. (1962) Immuno-electrophoretic demonstration of differences in serum proteins of newborn infants of normal and diabetic mothers. *Nature (Lond.)* **196**, 1214

SKIPPER, E. (1933) Diabetes mellitus and pregnancy. A clinical and analytical study. *Quart. J. Med.* **11**, 353

SPELLACY, W. N., GOETZ, F. C. (1963) Insulin antibodies in pregnancy. *Lancet*, **2**, 222

SPRAGUE, R. G. (1962) Comments on reports of the effect of hypophysectomy, of hypo-physeal stalk section and of adrenalectomy on diabetic retinopathy. *Diabetes*, **11**, 491

STIMMLER, L., BRANZIE, J., O'BRIEN, D. (1964) Plasma insulin levels in the newborn in-fants of normal and diabetic mothers. *Lancet*, **1**, 137

SUTHERLAND, J. M., OPPÉ, T. E., LUCEY, J. F., SMITH, C. A. (1959) Leg volume changes observed in hyaline membrane disease. *Amer. J. Dis. Child.* **98**, 24

TAKEUCHI, A., BENIRSCHKE, K. (1961) Renal venous thrombosis of the newborn and its relation to maternal diabetes. *Biol. Neonat.* **3**, 237

TAYLOR, K. W. (1963) Serum insulin in early cases of severe diabetes. *Brit. med. J.* **1**, 511

TEJNING, S. (1947) Dietary factors and quantitative morphology of the islets of Langer-hans. *Acta med. Scand., Suppl.* 198

THOMSON, J. (1956) Quoted by R. W. B. Ellis in *Child Health and Development*, 2nd Ed., Churchill, London

TROWELL, H. G., JELLIFFE, D. B. (1958) *Diseases of Children in the Subtropics and Tropics*, Arnold, London

VALLANCE-OWEN, J., HURLOCK, B., PLEASE, N. W. (1955) Plasma insulin activity in diabetes mellitus measured by the rat diaphragm technique. *Lancet*, **2**, 583

VERNET, A., SMITH, E. B. (1961) Lipoprotein patterns in diabetes and the changes occurring during pregnancy. *Diabetes*, **10**, 345

WALKER, J. (1954) Fœtal anoxia. *J. Obstet. Gynœc. Brit. Emp.* **61**, 162

WARREN, S., LE COMPTE, P. M. (1952) *Pathology of Diabetes*, 3rd Ed., Lea & Febiger, Philadelphia

WHITE, P. (1945) Pregnancy complicating diabetes. *J. Amer. med. Assoc.* **128**, 181

WHITE, P. (1952) In *Treatment of Diabetes Mellitus* by E. P. Joslin, 9th Ed., Lea & Febiger, Philadelphia

WHITE, P., KOSHY, P., DUCKERS, J. (1953) Subsequent course of children of diabetic mothers. *Med. Clin. N. Amer.* **37**, 1481

WIDDOWSON, E. M., SPRAY, C. M. (1951) Chemical development in utero. *Arch. Dis. Childh.* **26**, 205

WISLOCKI, G. B., DEMPSEY, E. W. (1955) Electron microscopy of the human placenta. *Anat. Rec.* **123**, 133

WOOLF, N., JACKSON, W. P. U. (1957) Maternal prediabetes and the fœtal pancreas. *J. Path. Bact.* **74**, 223

YOUNG, F. G. (1953) The growth hormone and diabetes. *Rec. Progr. Hormone Res.*, **8**, 471

YOUNG, F. G. (1961) Experimental research on diabetes mellitus. *Brit. med. J.* **2**, 1449

ZETTERSTRÖM, R., ABERG, B. (1955) Infants of diabetic mothers. II—Studies on the electrolyte metabolism and the effect of starvation during the first few days. *Acta pœdiat.* **44**, 1

ZETTERSTRÖM, R., ARNHOLD, R. G. (1958) Impaired calcium phosphate homeostasis in newborn infants of diabetic mothers. *Acta pœdiat.* **47**, 107

Acknowledgement: Figures 1, 10, 11 and 13 are reproduced by permission from *Archives of Diseases in Childhood*, figures 3 and 12 from *Postgraduate Medical Journal* and figure 7 from *The Lancet*.

CHAPTER 7

CHROMOSOMAL ABNORMALITIES

A. G. BAIKIE

SINCE 1959 when the first constitutional chromosomal abnormality in man was described, a bewildering number of further abnormalities have been reported, most of them of interest to pædiatricians. Some of the abnormalities have been found only in children, others like mongolism are still mainly of pædiatric concern, while the triple-X syndrome and XXY-Klinefelter's syndrome present a challenge to the pædiatrician as regards their detection in childhood. This chapter will be concerned with the clinical aspects of chromosomal abnormalities in pædiatrics. It is important not to forget the pædiatrician's opportunities for advancing our knowledge of these conditions by simple observations as well as by more esoteric research methods. The sensational advances in the field of human chromosome studies have tended to overshadow the general increase in interest in the genetic aspects of disease. Many of the common diseases due to environmental factors have in the past thirty years either been overcome or are now understood, although their control may depend on social and economic changes not yet accomplished. Consequently much research interest has been transferred to the rôle of genetic factors in disease, which formerly appeared so much more difficult to study. Thus we see a new interest in the inborn errors of metabolism, in population genetics and in congenital abnormalities, as well as in the application of the techniques of chromosome study. At present these different approaches are kept apart by the limitation of the methods of study which are available, but obviously this separation is unlikely to persist. When it is ended, the use of two or more research techniques where only one was formerly applicable must accelerate still further the rate of accession of knowledge of genetic factors in the causation of disease.

Technical Considerations

Details of the methods used in the making of chromosome preparations and the problems of chromosome analysis are outside the scope of this chapter. These subjects were recently reviewed by Clarke (1962) and Ford (1962). Nevertheless, an appreciation of some aspects of the methods is necessary for an understanding of the results, their significance and limitations.

Since interphase chromosomes are not usually visible as discrete bodies, chromosome studies are possible only on cells in division. Only bone marrow, and possibly testicular tissue, normally contain enough dividing cells to provide satisfactory chromosome preparations without culture. Even bone marrow is usually cultured for this purpose, although a direct method yielding good preparations without preliminary culture (Tjio and Whang

154

1962) is used, particularly in the study of leukæmia. For chromosome studies in all other conditions preliminary culture is employed. The materials most commonly cultured are peripheral blood leucocytes, of which the lymphocytes have been shown to divide (McKinney *et al.* 1962) and skin, from which the subcutaneous fibroblasts persist and divide. An adequate number of dividing cells for good chromosome preparations is ensured by the addition to the culture shortly before the dividing cells are harvested of either colchicine or the related alkaloid demecolcin (Colcemid, CIBA). This material arrests cell division at metaphase when chromosomes are most suitable for study. In so doing, it allows an accumulation of dividing cells to occur during the period between its addition and the making of the chromosome preparations. This use of colchicine or its related alkaloid does not seem to produce chromosome abnormalities *in vitro*, as was feared it might. A procedure entailing adminis-tration of demecolcin to the patient some time before the marrow biopsy so as to allow more divisions to accumulate *in vivo* (Bottura and Ferrari 1960, Kinlough *et al.* 1961) has not found general favour, partly because of persistent fears that it will produce chromosomal changes in the patient.

It may at first appear that chromosome preparations can only be made from tissues which normally have a high mitotic rate. This is probably not so. Peripheral blood lymphocytes do not normally divide, at least in the peripheral blood, and they will not divide in culture unless special steps are taken to induce them to do so. For chromosome studies this effect is achieved by the addition to culture of phytohæmagglutinin, an extract of the bean *Phaseolus vulgaris* (Nowell 1960). This technical success suggests that other cells which rarely or never divide *in vivo* may be induced to do so in culture, so that their chromosomes may be seen and studied.

The difference between merely counting the chromosomes in a dividing cell, and the much more skilled and time-consuming procedure of chromosome analysis must be understood. In actual analysis the chromosomes are paired and identified as far as is possible (Ford 1962). In so doing morphological abnormalities due to deletion and translocation may be detected and iso-chromosomes may be found. These significant abnormalities may pass undetected if the chromosomes are simply counted. To be significant, minor morphological abnormalities require to be found in all the cells present, or in a considerable proportion of those examined. Even in chromosome pre-parations from a normal individual not all the cells contain 46 chromo-somes. The frequency of occurrence and significance of cells with more or less than 46 chromosomes has been discussed by Jacobs and her colleagues (1961b and 1963).

It is important to appreciate that attempts at chromosome studies often fail, even in the hands of experienced workers and in optimal conditions, while because of the special requirements in the study of mosaicism it is often advisable to warn the patient that it may be necessary to sample a second or even a third tissue.

Morphological Abnormalities of Chromosomes

Abnormal chromosomes usually arise from breakage and rejoining of broken ends in new ways. The relationship of some morphologically abnormal chromosomes to normal chromosomes is shown in Fig. 1. The genesis of these abnormalities is discussed in detail by Swanson (1958) and by White (1961). These and other chromosomal aberrations were recognised and studied in other species before 1956. Consequently, their demonstration in man was not

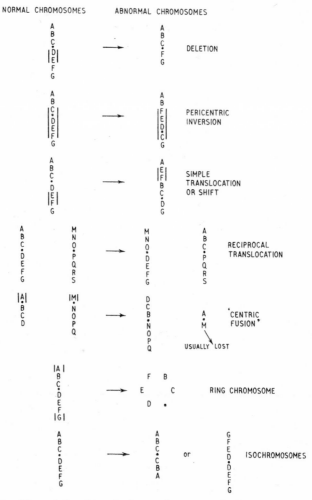

FIG. 1. The relationship of abnormal to normal chromosomes. The chromosomes are represented in the non-metaphase state, the centromere being indicated by a dot.

unexpected. In most instances of morphological abnormality rigid proof of the nature of the abnormality is lacking, and the decision as to the occurrence of a translocation or an isochromosome in man is best regarded as the most likely explanation, but no more than that. Proof may eventually come from study of the phenotypic associations of morphological chromosomal abnormalities, which may link deletion or triplication of this or that part of a chromosome with certain genetic characters. Since the situation of genic loci on the human chromosomes is unknown except as regards some loci carried on the X chromosome, this method is at present not generally applicable. In the current search for these genetic markers, the study of trisomic individuals, who have three homologous chromosomes instead of the normal two, is of particular importance (Huehns *et al.* 1964a and b).

It must be appreciated that small deletions and translocations may not be detectable by current methods. This is especially likely where larger chromosomes are involved. As with suspected mosaicism, the temptation to postulate such fine changes to explain abnormal clinical findings must often be resisted. Inversions are likely to be undetectable unless they involve the centromere and are asymmetrical with reference to it. Isochromosomes for metacentric chromosomes are obviously not identifiable.

Most chromosomal translocations described in man involve the acrocentric chromosomes of the groups 13–15 and 21–22. The most common is probably the translocation between chromosomes of these two groups in which the small centric fragment is commonly, but not invariably, lost. Individuals with this abnormality are of normal phenotype so the lost genetic material is thought to be unimportant. These translocation carriers are of medical importance because women amongst them are liable to produce unbalanced gametes at oögenesis which may give rise to mongol offspring (p. 162). In general, the phenotypic effect of a translocation will depend on the genic content of the material lost in the production of the translocation. This is unlikely to be the only factor operating. Pitt *et al.* (1964) have described a mother and two children with 45 chromosomes and a translocation, probably between two chromosomes of the group 13–15. The mother and one child were phenotypically normal but the other child had cerebral atrophy, clinodactyly and epicanthic folds. These authors discuss analogous reports in the literature and point out the fallacy of attributing the abnormal phenotype to the chromosomal translocation.

Ring chromosomes have been found in cultured cells of tumours (Levan 1956), in acute leukæmia (Baikie *et al.* 1959) and after X-irradiation (Tough *et al.* 1960). They are known to be unstable and liable to be lost at cell division. Nevertheless, they have been found as a constitutional chromosomal abnormality in man. As with translocations, their effect will depend, in part at least, on the amount of material lost in their formation. Turner *et al.* (1962) found a ring chromosome in a physically and mentally retarded boy, the ring chromosome having apparently been formed from one of the chromosomes of group 6–12. XO-Turner's syndrome with a ring chromosome has been described by Lindsten and Tillinger (1962) and by Lüers *et al.* (1963). In all three cases the liability to loss of ring chromosomes is reflected in the fact that each was a mosaic for cells with 46 chromosomes including the ring chromosome and cells with 45 chromosomes without it. The instability of ring chromosomes was further reflected in variation in the size of the ring from cell to cell in the patient of Lüers and her co-workers.

The formation of an isochromosome results in monosomy for one arm of a chromosome pair and trisomy for the other. Most instances in man have involved either chromosome 21 (Fraccaro *et al.* 1960b) or the X chromosome

(Fraccaro *et al.* 1960c). In the case of chromosome 21 the isochromosome for the long arm has the phenotypic effect apparently equivalent to triplication of the whole chromosome, so that a mongol results. The individuals with isochromosomes for the long arm of the X chromosome are abnormally chromatin-positive females with some of the phenotypic features of Turner's syndrome. A woman with an isochromosome for the short arm of the X chromosome had some of the features of Turner's syndrome but was not of notably short stature (Jacobs *et al.* 1960). Comparison of the phenotypic features of these patients provides an obvious opportunity to locate genes on the long or short arm of the X chromosome if monosomy and trisomy have different specific effects. The results of these studies have hitherto been disappointing.

Mosaics

An individual composed of two or more cell-lines of different chromosome constitution is said to be a chromosome mosaic. This abnormality commonly arises as a result of a divisional error at the first cleavage division of the embryo. If the error occurs later a triple cell-line mosaic may result. Thus a normally constituted zygote of 46 chromosomes will give rise to a chromosome mosaic with cell-lines of 45 and 47 chromosomes if the error arises at the first cleavage division. If the error occurs later, cells of 45 and 47 chromosomes may co-exist with normally constituted cells of 46 chromosomes. In such an individual the composition of the mixture of cells will depend not only on the stage of development at which the divisional error occurred but also on the relative viability of the cell-lines. Furthermore the composition of the mixture may not be the same throughout the body, if the divisional error occurs after embryological development is well advanced, or if the relative viability of a cell-line is different in different tissues. The range of possible constitutions of chromosome mosaics is further increased by the probability that an abnormally constituted zygote may be especially liable to mitotic error; and when one divisional error has once occurred, subsequent errors are rendered more likely. Paradoxically, the occurrence of one or more errors of division in an abnormally constituted zygote may sometimes result in the appearance of a normal cell-line.

Mosaicism may involve any tissue, yet it is demonstrable only if each cell-line is represented in the tissue or tissues studied. Since chromosome studies can at present be carried out on only three tissues, undetected mosaicism may be common. Nevertheless it should not be invoked as an explanation for otherwise unexplained phenotypic features. Because of the possible occurrence of mosaicism, it is often desirable to study more than one tissue e.g. subcutaneous fibroblasts or bone marrow, as well as peripheral blood lymphocytes. It is especially desirable to examine the chromosomes of two or more tissues when a chromosome abnormality has been found in one and the result indicates the presence of more than one cell-line. Another situation calling for examination of two or more tissues is where the chromosome abnormality found in a patient is apparently at variance with the clinical picture. Mosaicism involving a sex chromosome abnormality may be indicated by a discrepancy between the results of examination by buccal smear

(p. 172) and chromosome studies on a single tissue. In other cases evidence of mosaicism may be obtained by examination of a buccal smear alone. For example, a chromatin positive individual with some cells containing two chromatin bodies may be an XX/XXX mosaic or an XXY/XXXY mosaic. This same finding can of course arise in homogeneously constituted individuals with three or more X chromosomes. Differences between the results of examination of buccal smears and the drumsticks of peripheral blood polymorphs may also indicate mosaicism in abnormalities of the X chromosome.

It is now known that mosaicism occurs commonly in abnormalities of the X chromosomes. Thus, in 32 women with primary amenorrhœa studied by Jacobs *et al.* (1961a) 15 had X chromosome abnormalities and 5 of these were mosaics. Of 37 mentally deficient individuals with abnormalities of the X chromosome, 6 were found on final diagnosis to be chromosome mosaics (Maclean *et al.* 1962). In the autosomal abnormalities mosaicism is probably much less common.

Strictly speaking, individuals with leukæmia and other neoplasms who have cells of abnormal chromosome constitution as well as normally constituted cells may be regarded as mosaics. In fact, the term is used only where the chromosome abnormalities are constitutional in nature rather than acquired, or the abnormalities have been acquired at an early stage of development.

Mongolism

In 1932 Waardenberg, an ophthalmologist and geneticist, suggested that mongolism might be due to an abnormality of chromosome number. Adrien Bleyer, a pædiatrician, made a similar suggestion two years later. In both cases the hypothesis was based on a consideration of the features of mongolism and a knowledge of the consequences of abnormalities of chromosome number in other species. The validity of the analogy was recognised by Penrose (1939) but adequate techniques for examining human chromosomes were not available. Using the unsatisfactory methods then available Mittwoch (1952) examined spermatogonial metaphases in a mongol but concluded that the expected number of 48 chromosomes was present. We are thus reminded that the principles of cytogenetics revealed by the study of other species are applicable to man; and that the exploitation of cytogenetic knowledge in relation to human disease required only the development of an adequate method for the study of human chromosomes. It is surprising that after such a method became available three years should have elapsed before Lejeune *et al.* (1959) first reported the occurrence of 47 chromosomes in mongols. The independent demonstration of the chromosome abnormality in mongolism by Jacobs *et al.* (1959a) was prompted by different but nonetheless valid considerations; namely, the imperfect analogy with Klinefelter's syndrome in which the chromosome abnormality had already been discovered (Jacobs and Strong 1959), and the known liability of mongols to acute leukæmia in which chromosomal changes were known to occur.

The extra chromosome in mongolism is accepted as being a third chromosome 21, although chromosomes 21 and 22 cannot generally be distinguished. The possibility of some mongols being trisomic for chromosome 21 and others trisomic for 22 is discounted. Whether the mongol chromosome is ultimately shown to be one of the larger or smaller pair it seems likely that that pair will continue to be known as 21. There are good reasons for believing that the mongol chromosome is the same chromosome which undergoes partial deletion to give rise to the Philadelphia chromosome of chronic myeloid leukæmia. In mongolism, the extra chromosome almost certainly arises as a result of non-disjunction at gametogenesis. The known association of mongolism with advancing maternal age makes it likely that non-disjunction generally occurs at oögenesis, the possibility of non-disjunction at spermatogenesis occasionally giving rise to mongolism has not been excluded. Possible factors in the occurrence of non-disjunction at oögenesis have been discussed by Polani (1963). It is known that exposure to radiation may increase the frequency of non-disjunction at meiosis in Drosophila, but only equivocal evidence has been found to incriminate maternal radiation exposure as a factor in the occurrence of mongolism (Uchida and Curtis 1961).

Chromosome studies are usually unnecessary for a diagnosis of mongolism. At all ages a systematic assessment of the individual clinical features is more reliable than a decision based on the appropriateness or otherwise of the general appearance. Unfortunately, no single clinical sign can be accepted as diagnostic but special weight should be given to abnormalities of the palmar dermal ridges (Walker 1958, Uchida and Soltan 1963), and to the increases in the acetabular and iliac angles in pelvic radiographs which are common in mongols but rare in normal subjects (Caffey and Ross 1956). The abnormalities of the palmar dermatoglyphs common in mongolism are a transverse palmar crease, a single crease on the fifth finger, a triradius near to the centre of the palm, absence of pattern on the thenar eminence and a tendency for loops to occur on every finger rather than whorls or arches. Apart from these features many of the abnormalities which occur in mongolism are relatively unhelpful when the diagnosis is difficult. Nevertheless, a clinical diagnosis of mongolism is only rarely to be entertained in the absence of mental retardation, short stature and microcephaly. In patients lacking these features confirmation by chromosome studies is essential.

Where facilities for chromosome studies are freely available, diagnostic confirmation in mongolism may often be requested unnecessarily. If chromosome studies were required for diagnosis in all cases of mongolism, the facilities available for chromosome studies would in many centres be fully engaged with this problem alone. Cytological confirmation of the diagnosis is obviously required in any case of real doubt such as may arise in instances of partial trisomy (see below). In the newborn a diagnosis of mongolism may be difficult, particularly so in the case of negro children. The difficulties are often resolved after a few weeks, yet if doubts have been raised in the minds of the parents it is obviously desirable to allay these as quickly as possible by chromosome studies. In the various situations in which a familial liability to mongolism may be suspected, chromosome studies are important, not only to confirm the diagnosis, but to establish the cytological type of mongolism which in turn may influence the genetic counsel offered to the parents. These situations are discussed below.

Examinations of a buccal smear for sex chromatin can of course make no contribution to the investigation of mongolism *per se*. Nevertheless, this simple test should be carried out in all male mongols in view of the occasional simultaneous occurrence of trisomy 21 and Klinefelter's syndrome.

It is now obvious that a great variety of cytological findings may occur in mongolism (Table I). In all of them except perhaps the case reported by Hall (1962), effective trisomy for chromosome 21 occurs. The patients with chromosomal translocations and isochromosomes are not clinically distinguishable from those with simple trisomy. The experience of Dent *et al.* (1963) suggests that translocation mongols may be relatively mildly affected and that webbing of the neck may be a more frequent feature of these cases.

TABLE I

REPORTED CHROMOSOME FINDINGS IN MONGOLISM

Chromosome constitution	Chromosome number	Authors
Single cell line		
Trisomy 21	47	Lejeune *et al.* 1959
*Trisomy 21 + XXY	48	Ford *et al.* 1959
Trisomy 21 + XXX	48	Day *et al.* 1963
Trisomy 21 + trisomy 13–15	48	Becker *et al.* 1963
Trisomy 21 + large Y.	47	Bishop *et al.* 1962
Partial trisomy 21	46 and fragment	Dent *et al.* 1963
Translocation 13–15 : 21	46	Polani *et al.* 1960
Translocation 21 : 21 or isochromosome 21	46	Fraccaro *et al.* 1960b
?Normal	46	Hall 1962
Mosaics		
*Normal/trisomy 21	46/47	Clarke *et al.* 1961
Normal/trisomy 21/tetrasomy 21	46/47/48	Fitzgerald and Lycette 1961
Normal/heterosomy 21	46/47/48/49/50/51	Valencia *et al.* 1963
Translocation 21 : 22/translocation 21 : 22 and fragment	46/46 + fragment	Penrose *et al.* 1960
*Normal/trisomy 21/trisomy 21 + isochromosome 21	46/47/48	Gustavson and Ek 1961
*Normal/normal + fragment	46/46 + fragment	Ilbery *et al.* 1961
Isochromosome 21/isochromosome 21 + fragment	46/46 + fragment	Gray *et al.* 1962

* Atypical clinical features.

Although some of the genetic material from chromosome 21 is lost in the process of translocation and in the production of isochromosomes, this loss is apparently insufficient to have any more definite effects on the phenotype. The few patients with trisomy 21 and other constitutional chromosomal abnormalities as well, have generally presented as instances of mongolism or as mongols with some additional phenotypic abnormalities. The widest deviation from the usual mongol phenotype seems to occur in patients who have much less than a full three doses of the genes on chromosome 21. This can arise in two main ways: because the individuals are mosaics of normal and trisomic cells (Clarke *et al.* 1961 and 1963, Ilbery *et al.* 1961) or because of the loss of part of the third chromosome leaving only a fragment (Migeon *et al.* 1962, Dent *et al.* 1963). Only the patient described by Clarke *et al.* is of normal intelligence. Since chromosome studies became possible there have been no other reports of observations on the so-called mongols of normal intellect which were occasionally mentioned in the earlier literature.

Translocation mongols. Familial concentration of mongolism is not common. Nevertheless, it has been appreciated for some time (Penrose 1951) that when it occurs and a patient's maternal relative is affected, the mother's age at the birth of the mongol is usually lower than average. Investigation of some of those familial cases showed that the mongols had 46 chromosomes including a normal pair 21 and an abnormal chromosome replacing one of the 13–15 groups (Penrose *et al.* 1960, Carter *et al.* 1960). The mothers of these mongols are themselves phenotypically normal and have often had normal as well as mongol children. They have 45 chromosomes, including one normal 21 and an abnormal chromosome indistinguishable from that of their mongol offspring. The abnormal one is the result of a translocation between a chromosome of the 13–15 group and a chromosome 21. Since the translocation carriers are phenotypically normal, no essential genetic material can have been lost from either of the chromosomes in the course of translocation. The translocation mongol with two chromosomes 21 and the abnormal chromosome is effectively trisomic for 21. In a smaller number of cases of familial mongolism the abnormal chromosome found in both mongol and carrier is a metacentric chromosome resembling chromosomes 19–20 of the normal set (Fraccaro *et al.* 1960). It has been variously interpreted as a 21 : 22 translocation or as an isochromosome for the long arms of 21.

Many case reports have now been published of families with translocation mongols and translocation carriers. Edwards *et al.* (1963) have pointed out that the tendency to report familial cases may give the erroneous impression that, in all translocation mongols, familial occurrence of the translocation may be demonstrated. They (Edwards *et al.* 1963) have studied 25 mongols born to mothers under the age of 30. In the 25 cases were two instances of 13–15:21 translocation and two of 21:22 or isochromosome type. In all these cases the parents were of normal chromosome constitution. The 25 cases also include one mongol/normal mosaic and the partial mongol mentioned above (Dent *et al.* 1963). In another investigation (unpublished) all 47 mongol inmates of an institution for mental defectives were studied. Of these patients 1 was a Klinefelter-mongol, 1 had an unduly large Y chromosome and 1 had a 13–15:21 translocation. The parents of the translocation mongol had no chromosome abnormality. 11 of these 47 mongols were born to women below the age of 30.

In spite of the evident rarity of familial translocation mongolism it is important that translocation carriers should be found and genetic counsel offered. If a translocation mongol is found, a detailed family history should be taken and chromosome studies carried out in both parents. Chromosome studies are specifically indicated in any mongol born to a mother under the age of 30. A family history of mongolism or of unexplained abortions or neonatal deaths, especially if on the maternal side, may indicate a familial translocation, and so suggest a need for chromosome studies in a woman even before a first pregnancy. When two mongols have already occurred in a sibship the need for further investigation is obvious, whatever the mother's age. In these situations it is desirable to establish the chromosome constitution of both parents. If any parental chromosome abnormality is found it will usually be in the mother in the case of 13–15/21 translocation and in the father in the case of the much less common 21/22 or isochromosome type. Since exceptions to both rules have been described it is obviously desirable to study both parents (Sergovitch *et al.* 1962, Hamerton *et al.* 1961), whatever the chromosome findings in the mongol. Another good reason for examining both parents is provided by the occasional occurrence of normal/trisomy 21 mosaicism in apparently normal individuals (Smith *et al.* 1962a, Weinstein and Warkany 1963). Women with this abnormality are liable to have more than one mongol. The mongols born to such women are of course homogeneously trisomic for chromosome 21.

It is not generally necessary for the parents and child to attend at the place of chromosome studies for blood samples to be taken. If attendance is required, it is more often to ensure that all the relevant information available about the family has been obtained. Where distances are great, personal attendance by the parents may often be postponed until the results of chromosome studies are known. Attendance for genetic counselling is more necessary than attendance for the taking of blood samples. With all techniques of culture the samples can be taken and sent to the place of chromosome study after appropriate preliminary processing.

Apart from those families in which the occurrence of mongolism is to be attributed to a familial chromosomal translocation, there are others which seem to show a non-specific liability to errors of cell division. Many of these families have now been described and it seems likely that many more still pass undetected. Such families include some where mongolism, sex chromosome abnormality and leukæmia have occurred (Miller *et al.* 1961); mongolism and Klinefelter's syndrome (Benirschke *et al.* 1962); and mongolism, Klinefelter's syndrome and twinning (Wright *et al.* 1963).

Genetic counselling in mongolism. When a couple have had one mongol child they often decide to have no more children or they may ask about the risk of further children being similarly affected. Carter and Evans (1961) found that the risk is increased 50-fold for mothers who have had a mongol before the age of 25 and 5-fold for mothers in the age group 25–34. They found no increased risk for mothers whose mongol child had been born when she was 35 or older. These increased risks must of course be related to the overall risk that a mongol may result from any pregnancy. This overall risk is related to maternal age and is of the order of 1 in 2000 for the youngest age-group (Collman and Stoller 1962). The observations of Carter and Evans may with some reservations be accepted as a basis for genetic counselling when the results of chromosome studies are not available. One reservation is suggested by the probability that if Carter and Evans study had been on a larger scale they would have found some increased risk for a mother whose mongol had been born when she was 35 or older. Some translocation carriers must have their first live child at that age and for them the risk is very greatly increased regardless of age. This situation may be suggested by a pregnancy history of previous abortions or of the neonatal death of children not known to the parents to be mongols. A second reservation arises from the possibility of detecting such a family history indicative, with varying degrees of confidence, of a familial translocation. Apart from the mother's own pregnancy history, a history of mongolism and an excess of abortions or neonatal deaths should be sought in the mother's own sibship, in the pregnancy histories of her sisters, her mother's sisters and her maternal grandmother. If such a history is found in a woman who has had one mongol child, the risk of her having a second mongol should be regarded as that of a translocation carrier, until that possibility has been excluded by chromosome studies.

When the results of chromosome studies are available genetic counsel can be offered with greater confidence. If the mother is the carrier of a 13–15:21 translocation (and the affected child is a translocation mongol) then mongolism may be expected in about one-third of her offspring. When the father is a carrier of a 13–15:21 translocation the risk of mongolism is very much smaller (Hamerton and Steinberg 1962). When the father is the carrier of a 21:22 chromosomal fusion or an isochromosome 21 the risk of a mongol child is high and appears to increase with advancing paternal age (Penrose 1962). In about one-third of translocation mongols the parents are found to have an apparently normal chromosome constitution. The possibility of chromosomal mosaicism in either parent cannot be excluded and consequently the risk of the dual occurrence of mongolism must be rated as high. There is evidence that where a mongol with 47 chromosomes and trisomy 21 is born to normal parents, if the mother is under 35, the risk of recurrence is several times greater than the random risk at that age (Hamerton 1962). It may be that the increased risk in this situation is due entirely to the existence of families with non-specific liability to errors of cell division, the carriers of the trait being of apparently normal chromosome constitution. In any case, the birth of one mongol in a family in which sex chromosome abnormalities or familial leukæmia is known to occur should not be regarded as a random occurrence: the risk of recurrence is probably high.

When the mother herself is a mongol, genetic advice is unlikely to be sought. Of the 11 reported live born children of mongol mothers 5 have been mongols and 2 others mentally subnormal (Penrose 1963). The risk is obviously high in the first or subsequent pregnancies.

Chromosome 21. No genetic marker for chromosome 21 has yet been identified. The familial occurrence of chromosomal translocations involving chromosome 21 provides a special opportunity for finding a marker. Using this approach Shaw and Gershowitz (1962) found some evidence that chromosome 21 may carry the ABO blood group locus. This finding is still unsubstantiated. Wherever the Rh locus occurs it seems unlikely that it is on chromosome 21 (Day *et al.* 1963). Some evidence has been adduced to suggest that chromosome 21 may carry the locus that determines the activity of galactose-1-phosphate-uridyl-transferase in the blood (Brandt 1963) and the locus for polymorphonuclear leucocyte alkaline phosphatase activity. Consideration of all the evidence bearing on polymorph alkaline phosphatase activity from cases of chronic myeloid leukæmia and from mongols indicates a complex genetic control for this enzyme (King *et al.* 1962).

Evidence of an interesting abnormality of tryptophan metabolism in mongols (Jerome 1962) has not yet been fully investigated as a possible chromosome marker. Mongols excrete increased amounts of β-amino-iso-butyric acid (Lundin and Gustavson 1962) but the significance of this is uncertain.

Hirschsprung's Disease

There is an apparent association between Hirschsprung's disease and mongolism in that 3 of 207 children with Hirschsprung's disease were mongols (Bodian and Carter 1963). Hirschsprung's disease has also been reported in a child with XO/XX/XXX mosaicism (Hayward and Cameron 1961); and in a child with multiple congenital abnormalities and an unidentified extra chromosome (Butler et al. 1962). It is unlikely that this association with chromosomal abnormalities is a causal one.

Trisomy 22

It is generally agreed that chromosomes of the pairs 21 and 22 cannot be distinguished with certainty by the cytogenetic methods at present available. Consequently, examples of apparent trisomy 21–22 which lack the phenotype of mongolism have usually been interpreted as instances of trisomy 22. Less commonly, the extra chromosome has been accepted as either chromosome 22 or a Y chromosome. In many of the cases reported other interpretations seem possible, such as partial trisomy for a larger chromosome with loss of material due to deletion, an interpretation mentioned by Ferguson and Pitt (1963). The small group of cases reported as instances of trisomy 22 may therefore be heterogeneous as regards chromosome constitution. Consequently, it is not surprising that the group shows no characteristic clinical picture such as is obvious for trisomy 13–15, 17–18 and 21. Nevertheless, in 4 of 8 cases, muscular hypotonia was a prominent feature.

The single instance of the Sturge-Weber syndrome regarded as trisomic for chromosome 22 (Hayward and Bower 1960) is discussed later (p. 180). Turner and Jennings (1961) reported a schizophrenic boy without other abnormalities. A pair of mentally retarded twin girls of schizoid personalities but without physical abnormality was described by Biesele et al. (1962). Because of the possible association of trisomy 22 with schizophrenia, Biesele and his colleagues examined the chromosomes of 10 schizophrenic children but with normal results. Dunn et al. (1961) found possible trisomy for chromosome 22 in association with benign congenital hypotonia (Walton 1957). Muscular hypotonia, hepatomegaly and cardiac abnormalities were found in a child who died at the age of 2 months and was regarded as an instance of trisomy 22 (Koulischer and Perier 1962). Other instances of possible trisomy 22 in children with multiple congenital abnormalities including muscular hypotonia have been reported by Hall (1963) and by Ferguson and Pitt (1963).

The finding of possible mosaicism for normal cells and cells containing an extra small acrocentric chromosome in patients with dystrophia myotonica (Fitzgerald and Caughey, 1962) is discussed in p. 180. One of the interpretations they consider is that the extra acrocentric chromosome is a chromosome 22.

Trisomy 17–18 (E₁-trisomy)

The first recognised example of this autosomal trisomic state was reported by Edwards and his colleagues in 1960, who at first regarded the extra chromosome as No. 17. Patau *et al.* (1960), who described the second case, thought the extra chromosome to be No. 18. It is only rarely and that with a low degree of confidence that these two chromosome pairs can be distinguished in the average preparations, so that it is best described as trisomy 17–18. Since the chromosome group 16–18 is collectively known as E, this trisomic state is sometimes called E₁-trisomy to denote the first described trisomy for this chromosome group. 32 cases of this condition reported up to December 1962 have been reviewed by Hecht *et al.* (1963).

The clinical picture is a fairly characteristic one (Fig. 2), so that a diagnosis can often but not invariably be made on clinical features alone. It seems remarkable that it was not recognised as a syndrome before chromosome studies became practicable. That it can now be recognised on clinical examination illustrates the importance of systematic analysis and listing of the components in the multiple congenital abnormality states. The child is usually of low birth weight after a normal gestation. Evidence of mental retardation is present and muscular hypertonia occurs. The face is abnormal with malformed and low-set ears, micrognathia and a small mouth. Neck webbing and a broad flat chest are common. The hands are usually held in the "surrender position" with the fingers flexed and the index finger overlapping the others (Fig. 3). Short big toes are common (Fig. 4), and the finger nails are often defective. Equinovarus deformity of feet with a "rocker-bottom" shape is frequent. Other abnormalities may occur, but a diagnosis can often be made on the coincidence of some of these common features. As with mongolism, the dermatoglyphs are characteristic and possibly provide the most reliable single sign (Uchida *et al.* 1962): both finger and toe prints show a preponderance of simple arches, which results in a low ridge count with no triradii.

The longest survival reported in trisomy 17–18 is 23 months (Weiss *et al.* 1962). Death commonly occurs after a few weeks of life. There are several reports of autopsy findings. Amongst the most common features are the co-existence of a high ventricular septal defect and a bicuspid pulmonary valve; this combination of cardiac abnormalities may be a specific consequence of the chromosome abnormality. Other common pathological findings include an unfixed mesentery, heterotopic pancreatic tissue, a defective falx cerebri and absence or hypoplasia of the corpus callosum. It is interesting that all these defects arise in organs which are embryologically midline structures.

As with mongolism, it is obvious that patients with different chromosomal abnormalities resulting in effective trisomy 17–18 may be phenotypically indistinguishable from those with 47 chromosomes and simple trisomy. Koulischer *et al.* (1963) have described mosaicism for normal cells and cells trisomic for chromosome 17–18 in a child who died at the age of 11 months. Five cases of trisomy 17–18 in which a clinical diagnosis was confirmed by chromosome studies were reported by Weiss *et al.* (1962); one of their patients

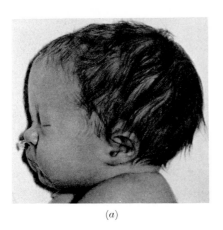

(a)

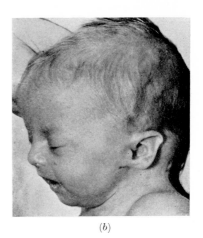

(b)

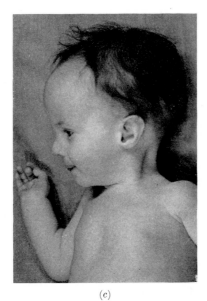

(c)

FIG. 2. Three examples of the facies in trisomy 17–18. (a) and (b) show the low set and deformed ears, and (c) "surrender" position of the hands.

(Fig. 2 (a) by courtesy of Dr J. H. Edwards.)

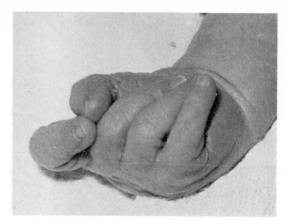

FIG. 3. Trisomy 17–18. Overlapping of index finger.

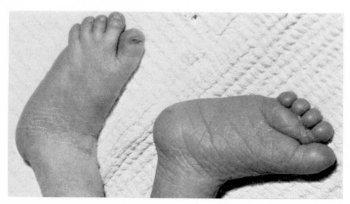

FIG. 4. Trisomy 17–18. Foot, to show short hallux (the "rocker-bottom" deformity is less well displayed).

(Figs. 3 and 4 by courtesy of Dr J. H. Edwards.)

was a mosaic of normal and trisomic cells, yet she was clinically indistinguishable from the others. One child with a translocation between a chromosome 17–18 and one of the 13–15 group as well as four normal chromosomes of the pairs 17–18 has been described by Hecht *et al.* (1963). The parents of this child were apparently of normal chromosome constitution, in contrast to the parents of a child with a similar translocation described by Brodie and Dallaire (1962), where the mother was the carrier of a balanced translocation.

The tendency to multiple chromosomal changes, notable in mongolism and in abnormalities of the X chromosome, may also be present in trisomy 17–18. However, the only instance of multiple chromosomal abnormality yet reported is one of double trisomy for both the X chromosome and chromosome 17–18 (Uchida *et al.* 1962). The clinical features in this child were indistinguishable from those of uncomplicated trisomy 17–18.

No reliable measure is yet available of the frequency of trisomy 17–18 at birth. Smith (1963) suggests an incidence as high as 0·23 per 1000 live births, and Edwards (personal communication) thinks it likely to be between 0·1 and 0·2 per 1000 births. Delay in recognition and the shortened expectation of life must weigh heavily against complete ascertainment of the frequency of the condition. Carr's finding (p. 178) of two instances of trisomy 17–18 in 54 spontaneous abortions suggests a much higher incidence of the abnormality at conception than at birth. In the small number of liveborn cases so far known there has been an apparent excess of females. It may be that trisomy 17–18 is less well tolerated by a male fœtus with a consequent increase in the likelihood of abortion.

There is no known cause for the meiotic non-disjunction resulting in trisomy 17–18, although in two cases the mothers had received diagnostic X-irradiation to the abdomen in pregnancy. As with mongolism, there is a relationship to advancing maternal age, but in the case of trisomy 17–18 it is less marked and much less well established. It certainly has not yet been possible in trisomy 17–18 to show that the condition is associated with advancing maternal age *per se* and not with advancing paternal age. There has been no reported instance of two cases of trisomy 17–18 in a sibship, although the child effectively trisomic for chromosome 17–18 described by Hecht *et al.* (1963) had sibs who died soon after birth and who may have been affected. On the other hand, trisomy 17–18 probably occurs with increased frequency in families with a non-specific liability to chromosomal abnormalities due to meiotic non-disjunction. Turner *et al.* (1964) and Hecht *et al.* have both described cases with mongol sibs. Recently, an instance of possible clustering in time and place of cases of trisomy 17–18 and mongolism has been reported by Heinrichs *et al.* (1963). If confirmed, this observation would suggest the operation of an environmental factor, such as infection, predisposing to meiotic non-disjunction in a community.

Early diagnosis of trisomy 17–18 is desirable for prognosis; to forestall surgical correction of anomalies other than those presenting an immediate threat to life (Smith 1963); and as a basis for genetic counselling. Parents may be told that the condition is not generally familial, and that the chance of having a second abnormal child is only slightly greater than it otherwise would be.

No certain genetic marker for chromosome 17–18 has yet been identified, in spite of the study of a range of possible markers in some cases, notably those of Hecht and his colleagues (1963). A defect of thyroxine synthesis has been found in a child who is probably partially monosomic for a chromosome of the 17–18 group (Bühler *et al.* 1964).

Trisomy 13–15 (D_1-trisomy)

This chromosomal abnormality was first described by Patau *et al.* in 1960. The chromosomes of the pairs 13, 14 and 15 (group D) cannot be individually identified and so the condition has been called D trisomy. Since it must now be certain that trisomy for the same chromosome is concerned in all the reported cases of similar phenotypes the chromosome is sometimes designated D_1 and the syndrome, the D_1 syndrome (Smith *et al.* 1963). The findings in 14 cases have recently been reviewed (Smith 1963).

The clinical syndrome now associated with trisomy 13–15 was probably recognised by Kundrat as long ago as 1882, but did not gain general recognition. At birth, affected children are much more obviously abnormal (Fig. 5) than either mongols or instances of trisomy 17–18. All the infants have been apparently deaf and mentally retarded, some were hypertonic and many had episodic apnœa. Malformed and low-set ears are common. Some ocular abnormality such as anophthalmia, microphthalmia or colobomata has been found in most cases. A sharply sloping forehead and microcephaly are associated with absence of the olfactory bulbs and tracts. Cleft lip, usually with cleft palate, has been present in most cases; the absence of this conspicuous feature may however be allowed to weigh too heavily against a diagnosis thoroughly justified by the presence of other features. Cutaneous hæmangiomata occur. Polydactyly of feet and hands is common and many cases have had retroflexible thumbs. A variety of congenital heart lesions have been found including dextrocardia and ventricular septal defects. Some confusion has arisen from the description of equinovarus or "rocker-bottom" deformity of the feet in both trisomy 13–15 and in trisomy 17–18. It does occur in trisomy 17–18; in trisomy 13–15 posterior prominence of the heel is often conspicuous. Cryptorchidism and abnormalities of the relationship of penis to scrotum may be found. The dermatoglyphic patterns are abnormal but, unlike those of trisomy 17–18, they are not specific (Uchida and Soltan 1963). The patterns on palms resemble those of mongolism and simian creases are common. A possible simple aid to diagnosis has recently been reported by Huehns *et al.* (1964b). In 6 cases with trisomy 13–15 they found from 1 to 6 anomalous nuclear projections and other nuclear abnormalities in neutrophil polymorphs in blood films.

In trisomy 13–15 the mean survival appears to be shorter than in trisomy 17–18 although one child surviving for almost 5 years has been mentioned (Huehns *et al.* 1964b). At autopsy some lesions which are not clinically obvious may be found, including accessory spleens, an unusually large gallbladder and hydronephrosis. The autopsy findings as regards the brain defect have been described by Miller *et al.* (1963). Some female infants have been found to have a partially septate uterus.

Individuals with abnormalities of chromosomes 13–15, other than simple

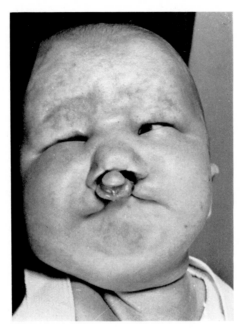

Fig. 5. Trisomy 13–15, showing microphthalmia and bilateral cleft palate.

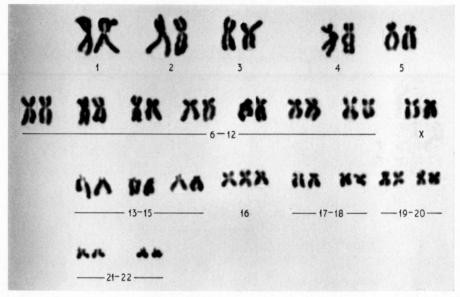

FIG. 6. Trisomy 16, karyotype (Lewis *et al*. 1963).

trisomy, do not apparently have the characteristic phenotype of the trisomic state. A case of double trisomy for chromosome 21 and the 13–15 group has been reported by Becker *et al.* (1963). The child was aged 4 and regarded as a mongol with some unusual features which were not typical of trisomy 13–15. A second case of double trisomy has been reported (Gustavson *et al.* 1962) where the other chromosome involved was an unidentified small acrocentric. The features of trisomy 13–15 noted in this child were microphthalmia, polydactyly and a ventricular septal defect. No certain example of mosaicism in trisomy 13–15 has been reported. Warkany *et al.* (1962b) have described a child with mental retardation and absence of the patellæ. The clinical picture was not suggestive of trisomy 13–15. Chromosome studies indicated a mosaic of normally constituted cells and cells with 47 chromosomes. The extra chromosome in these cells resembled one of the 13–15 group but other interpretations were possible. In this case the absence of features of the recognised phenotype weighed against accepting the additional chromosome as one of the group 13–15. Atkins and Rosenthal (1961) described one case of trisomy 13–15, having relatively few of the phenotypic features of the condition. It has been suggested by Smith *et al.* (1963) that this case may be an example of mosaicism. This possibility can never of course be completely excluded, but chromosome studies were carried out on only one tissue and the cytological findings did not suggest mosaicism.

The frequency of trisomy 13–15 at birth is unknown. It is certainly less common than mongolism and probably less common than trisomy 17–18. As with trisomy 17–18, the frequency of stillbirth, the short expectation of life of those cases born alive, and delay in diagnosis must all militate against complete ascertainment. The finding of 3 instances of trisomy 13–15, 2 of trisomy 17–18 and one of mongolism in 54 spontaneous abortions (Carr 1963) is in inverse proportion to the apparent frequency of these conditions at birth. Carr's results (p. 178) may indicate that, of the three common autosomal trisomic states, mongolism is most and trisomy 13–15 least compatible with intra-uterine life.

As with the other autosomal trisomic states, there is evidence that advancing maternal age may predispose to the meiotic non-disjunction resulting in trisomy 13–15. This is however, not as well established as in the case of mongolism, or even as strongly suggestive as in trisomy 17–18 (Smith 1963). There is a possible female preponderance of cases but so far the total number of reported cases is small. Apart from maternal age no other causal factor is discernible. A single sibship in which one member had trisomy 13–15 and another XO-Turner's syndrome suggests a special liability to meiotic non-disjunction in one of the parents (Therman *et al.* 1961). Were it not for the occurrence of such families the parents of a child with trisomy 13–15 might be told that the risk of abnormality in subsequent children is not increased. As it is, they may be told that the condition is not familial, has no known cause and that the chance of abnormality in subsequent children is only slightly increased.

No certain genetic marker for chromosomes 13–15 has yet been identified, but unusual persistence of hæmoglobins Gower-2 and $\gamma4$ have been reported (Huehns *et al.* 1964a). This may indicate that genes influencing the synthesis of γ chains as well as the postulated ε chains of hæmoglobin occur on the triplicated chromosome.

Trisomy 16

Lewis and his colleagues (1963) have reported the only instance of trisomy for chromosome 16. The patient was a normally chromatin-positive female aged 59 with multiple congenital abnormalities including mental defect, hypogonadism, facial appearance suggestive of precocious senility, osteoporosis and widespread calcification of soft tissues (personal communication). The karyotype of the cells with 47 chromosomes (Fig. 6) is highly suggestive of trisomy-16. Lewis and his co-workers have carried their attempt at identification further by interesting observations on variance and means of the chromosome arm ratios, which seem to exclude the possibility of the extra chromosome being either one of the 17–18 group or an isochromosome of X.

Trisomy 6–12

Possible trisomy for chromosomes in this group has been reported by Jacobs et al. (1961), Pfeiffer et al. (1962), and Stalder et al. (1963). In all of these cases the sex chromatin findings were inconsistent with the extra chromosome being an X chromosome. In a fourth case El-Alfi et al. (1963) used autoradiographic techniques to exclude this possibility. Of these 4 cases, 3 had mental retardation and genital abnormalities, and 3 had flexion deformities of the fingers.

Sex Chromosome Abnormalities

Numerical abnormalities of the X chromosome are the commonest of human chromosome abnormalities, XXY-Klinefelter's syndrome alone being as frequent at birth as mongolism. At first glance it is surprising that so few examples of abnormalities of the X chromosome have been recognised and reported in children. This results from the absence in childhood of those features which most commonly lead adult patients to seek medical advice. The usual presenting manifestations in adults are infertility, gynæcomastia and sometimes mental retardation in the XXY-Klinefelter's syndrome; primary amenorrhœa and short stature in the XO-Turner's syndrome and its variants; and secondary amenorrhœa or mental retardation in the few cases of the triple-X syndrome which are diagnosed. It is not surprising that XO-Turner's syndrome, usually in patients presenting on account of short stature, is the only X chromosome abnormality commonly diagnosed in childhood. The pre-pubertal XXY male, if not mentally retarded, may appear normal; and triple-X females are detected only infrequently even amongst adults, because amenorrhœa and mental retardation are not constant features (Close 1963). Some instances of these occult X chromosome abnormalities in children have been detected by the examination of groups of mentally retarded children using the buccal smear technique for sex chromatin. Case reports of patients found in such studies have led to an erroneous impression that most individuals with X chromosome abnormalities are mentally subnormal. In fact, while the XXY and triple-X states are more common amongst mental defectives than in the general population (Maclean et al. 1962), most XXX and XXY individuals are mentally normal.

The best measure of the frequency of X chromosome abnormalities found at birth is provided by the survey carried out in Edinburgh by Maclean and his colleagues (1964). Using the buccal smear method they examined 20,725 consecutive live births in hospital. When discrepancy was found between the phenotypic sex and the nuclear sex, chromosome studies were carried out where possible (Table II). Surveys of this kind indicate only the minimum incidence of abnormalities of the X chromosome. Abnormalities of the Y

TABLE II

RESULTS OF A BUCCAL SMEAR SURVEY FOR SEX CHROMATIN IN 20,725 CONSECUTIVE BIRTHS, WITH CHROMOSOME STUDIES IN DISCREPANT CASES (MACLEAN *et al.* 1964)

Males—10,725 *examined*		*Per* 1000 *live births*
Abnormal	21	1·96
XXY	15*	1·40
XY/XXY	3	0·28
XXYY	1	—
XY/probably XXY	2	—
Females—10,000 *examined*		
Abnormal	16	1·6
XXX	12*	1·2
XO	3	0·3
XO/deletion of long arm of X	1	—

* Unconfirmed by chromosome studies in 3 cases.

chromosome and the autosomes are of course undetected, as are those mosaics in whom cells with abnormality of the X chromosome are either absent from the buccal mucosa or poorly represented. There is no reason to believe that the population studied in Edinburgh was not representative of liveborn children in a European community. The results obtained are in agreement with those of the very much smaller surveys by Moore (1959) in Canada, and by Bergeman (1961) in Switzerland. Amongst Japanese schoolgirls Nakagome *et al.* (1963), found a comparable incidence of XO-Turner's syndrome. On the other hand, Naik and Shah (1962) examined 3890 newborn children in India without finding any abnormalities of nuclear sex. Further studies of this kind in different countries and at other ages are desirable.

There is an obvious need for follow-up of children found to have X chromosome abnormalities at birth. Observations on growth and development as well as on morbidity and mortality are required. Such a study is not easily organised. Of the children with X chromosome abnormalities found in the Edinburgh survey, all the triple-X females, and all the XXY males except one with a small scrotum, were of normal appearance. It is difficult to decide what, if anything, should be told the parents of such children. Since triple-X females may be apparently normal (Close, 1963) the parents of these children should not be told of abnormality. The short stature and probable infertility of XO females may be mentioned. An XXY male can be regarded as probably infertile. There can be no justification for telling the parents of infants with X chromosome abnormalities of the risk of mental defect, even in the XXY state.

Sex chromatin. Large scale surveys of many people for X chromosome abnormalities depend on the simplicity and reliability of examination of a buccal smear for sex chromatin. The Lyon hypothesis (Lyon 1962) dealing with the mechanism and significance of inactivation of a second or third X chromosome is at present the centre of much controversy. None of this controversy casts any doubt on the reliability of examination for sex chromatin as a diagnostic test. The number of sex chromatin or Barr bodies (Barr and Bertram 1949) which may be demonstrable in a diploid cell is one less than its number of X chromosomes. Polyploid cells prove an exception to this rule (Harnden 1962b) but this is rarely of diagnostic importance. It should be appreciated that this X − 1 relationship refers to the number of Barr bodies which may be seen, and not to the number invariably demonstrable in every cell. Just as a normal female may have only 40% of chromatin positive cells, a triple-X female may have only 15% doubly positive cells. This point is of importance in making plain the need to examine at least 100 cells in a diagnostic buccal smear, even when there is no special reason to suspect mosaicism. In suspected mosaicism it may be desirable to examine buccal smears from both sides of the mouth; and to look for drumsticks and double drumsticks in peripheral blood films or, better still buffy coat preparations. There is now little doubt that the drumstick of the polymorphonuclear leucocyte is the equivalent of the Barr body of other cells. Its lower frequency of obvious occurrence is probably accounted for by the fact that it must be extruded from the polymorph nucleus before it can be seen. In the triple-X states double drumsticks are very rare and polymorphs with three drumsticks have not been described in individuals with four X-chromosomes. These limitations, and the difficulty of differentiating between the true drumstick and nuclear appendages without known significance, makes examination for polymorph drumsticks unsuitable for routine use.

An unexpectedly low incidence of chromatin-positive cells has been found in buccal smears made from normal female newborn children (Smith *et al.* 1962b; Taylor 1963). This phenomenon has been described only in the first two days of life when the sex chromatin present may be diffuse and stain with difficulty. In practice this variation, which is thought to be due to hormones of maternal origin, is probably of little importance. Variation in the size of the chromatin body during treatment with antibiotics (Sohval and Casselman 1961) and corticosteroids does not commonly give rise to diagnostic difficulty.

Pseudohermaphrodites and Hermaphrodites

The generic term *pseudohermaphroditism* is applied to all individuals in whom ambiguity of the external genitalia is associated with gonads of one sex. Such abnormalities occur only exceptionally in the commoner numerical abnormalities of the X chromosome, the XXY, XO and XXX states. Similarly, cases of pure gonadal dysgenesis (Harnden and Stewart 1959) whether of XX or XY chromosomes constitution are, before puberty, accepted as normal females. Ambiguity of the external genitalia may range from simple clitoral enlargement in an otherwise normal female, through clitoral enlargement with a phallic urethra and fusion of the labia, to appearances indistinguishable from those of a male with bilateral cryptorchidism. Various degrees of masculinisation of non-constitutional ætiology, usually manifest as simple clitoral enlargement, may occur in newborn females. This may be found in the adrenogenital syndrome; where the mother has been treated during pregnancy with masculinising drugs; or even because of a maternal masculinising tumour such as an arrhenoblastoma. The detection of these situations is usually simple, depending on the maternal history or on hormone excretion studies in the virilising adrenogenital syndrome.

If hormonal factors in mother or child cannot be blamed for sexual ambiguity, the next appropriate step in investigation is the determination of the nuclear sex on a buccal smear. Chromatin-positive children with ambiguous external genitalia in whom abnormal hormonal factors cannot be implicated are usually true hermaphrodites. A diagnosis of true hermaphroditism requires the presence of either ovo-testes or discrete masses of gonadal tissue of both kinds. True hermaphroditism has now been described with a variety of chromosomal constitutions (Table III), but the most common is probably

TABLE III

REPORTED SEX CHROMATIN AND CHROMOSOME FINDINGS
IN TRUE HERMAPHRODITES

Sex chromatin	Sex chromosomes	Authors
+ive	XX	Harnden and Armstrong 1959
+ive	XX	Hungerford et al. 1959
+ive	XX/XXX	Ferguson-Smith et al. 1960
−ive	XY/XO	Hirschhorn et al. 1960
+ive	XX/XY	Waxman et al. 1962
+ive	XX/XXY/XXYYY	Fraccaro et al. 1962b

XX. Wilkins (1960) recommends that a true hermaphrodite child should be reared as of the sex for which both its external genitalia and its gonadal morphology are most apt, regardless of its chromosomal sex. If well-developed ovary, uterus and tubes are present the removal of testes or ovo-testis may be expected to result in normal female development. Unless the phallus is adequate for a male the child should be reared as a female.

The chromatin-negative cases will be mainly accounted for by cryptorchid males with hypospadias. They will also include cases of a rare but apparently distinct form of pseudohermaphroditism (Table IV) recently reviewed by Sohval (1963), the XO/XY syndrome. The reported cases have presented as males or females and buccal smears in all have been chromatin-negative. Chromosome studies have usually shown these individuals to be XO/XY mosaics (Willemse et al. 1962), but one was a triple mosaic XO/XY/XX (Schuster and Motulsky 1962). Not surprisingly, where only a single tissue has been studied, some of these children have been thought to be of chromosome constitution XO (Bloise *et al.* 1960) and some XY (Alexander and Ferguson-Smith 1961). Most of these patients have had an enlarged clitoris or a small penis with an urethral meatus at its base, vagina, uterus, fallopian tubes, an intra-abdominal testis on one side and a vestigial gonad on the other. Because of the character of the second gonad these patients cannot be classified as true hermaphrodites. Clinical features helpful in diagnosis include the occurrence of a vagina in a chromatin-negative individual with ambiguous external genitalia. Laparotomy may be necessary for conclusive diagnosis. Sohval (1964) has discussed the occurrence of gonadal neoplasms in this group of patients.

TABLE IV

REPORTED SEX CHROMATIN AND SEX CHROMOSOME FINDINGS
IN PSEUDOHERMAPHRODITES

Syndrome	Sex chromatin	Sex chromosomes	Authors
Testicular feminisation	−ive	XY	Jacobs *et al.* 1959b
?XO/XY syndrome	−ive	XO	Bloise *et al.* 1960
XO/XY syndrome	−ive	XO/XY	Blank *et al.* 1960
?XO/XY syndrome	−ive	XY	Alexander and Ferguson-Smith 1961
XO/XY syndrome	−ive	XO/XY	Willemse *et al.* 1962
?XO/XY syndrome	−ive	XO/XY/XX	Schuster and Motulsky 1962
?XO/XY syndrome	−ive	XO/XxY	Miles *et al.* 1962
—	+ive	XX	Shah *et al.* 1961
—	−ive	XO/Xy/XXXy	Fraccaro *et al.* 1962a
—	++ive	XO/XXXY	Warkany *et al.* 1962a
—	+ive	XX	Franks and Northcutt 1963

Not all XO/XY individuals are of this type. Some have presented as actual females of short stature with primary amenorrhœa and without clitoral enlargement. In these patients only streak gonads without testicular tissue were found at laparotomy (Jacobs *et al.* 1961).

Testicular Feminisation Syndrome

The term male pseudohermaphroditism is sometimes used as a synonym for the testicular feminisation syndrome. The latter term is to be preferred since it indicates a definite separation of this condition from the spectra of true and pseudohermaphroditism. Such a separation appears to be justified. The condition was recognised and extensively studied before human chromosome studies became practicable. It is probably a rare condition which is seldom undiagnosed. There were no cases amongst the 10,000 female newborn studied by Maclean *et al.* (1964). Similarly, although primary amenorrhœa is a constant feature, there were only two cases of testicular feminisation amongst 32 women with primary amenorrhœa (Jacobs *et al.* 1961). In contrast, in the same group there were 6 cases of XO-Turner's syndrome and 5 patients with one normal and one abnormal X chromosome.

Children with the testicular feminisation syndrome appear to be normal females unless they present with inguinal hernia, when testes may be found in one or both inguinal canals. In other cases the testes remain in the abdominal cavity or come to lie in a labial position analogous to the scrotal position in males. The diagnosis may be suggested after puberty by a history of disproportionate pain occasioned by a blow in the groin. The uterus and the upper-third of the vagina are lacking; and the testes are the only gonads. At puberty, normal breast development may occur, although pubic and axillary hair are absent and there is no menarche. These individuals are chromatin-negative and have 46 chromosomes, including morphologically normal X and Y chromosomes (Jacobs *et al.* 1959). They are in fact sex-reversed males. The condition is familial and is transmitted through the female line. It has been shown that in affected families the sum of the normal males and the apparent females with testicular feminisation is not significantly different from the number of true females. The mode of inheritance is either as a sex-linked recessive or as a sex-limited autosomal dominant.

No attempt should be made to reverse the social sex of these apparently female children and the true sex should probably not be communicated to the parents. The testes should not be removed until feminisation is complete (Wilkins 1960) but, if they are removed, cyclical œstrogen therapy may be given at puberty. When feminisation is complete the testes should be removed, regardless of their position, because of the very high risk of malignant tumours arising in these organs (Morris 1953). The patients are psychologically female and many are happily married although childless. The problem of whether or not the true sex should be communicated to an adult patient contemplating marriage is a difficult one. It is easy to allow the interests of the patient to overshadow the interests and rights of the future husband. This and other legal issues relating to the true sex of these apparent females have still to be raised in law.

XO-Turner's Syndrome

This is the only X-chromosome abnormality commonly diagnosed in childhood. Diagnosis is suggested by the obvious physical abnormalities which occur in this condition. The clinical features of 25 cases, most of which were diagnosed in childhood, have been reviewed by Lemli and Smith (1963). All were of short stature and all had at least 5 other obvious abnormalities. Of these abnormalities, the most helpful in diagnosis were the occurrence of pigmented nævi, a low posterior hair line, a broad chest with widely spaced nipples, a history of congenital lymphœdema, and abnormal fingernails. Webbing of the neck was present in 13 of 25 patients and coarctation of the aorta in 9. In contrast, renal anomalies, which are much less often mentioned as part of the syndrome, were detected in 9 of the 14 patients who were appropriately investigated. The so-called congenital lymphœdema of Turner's syndrome is probably not true lymphœdema. It generally disappears in early childhood leaving in some children a puffiness of the backs of fingers and toes. The abnormality of fingernails consists of small nails with relatively wide nail-folds, a deeply set base and increased transverse curvature. Abnormalities of the external genitalia do not occur in the simple XO state, but genital hypoplasia and primary amenorrhœa are probably invariable. The Bonnevie-Ulrich syndrome is to be regarded as synonymous with Turner's syndrome observed in early childhood.

The majority of females with the clinical features of Turner's syndrome are of course chromatin-negative, having 45 chromosomes and the sex chromosome constitution XO. In chromatin-positive cases, even where 46 chromosomes including two X chromosomes have been demonstrated, a suspicion of occult mosaicism with some XO cells must exist. Mosaics in whom one cell line has the sex chromosome constitution XO appear to be particularly common. In these patients the phenotype is generally indistinguishable from that of XO individuals (Jacobs et al. 1961). The chromosome findings which have been described in patients with the clinical picture of the XO state are listed in Table V. It seems that whenever less than two

TABLE V

REPORTED SEX CHROMATIN AND SEX CHROMOSOME FINDINGS IN PATIENTS
WITH SOME CLINICAL FEATURES OF TURNER'S SYNDROME

Sex chromosome constitution	Chromosome number	Sex chromatin	Authors
Single cell line			
XO	45	−ive	Ford et al. 1959b
XX	46	+ive	Fraccaro et al. 1960a
XX	46	Abnormally +ive	Fraccaro et al. 1960c
Xx	46	Abnormally +ive	Jacobs et al. 1960
XX	46	Abnormally +ive	Jacobs et al. 1961
XY	46	−ive	Oikawa and Blizzard 1961
Mosaics			
XO/XX	45/46	+ive	Ford 1960
XO/XY	45/46	−ive	Blank et al. 1960
XO/XXX	45/47	Abnormally +ive	Jacobs et al. 1960
XO/XYY	45/47	−ive	Jacobs et al. 1961
XO/XX	45/46	Abnormally +ive	Blank et al. 1961
XO/XX/XXX	45/46/47	Abnormally +ive	Hayward and Cameron 1961

normal X chromosomes occur in a female she is liable to be of short stature, with genital hypoplasia. In mosaics, the degree of effect may depend on the proportion of XO cells present. The XO female with a normal menstrual history who had borne a normal child (Bahner et al. 1960) must be suspected of having undemonstrated XX cells, if only in the genital tract. The difference between XO/XY females with Turner's syndrome and XO/XY pseudohermaphrodites (p. 174) may depend on the relative proportion of the two cell lines in gonadal tissues.

Males with some of the clinical features of XO-Turner's syndrome have been described. With one exception all have been found to have a normal male karyotype. A phenotypic male with testes, neck webbing, congenital lymphœdema and hypoplastic fingernails was found by Oikawa and Blizzard (1961) to be chromatin positive and of apparently normal female chromosome constitution.

No cause is known for the non-disjunction leading to the XO state. No relationship to parental age was found by Boyer et al. (1961).

The XO syndrome does not lend itself to treatment. The female sex of the patient should never be questioned. Since it is doubtful if the failure of growth is due to any endocrine deficiency (Lemli and Smith 1963), hormone therapy is unlikely to have any effect, although there is a need for further study of this possibility. At the time of the expected menarche œstrogen therapy may be used to produce psychologically beneficial breast development and even uterine bleeding on withdrawal.

The Y Chromosome

Before 1959 it was generally held that the human Y chromosome, by analogy with the Y chromosome of Drosophila, was genetically almost inactive (Stern 1960). It soon became evident that this was not so. The absence of a Y chromosome in XO individuals is associated with femaleness. In XXY, XXXY and XXXXY individuals, the single Y chromosome is not out-balanced by even four X chromosomes and they are males, although abnormal males. On the other hand, the presence of two Y chromosomes as in the XYY individual described by Hauschka et al. (1962) was not associated with unusual maleness, or indeed with any obvious phenotypic abnormality. The frequency of occurrence of such XYY individuals is unknown because their normal phenotype does not prompt chromosome studies and they show no abnormality of sex chromatin. That the presence of more than one Y chromosome is not associated with unusual maleness is shown by the XXYY individuals described by Carr et al. (1961) and by Ellis et al. (1961). These patients were clinically indistinguishable from XXY males except that one showed absence of the head and body of one epididymis.

The Y chromosome may show rather more individual variation in length than other chromosomes, and Bender and Gooch (1961) have advised caution in attributing clinical manifestations to such variations. In a family with a very long Y chromosome the condition was apparently heritable and not necessarily associated with any developmental abnormality (Bishop et al. 1962). The propositus in this family with the unusually long Y chromosome was a mongol. Unusually small Y chromosomes have been found in patients with oligospermia and azoospermia (van Wijck et al. 1962); in a pseudohermaphrodite of chromosome constitution XO/XY (Conen et al. 1961); and in a family with muscular dystrophy and hypospadias (Muldal and Ockey 1962). It seems that in all these cases phenotypic abnormality led to chromosome studies, and in none can the abnormality be definitely associated with the unusual Y chromosome. Assessment of the significance of these cases will only be possible when the limits of variation in the length of the Y chromosome have been established in a sample of the general population.

Apart from its function in sex determination no genetic activity of the human Y chromosome is known. Dronamraju (1961) has suggested that a mutant gene for hairy ears may be carried on the Y chromosome. On first consideration the XY testicular feminisation syndrome may seem to imply an abnormality of the Y chromosome, but this is excluded by its known inheritance through the female line and by the occurrence of normal males in the affected sibships.

Exceptions to Sex-linked Recessive Inheritance

The occasional occurrence in females of diseases inherited as sex-linked recessives may be due to the apparent female having an abnormal sex chromosome constitution. A sex-linked recessive character may be expressed in a female of chromosome constitution XO, or XY as in the testicular feminisation syndrome. Walton (1956) found a female with Duchenne-type muscular dystrophy to be chromatin negative. A child with female external genitalia and hæmophilia had the sex chromosome constitution XY (Nilsson et al. 1959) as had also an apparent female with red-green colour vision defect (Stewart 1959). A sex-linked recessive character might also be expressed in a triple-X female who had acquired two abnormal maternal X chromosomes by non-disjunction at gametogenesis. Examination of the sex chromatin status is obviously indicated in any female manifesting a sex-linked recessive character. Explanations for such occurrences, other than as a consequence of abnormalities of the sex chromosomes, are discussed by Mellman et al. (1961) and de la Chappelle (1961).

Abortuses and Stillborn Infants

The reduced expectation of life of individuals with chromosomal abnormalities, particularly those with autosomal trisomies, has naturally led to a search for chromosome abnormalities in abortuses and stillbirths. There have been case reports of triploidy (Penrose and Delhanty 1961), chromatin-positive males (Maclean et al. 1961) and of XY/XXY mosaicism. Some measure of the frequency of chromosomal abnormality in fœtal wastage is provided by the studies of Delhanty et al. (quoted by Carr 1963) and of Carr (1963). In 34 spontaneous abortions Delhanty found the 2 instances of triploidy mentioned above and 2 with appearances suggestive of trisomy 13–15. The findings of Carr in 54 essentially unselected spontaneous abortions are shown in Table VI. The total incidence of chromosome abnormality

TABLE VI

Major Chromosomal Abnormalities in Spontaneous Abortuses (Carr 1963)

54 abortuses	12 with abnormality
XO	3
Trisomy 13–15	3
17–18	2
21	1
Triploid	2
Tetraploid	1

in 54 cases is surprising, as is the relatively low incidence of mongolism compared to the 2 other autosomal trisomic states. The absence of any XXY or XXX fœtuses from the series and the presence of 3 of an XO constitution may in part explain the relatively infrequency of the latter condition at birth (Maclean *et al.* 1964). No chromosome studies have been reported in the mothers from whom Carr's material was obtained. It is notable that of the first 7 mothers 6 had had normal children and 4 had had previous abortions. These findings are of obvious interest in relation to the management of habitual abortion.

Since no instances of monosomy for autosomes were found in Carr's series, it seems possible that a zygote monosomic for a chromosome other than X either does not occur or is not implanted. On the other hand Cowie and Slater (1963) have found a history of a significant excess of miscarriages in the mothers of mongols. The excess is obvious only in the case of mothers having mongol children at the age of 37 onwards. It has been interpreted as evidence that the mothers of mongols may produce ova lacking chromosome 21 but nevertheless able to be fertilized and transplanted. This may be confirmed or refuted by further work like that of Carr.

Congenital Heart Disease

Cardiac abnormalities occur in several of the recognised syndromes associated with chromosomal abnormalities, notably mongolism (Berg *et al.* 1960), XO-Turner's syndrome (Lemli and Smith 1963), trisomy 13–15 (Smith *et al.* 1963) and trisomy 17–18 (Townes *et al.* 1963). Only in Turner's syndrome and in trisomy 17–18 are particular cardiac lesions found. Aortic coarctation or hypoplasia is commonly found in Turner's syndrome but other abnormalities do occur. A high proportion of cases of trisomy 17–18 have bicuspid pulmonary valves and a high ventricular septal defect of triangular form. Rosenfield *et al.* (1962) have drawn attention to the occurrence of infantile arteriosclerosis in trisomy 17–18.

In Marfan's syndrome Tjio *et al.* (1960) found enlarged chromosomal satellites on different chromosomes in two unrelated familial cases. Normal chromosomes were found in a third case without a family history of the condition. These observations have not been confirmed and McKusick (1960) questioned the diagnosis of Marfan's syndrome in the 2 patients with enlarged satellites. More recently Källen and Levan (1963) have found an unusual variation in the length of chromosomes 21, 22 and the Y chromosome in males with Marfan's syndrome. These authors discount the possibility of a causal relationship between the chromosome changes and the syndrome. Instead they suggest that the variation they found is due to an affect on the phenotype of the chromosomes, analogous to the complex effects on the general body phenotype in Marfan's syndrome. This work suggests a need for further study of the chromosomes in this condition. The fine changes described by Källen and Levan may well have been overlooked by others who have reported a normal chromosome constitution in Marfan's syndrome.

Association between some instances of familial atrial septal defect and chromosome abnormalities has been reported by Böök *et al.* (1961). In one family with septal defects of the secundum type there was a translocation between chromosome 2 and a chromosome of the 6–12 group. In another family mother and son both had atrial septal defects. The mother was apparently a mosaic of normal cells and cells trisomic for either chromosome

19 or 20. The son was trisomic for the same chromosome but was also apparently monosomic for chromosome 21 or 22. Other interpretations of the findings in this family are possible. It seems likely that the relationship between these chromosome changes and the cardiac abnormality is not a causal one. Nevertheless, it is interesting that Palmer (1963) has found partial trisomy for chromosome 19 or 20 in a child with congenital abnormalities which included supravalvular aortic stenosis, abnormal facies, mental defect and inguinal hernia. Other patients with supravalvular aortic stenosis, with and without the other clinical features, had no chromosome abnormalities.

Normal chromosome constitutions have been found in association with other cardiac abnormalities. No chromosome abnormality has as yet been found in any patient with congenital heart disease who did not have either extra-cardiac abnormalities or a family history of congenital heart disease. In a remarkable family with Fallot's tetrad and other cardiac abnormalities no chromosome changes were found in affected or unaffected members (Pitt 1962).

Nervous System

No certain association has been established between any disease confined to the nervous system and a chromosomal abnormality. Of the established autosomal trisomic states specific cerebral anomalies occur in trisomy 13–15 and trisomy 17–18, but mongolism is surprisingly without demonstrable specific change.

Hayward and Bower (1960) reported trisomy for a small acrocentric chromosome in a typical example of the Sturge-Weber syndrome without additional abnormalities. They thought the child to be trisomic for chromosome 22. They (Hayward and Bower 1961) later investigated 7 other cases of the disease with negative results and mentioned similar findings by other workers. 3 typical cases were studied by Patau et al. (1961) with negative results in 2, but in their third patient they found a normal chromosome number with one abnormal chromosome apparently replacing one of the group 13–15: this they interpreted as due to the translocation of a segment from an unknown chromosome to one of the 13–15 group. Consideration of this case led to the hypothesis that all cases of Sturge-Weber syndrome are due to partial trisomy. Patau et al. suggest that the extra genetic material exists commonly not as a separate chromosome but as a translocation to a chromosome which is not thereby rendered visibly abnormal. According to this theory, the cases described by Hayward and Bower and by Patau et al. are exceptional only in having chromosomal changes which are visible. Patau and his colleagues suggest that this sort of occult partial trisomy may be present in many cases of multiple congenital abnormalities, including some of those in which chromosome studies have been reported as yielding negative results. Apart from the patient of Hayward and Bower with 47 chromosomes, or the one with a visible chromosomal translocation described by Patau et al., there have been no reports of chromosomal abnormality in the Sturge-Weber syndrome.

Dystrophia myotonica was the subject of early chromosome studies. Its familial incidence and the variety of tissues in which abnormalities may occur seemed consistent with a chromosomal aberration. The earlier results were negative (unpublished observations), but more recently Fitzgerald and Caughey (1962) have found an extra small acrocentric chromosome in some of the cells of 5 out of 7 cases. It is suggested that these chromosomes are supernumerary chromosomes (White 1961), the existence of which is known in plants and animals, but which have not been shown unequivocally to occur in man. In other species they are small chromosomes which do not appear in every individual of the species, and which are believed to have relatively little phenotypic effect. The known behaviour of these chromosomes in other species would be consistent with the inconstant occurrence of the extra chromosome found by Fitzgerald and Caughey in dystrophia myotonica; and the difference from patient to patient they found as regards the number of cells having the extra chromosome might explain the case-to-case variation in the severity of the disease.

A single family with limb-girdle muscular dystrophy (Nattrass 1957) has been reported by Muldal and Ockey (1962). Both males and females were affected by the muscular dystrophy and some of the males of the family had hypospadias. A partially deleted Y chromosome was found in some of the males. Muldal and Ockey believe this chromosome abnormality to be related to the occurrence of hypospadias in the family but not to the muscular dystrophy.

The occasional occurrence of fibrosarcomatous change in the neuro-fibromata of von Recklinghausen's disease suggested an analogy with the development of acute leukæmia in mongols, but chromosome studies in von Recklinghausen's disease yielded negative results. A similar analogy between mongolism and epiloia with regard to the development of gliomata and adenomata of heart and kidneys in the latter condition led to chromosome studies in epiloia, also with negative results (Harnden 1961a).

A variety of neurological abnormalities have been described in individuals, mostly children, with chromosomal translocations. Little evidence has as yet emerged to indicate any specific relationship between these particular chromosomes and the normal development and function of the nervous system.

Leukæmia

Leukæmia was one of the first diseases studied when methods became available for observations on human chromosomes. The first widely used method for the making of chromosome preparations from bone marrow (Ford *et al.* 1958) was developed especially for the study of leukæmia. It was then thought that a particularly promising situation for investigation existed in childhood acute leukæmia. If a chromosome abnormality could be demonstrated in an untreated patient, important correlations with natural history and response to treatment might be established by serial study during therapeutic remission and in subsequent relapse. This hope has not been realised, probably because a summation of technical difficulties weighs against consistent success in serial studies.

In acute leukæmia in children no specific chromosome abnormality has been found and it is in fact doubtful if the same abnormality has been observed in any two cases (Sandberg *et al.* 1960, Hungerford 1961). The abnormalities found have been of both chromosome number and morphology. In their nature and frequency of occurrence they are not obviously different from those found in acute leukæmia in adults (Baikie *et al.* 1961). Hungerford (1961) gives reasons for considering the chromosome changes he found as secondary phenomena, and their occurrence to be related to the duration and treatment of the disease. If a specific chromosome abnormality does exist in childhood acute leukæmia, analogous to that of chronic myeloid leukæmia, it has not yet been demonstrated. There have been few reports of the Philadelphia (Ph¹) chromosome in cases of chronic myeloid leukæmia in childhood. This probably reflects the rarity of this disease in children. Nevertheless, it has been described by Fortune *et al.* (1962) in a child aged $2\frac{1}{2}$ years and more recently by Reisman and Trujillo (1963) in five patients aged 10 months to 10 years. The latter authors were unable to demonstrate the Ph¹ chromosome in four children whose ages ranged from 7 months to 3 years with a variety of chronic myeloid leukæmia which they referred to as the infantile type. For some time it has been recognised that the clinical and hæmatological features of chronic myeloid leukæmia as it occurs in children may differ from the characteristics of the disease in adults (Cooke 1953). It is a matter of some interest if the findings of Reisman and Trujillo are confirmed and two varieties of chronic myeloid leukæmia are to be found in children, one with the Ph¹ chromosome and one without.

The special ætiological importance of the occurrence of acute leukæmia in mongols has prompted chromosome studies in many cases. Where additional chromosome abnormalities have been found they appear to be non-specific. With or without additional chromosome abnormalities, the trisomy 21 (Tough *et al.* 1961) or the chromosomal translocation (German *et al.* 1962) seems to be unchanged. No case of chronic myeloid leukæmia in a mongol has yet been reported. Such an occurrence would be of great ætiological significance because of the relationship between the Ph¹ chromosome and the basic chromosomal abnormality of mongolism. It has been suggested by Dent *et al.* (1963) that mongols may, by virtue of their trisomic state for the chromosome in question, be especially protected against the development of the disease which is associated with the occurrence of a cell line having less than the normal two doses of the genetic material of chromosome 21.

There are no reports of chromosome studies in the cases of childhood leukæmia occurring in a possibly epidemic form at Niles, Illinois in the U.S.A. (Heath and Hasterlik 1963). In a family with 3 cases of congenital acute leukæmia reported by Campbell *et al.* (1962) no chromosome abnormality was found in one of the affected children nor in the apparently unaffected parents. In identical twins with acute leukæmia chromosome studies on bone marrow yielded dissimilar results (Pearson *et al.* 1963).

Negative Chromosome Studies in Various Clinical States
In rare diseases and unusual combinations of congenital abnormalities the desirability of chromosome studies is often raised. The more localised the defect or the more specific its functional effect the less likely is it to be associated with a visible chromosomal abnormality. Furthermore, in most of the conditions encountered chromosome studies have already been carried

out with negative results. The best records of negative results are to be found in The Human Chromosome Newsletter which is privately prepared and circulated by the Medical Research Council Clinical Effects of Radiation Research Unit, Edinburgh. This publication is in the hands of most people active in the field of human chromosome studies.

REFERENCES

ALEXANDER, D. S., FERGUSON-SMITH, M. A. (1961) Chromosomal studies in some variants of male pseudohermaphroditism. *Pediatrics*, **28**, 758

ATKINS, L., ROSENTHAL, M. K. (1961) Multiple congenital abnormalities associated with chromosomal trisomy. *New Engl. J. Med.* **265**, 314

BAHNER, F., SCHWARTZ, G., HARNDEN, D. G., JACOBS, P. A., HEINZ, H. A., WALTER, K. (1960) A fertile female with XO sex chromosome constitution. *Lancet*, **2**, 100

BAIKIE, A. G., BROWN, W. M. C., JACOBS, P. A., MILNE, J. S. (1959) Chromosomal studies in human leukæmia. *Lancet*, **2**, 425

BAIKIE, A. G., JACOBS, P. A., McBRIDE, J. A., TOUGH, I. M. (1961) Cytogenetic studies in acute leukæmia. *Brit. med. J.* **1**, 1564

BARR, M. L., BERTRAM, E. G. (1949) A morphological distinction between neurones of the male and female, and the behaviour of the nucleolar satellite during accelerated nucleoprotein synthesis. *Nature, Lond.* **163**, 676

BECKER, K. L., BURKE, E. C., ALBERT, A. (1963) Double autosomal trisomy (D trisomy plus mongolism). *Proc. Mayo Clin.* **38**, 242

BENDER, M. A., GOOCH, P. C. (1961) An unusually long human Y chromosome. *Lancet*, **2**, 463

BENIRSCHKE, K., BROWNHILL, L., HOEFNAGEL, D., ALLEN, F. H. (1962) Langdon Down anomaly (mongolism) with 21/21 translocation and Klinefelter's syndrome in the same sibship. *Cytogenetics*, **1**, 75

BERG, J. M., CROME, L., FRANCE, N. E. (1960) Congenital cardiac malformations in mongolism. *Brit. Heart. J.* **22**, 331

BERGEMAN, E. (1961) Geschlechts-chromatinbestimmungen am Neugeboren. *Schweiz. med. Wschr.* **91**, 292

BIESELE, J. J., SCHMID, W., LAWLIS, M. G. (1962) Mentally retarded schizoid twin girls with 47 chromosomes. *Lancet*, **1**, 403

BISHOP, A., BLANK, C. E., HUNTER, H. (1962) Heritable variation in the length of the Y chromosome. *Lancet*, **2**, 18

BLANK, C. E., BISHOP, A., CALEY, J. P. (1960) Examples of XY/XO mosaicism. *Lancet*, **2**, 1450

BLANK, C. E., GORDON, R. R., BISHOP, A. (1961) Atypical Turner's syndrome. *Lancet*, **1**, 947

BLEYER, A. (1934) Indications that mongoloid idiocy is a gametic mutation of a degressive type. *Amer. J. Dis. Child.* **47**, 342

BLOISE, W., DE ASSIS, L. M., BOTTURA, C., FERRARI, I. (1960) Gonadal dysgenesis ('Turner's syndrome) with male phenotype and XO chromosomal constitution. *Lancet*, **2**, 1059

BODIAN, M., CARTER, C. O. (1963) A family study of Hirschsprung's disease. *Ann. hum. Genet.* **26**, 261

BÖÖK, J. A., SANTESSON, B., ZETTERQVIST, P. (1961) Association between congenital heart malformation and chromosomal variations. *Acta pœdiat.* **50**, 217

BOTTURA, C., FERRARI, I. (1960) A simplified method for the study of chromosomes in man. *Nature, Lond.* **186**, 904

BOYER, S. H., FERGUSON-SMITH, M. A., GRUMBACH, M. M. (1961) The lack of influence of parental age and birth order in the ætiology of nuclear sex chromatin-negative Turner's syndrome. *Ann. hum. Genet.* **25**, 215

BRANDT, N. J., FRØLAND, A., MIKKELSEN, M., NIELSEN, A., TOLSTRUP, N. (1963) Galactosæmia locus and the Down's syndrome chromosome. *Lancet*, **2**, 700

BRODIE, H. R., DALLAIRE, L. (1962) The E syndrome (trisomy 17–18) resulting from a maternal chromosomal translocation. *Canad. med. Ass. J.* **87**, 559

BÜHLER, E. M., BÜHLER, U. K., STALDER, G. R. (1964) Partial monosomy 18 and anomaly of thyroxine synthesis. *Lancet*, **1**, 170

BUTLER, L. J., FRANCE, N. E., RUSSELL, A., SINCLAIR, L. (1962) A chromosomal aberration associated with multiple congenital abnormalities. *Lancet*, **1**, 1242

CAFFEY, J., ROSS, S. (1956) Mongolism (mongoloid deficiency) during early infancy— some newly recognised diagnostic changes in the pelvic bones. *Pediatrics*, **17**, 642

CAMPBELL, W. A. B., MACAFEE, A. L., WADE, W. G. (1962) Familial neonatal leukæmia. *Arch. Dis. Childh.* **37**, 93

CARR, D. H., BARR, M. L., PLUNKETT, E. R. (1961) A probable XXYY sex determining mechanism in a mentally defective male with Klinefelter's syndrome. *Canad. med. Assoc. J.* **84**, 873

CARR, D. H. (1963) Chromosome studies in abortuses and stillborn infants. *Lancet*, **2**, 603

CARTER, C. O., HAMERTON, J. L., POLANI, P. E., GUNALP, A., WELLER, S. D. V. (1960) Chromosomal translocation as a cause of familial mongolism. *Lancet*, **2**, 678

CARTER, C. O., EVANS, J. A. (1961) Risk of parents who have had one child with Down's syndrome (mongolism) having another child similarly affected. *Lancet*, **2**, 785

CLARKE, C. M., EDWARDS, J. H., SMALLPEICE, V. (1961) 21-trisomy/normal mosaicism, in an intelligent child with some mongoloid characters. *Lancet*, **2**, 1028

CLARKE, C. M. (1962) Techniques in the study of human chromosomes in *Chromosomes in Medicine*, ed. J. L. Hamerton, Heinemann, London

CLARKE, C. M., FORD, C. E., EDWARDS, J. H., SMALLPEICE, V. (1963) 21-trisomy/normal mosaicism in an intelligent child with some mongoloid characters. *Lancet*, **2**, 1229

CLOSE, H. G. (1963) Two apparently normal triple-X females. *Lancet*, **2**, 1358

COLLMAN, R. D., STOLLER, A. (1962) A survey of mongoloid births in Victoria, Australia, 1942–1957. *Amer. J. publ. Hlth.* **52**, 813

CONEN, P. E., BAILEY, J. D., ALLEMANG, W. H., THOMPSON, D. W., EZRIN, C. (1961) A probable partial deletion of the Y chromosome in an intersex patient. *Lancet*, **2**, 294

COOKE, J. V. (1953) Chronic myelogenous leukemia in children. *J. Pediat.* **42**, 537

COWIE, V., SLATER, E. (1963) Maternal age and miscarriage in the mothers of mongols. *Acta genet.* **13**, 77

DAY, R. W., DUPUY, M. E., ELLIOT, M., MASOUREDIS, S. P. (1963a) D-antigen content of red cells in Down's syndrome. *Lancet*, **1**, 721

DAY, R. W., WRIGHT, S. M., KOONS, A., QUIGLEY, M. (1963b) XXY 21-trisomy and retinoblastoma. *Lancet*, **2**, 154

DE LA CHAPELLE, A., IKKALA, E., NEVANLINNA, H. R. (1961) Hæmophilia in a girl: a probable exception from sex-linked recessive inheritance. *Lancet*, **2**, 578

DENT, T., EDWARDS, J. H., DELHANTY, J. (1963) A partial mongol. *Lancet*, **2**, 484

DRONAMRAJU, K. R. (1961) Hypertrichosis of the pinna of the human ear, Y-linked pedigrees. *J. Genet.* **57**, 230

DUNN, H. G., FORD, D. K., AUERSPERG, N., MILLER, J. R. (1961) Benign congenital hypotonia with chromosomal anomaly. *Pediatrics*, **28**, 578

EDWARDS, J. H., HARNDEN, D. G., CAMERON, A. H., CROSSE, V. M., WOLFF, O. H. (1960) A new trisomy syndrome. *Lancet*, **1**, 787

EDWARDS, J. H., DENT, T., GULI, E. (1963) Sporadic mongols with translocations. *Lancet*, **2**, 902

EL-ALFI, O. S., POWELL, H. C., BIESELE, J. J. (1963) Possible trisomy in chromosome group 6–12 in a mentally retarded patient. *Lancet*, **1**, 700

ELLIS, J. R., MILLER, O. J., PENROSE, L. S., SCOTT, G. E. B. (1961) A male with XXYY chromosomes. *Ann. hum. Genet.* **25**, 145

FERGUSON, J., PITT, D. (1963) Another child with 47 chromosomes. *Med. J. Austr.* **1**, 545

FERGUSON-SMITH, M. A., JOHNSTON, A. W., WEINBERG, A. N. (1960) The chromosome complement in true hermaphroditism. *Lancet*, **2**, 126

FITZGERALD, P. H., LYCETTE, R. R. (1961) Mosaicism in man, involving the autosome associated with mongolism. *Heredity*, **16**, 509

FITZGERALD, P. H., CAUGHEY, J. E. (1962) Chromosome and sex chromatin studies in cases of dystrophia myotonica. *New Zeald. med. J.* **61**, 410

FORD, C. E., JACOBS, P. A., LAJTHA, L. G. (1958) Human somatic chromosomes. *Nature, Lond.* **181**, 1565

FORD, C. E., JONES, K. W., MILLER, O. J., MITTWOCH, U., PENROSE, L. S., RIDLER, M., SHAPIRO, A. (1959a) The chromosomes in a patient showing both mongolism and the Klinefelter syndrome. *Lancet*, **1**, 709

FORD, C. E., JONES, K. W., POLANI, P. E., DE ALMEIDA, J. C., BRIGGS, J. H. (1959b) A sex-chromosome anomaly in a case of gonadal dysgenesis (Turner's syndrome). *Lancet*, **1**, 711

FORD, C. E. (1960) Human cytogenetics: its present place and future possibilities. *Amer. J. hum. Genet.* **12**, 104

FORD, C. E. (1962) Human chromosomes in *Chromosomes in Medicine*, ed. Hamerton, J. L., Heinemann, London

FORTUNE, D. W., LEWIS, F. J. W., POULDING, R. H. (1962) Chromosome pattern in myeloid leukæmia in a child. *Lancet*, **1**, 537

FRACCARO, M., KAIJSER, K., LINDSTEN, J. (1960a) Further cytogenetical observations in gonadal dysgenesis. *Ann. hum. Genet.* **24**, 205

FRACCARO, M., KAIJSER, K., LINDSTEN, J. (1960b) Chromosomal abnormalities in father and mongol child. *Lancet*, **1**, 724

FRACCARO, M., IKKOS, D., LINDSTEN, J., LUFT, R., KAIJSER, K. (1960c) A new type of chromosomal abnormality in gonadal dysgenesis. *Lancet*, **2**, 1144

FRACCARO, M., GLEN-BOTT, M., SALZANO, F. M., RUSSELL, R. W. R., CRANSTON, W. I. (1962a) Triple chromosomal mosaic in a woman with clinical evidence of masculinisation. *Lancet*, **1**, 1379

FRACCARO, M., TAYLOR, A. I., BODIAN, M., NEWNS, G. H. (1962b) A human intersex ("true hermaphrodite") with XX/XXY/XXYYY sex chromosomes. *Cytogenetics*, **1**, 104

FRANKS, R. C., NORTHCUTT, R. (1963) Female pseudohermaphroditism and renal anomalies. *Amer. J. Dis. Child.* **105**, 490

GERMAN, J. L., DE MAYO, A. P., BEARN, A. G. (1962) Inheritance of an abnormal chromosome in Down's syndrome (mongolism) with leukemia. *Amer. J. hum. Genet.* **14**, 31

GRAY, J. E., MUTTON, D. E., ASHBY, D. W. (1962) Pericentric inversion of chromosome 21: a possible further cytogenetic mechanism in mongolism. *Lancet*, **1**, 21

GUSTAVSON, K.-H., EK, J. I. (1961) Triple stem-line mosaicism in mongolism. *Lancet*, **2**, 319

GUSTAVSON, K.-H., IVEMARK, B. I., ZETTERQVIST, P., BÖÖK, J. A. (1962) Postmortem diagnosis of a new double-trisomy associated with cardiovascular and other anomalies. *Acta pædiat.* **51**, 686

HALL, B. (1962) Down's syndrome (mongolism) with normal chromosomes. *Lancet*, **2**, 1026

HALL, B. (1963) Mongolism and other abnormalities in a family with trisomy 21–22 tendency. *Acta pædiat., suppl.* **146**, 77

HAMERTON, J. L., COWIE, V. A., GIANNELLI, F., BRIGGS, S. M., POLANI, P. E. (1961) Differential transmission of Down's syndrome (mongolism) through male and female translocation carriers. *Lancet*, **2**, 956

HAMERTON, J. L. (1962) Cytogenetics of mongolism, in *Chromosomes in Medicine*, ed. Hamerton, J. L., Heinemann, London

HAMERTON, J. L., STEINBERG, A. G. (1962) Progeny of D/G translocation heterozygotes in familial Down's syndrome. *Lancet*, **1**, 1408

HARNDEN, D. G., ARMSTRONG, C. N. (1959) The chromosomes of a true hermaphrodite. *Brit. med. J.* **2**, 1287

HARNDEN, D. G., STEWART, J. S. S. (1959) The chromosomes in a case of pure gonadal dysgenesis. *Brit. med. J.* **2**, 1285

HARNDEN, D. G. (1961a) Congenital abnormalities with an apparently normal chromosome complement, in *Human Chromosomal Abnormalities*, ed. Davidson, W. M., Smith, D. R., Staples, London

HARNDEN, D. G. (1961b) Nuclear sex in triploid XXY human cells. *Lancet*, **2**, 488

HAUSCHKA, T. S., HASSON, J. E., GOLDSTEIN, M. N., KOEPF, G. F., SANDBERG, A. A. (1962) An XYY man with progeny indicating familial tendency to non-disjunction. *Amer. J. hum. Genet.* **14**, 22

HAYWARD, M. D., BOWER, B. D. (1960) Chromosomal trisomy associated with the Sturge-Weber syndrome. *Lancet*, **2**, 844

HAYWARD, M. D., BOWER, B. D. (1961) The chromosomal constitution of the Sturge-Weber syndrome. *Lancet*, **1**, 558

HAYWARD, M. D., CAMERON, A. H. (1961) Triple mosaicism of the sex chromosomes in Turner's syndrome and Hirschsprung's disease. *Lancet*, **2**, 623

HEATH, C. W., HASTERLIK, R. J. (1963) Leukemia among children in a suburban community. *Amer. J. Med.* **34**, 796

HECHT, F., BRYANT, J. S., MOTULSKY, A. G., GIBLETT, E. R. (1963) The No. 17–18 (E) trisomy syndrome. *J. Pediat.* **63**, 605

HEINRICHS, E. H., ALLEN, S. W., NELSON, P. S. (1963) Simultaneous 18-trisomy and 21-trisomy cluster. *Lancet*, **2**, 468

HIRSCHHORN, K., DECKER, W. H., COOPER, H. L. (1960) Human intersex with chromosome mosaicism of type XY/XO. *New Engl. J. Med.* **263**, 1044

HUEHNS, E. R., HECHT, F., KEIL, J. V., MOTULSKY, A. G. (1964a) Developmental hemoglobin anomalies in a chromosomal triplication: D_1 trisomy syndrome. *Proc. nat. Acad. Sci., Wash.* **51**, 89

HUEHNS, E. R., LUTZNER, M., HECHT, F. (1964b) Nuclear abnormalities of the neutrophils in D_1 (13–15)-trisomy syndrome. *Lancet*, **1**, 589

HUNGERFORD, D. A., DONNELLY, A. J., NOWELL, P. C., BECK, S. (1959) The chromosome constitution of a human phenotypic intersex. *Amer. J. hum. Genet.* **11**, 215

HUNGERFORD, D. A. (1961) Chromosome studies in human leukemia I. Acute leukemia in children. *J. nat. Cancer Inst.*, **27**, 983

ILBERY, P. L. T., LEE, C. W. G., WINN, S. M. (1961) Incomplete trisomy in a mongoloid child exhibiting minimal stigmata. *Med. J. Austr.* **2**, 182

JACOBS, P. A., STRONG, J. A. (1959) A case of human intersexuality having a possible XXY sex determining mechanism. *Nature, Lond.* **183**, 302

JACOBS, P. A., BAIKIE, A. G., BROWN, W. M. C., STRONG, J. A. (1959a) The somatic chromosomes in mongolism. *Lancet*, **1**, 710

JACOBS, P. A., BAIKIE, A. G., BROWN, W. M. C., FORREST, H., ROY, J. R., STEWART, J. S. S., LENNOX, B. (1959b) Chromosomal sex in the syndrome of testicular feminisation. *Lancet*, **2**, 591

JACOBS, P. A., HARNDEN, D. G., BROWN, W. M. C., GOLDSTEIN, J., CLOSE, H. G., MACGREGOR, T. N., MACLEAN, N., STRONG, J. A. (1960) Abnormalities involving the X chromosome in women. *Lancet*, **1**, 1213

JACOBS, P. A., HARNDEN, D. G., BUCKTON, K. E., BROWN, W. M. C., KING, M. J., MCBRIDE, J. A., MACGREGOR, T. N., MACLEAN, N. (1961a) Cytogenetic studies in primary amenorrhœa. *Lancet*, **1**, 1183

JACOBS, P. A., BROWN, W. M. C., DOLL, R. (1961b) Distribution of human chromosome counts in relation to age. *Nature, Lond.* **191**, 1178

JACOBS, P. A., BRUNTON, M., BROWN, W. M. C., DOLL, R., GOLDSTEIN, H. (1963) Change of human chromosome count distribution with age: evidence for a sex difference. *Nature, Lond.* **197**, 1080

JEROME, H. (1962) Anomalies du métabolisme du tryptophane dans la maladie mongolienne. *Bull. Soc. méd. Hôp. Paris*, **113**, 168

KÄLLÉN, B., LEVAN, A. (1962) Abnormal length of chromosomes 21 and 22 in four patients with Marfan's syndrome. *Cytogenetics*, **1**, 5

KING, M. J., GILLIS, E. M., BAIKIE, A. G. (1962) Alkaline-phosphatase activity of polymorphs in mongolism. *Lancet*, **2**, 1302

KINLOUGH, M. A., ROBSON, H. N., HAYMAN, D. L. (1961) A simplified method for the study of chromosomes in man. *Nature, Lond.* **189**, 420

KOULISCHER, L., PERIER, J. (1962) A propos d'un cas de trisomie 22. *Bull. Acad. roy. Méd. Belg.* **7**, 329

KOULISCHER, L., PELC, S., PÉRIER, O. (1963) A case of trisomy-18 mosaicism. *Lancet*, **2**, 945

KUNDRAT, H. (1882) *Arrhinencephalic als typische Art von Missbildung.* von Leuschner and Lubensky, Graz

LEJEUNE, J., GAUTHIER, M., TURPIN, R. (1959) Les chromosomes humaine en culture de tissues. *C.R. Acad. Sci., Paris*, **248**, 602

LEMLI, L., SMITH, D. W. (1963) The XO syndrome: a study of the differential phenotype in 25 patients. *J. Pediat.* **63**, 577

LEVAN, A. (1956) Self-perpetuating ring chromosomes in two human tumours. *Hereditas*, **42**, 366

LEWIS, F. J. W., HYMAN, J. M., MACTAGGART, M., POULDING, R. H. (1963) Trisomy of autosome 16. *Nature, Lond.* **199**, 404

LINDSTEN, J., TILLINGER, K.-G. (1962) Self-perpetuating ring chromosome in a patient with gonadal dysgenesis. *Lancet*, **1**, 593

LÜERS, T., STRUCK, E., NEVINNY-STICKEL, J. (1963) Self-perpetuating ring chromosome in gonadal dysgenesis. *Lancet*, **2**, 887

LUNDIN, L.-G., GUSTAVSON, K.-H. (1962) Urinary BAIB excretion in Down's syndrome (mongolism). *Acta genet.* **12**, 156

LYON, M. F. (1962) Sex chromatin and gene action in the mammalian X-chromosome. *Amer. J. hum. Genet.* **14**, 135

MCKINNEY, A. A., STOHLMAN, F., BRECHER, G. (1962) The kinetics of cell proliferation in human peripheral blood. *Blood*, **19**, 349

MCKUSICK, V. A. (1961) *Medical Genetics 1958–1960*, Mosby, St. Louis

MACLEAN, N., HARNDEN, D. G., BROWN, W. M. C. (1961) Abnormalities of sex chromosome constitution in newborn babies. *Lancet*, **2**, 406

MACLEAN, N., MITCHELL, J. M., HARNDEN, D. G., WILLIAMS, J., JACOBS, P. A., BUCKTON, K. E., BAIKIE, A. G., BROWN, W. M. C., MCBRIDE, J. A., STRONG, J. A., CLOSE, H. G., JONES, D. C. (1962) A survey of sex-chromosome abnormalities among 4514 mental defectives. *Lancet*, **1**, 293

MACLEAN, N., HARNDEN, D. G., BROWN, W. M. C., BOND, J., MANTLE, D. J. (1964) Sex-chromosome abnormalities in newborn babies. *Lancet*, **1**, 286

MELLMAN, W. J., WOLMAN, I. J., WURZEL, H. A., MOORHEAD, P. S., QUALLS, D. H. (1961) A chromosomal female with hemophilia A. *Blood*, **17**, 719

MIGEON, B. R., KAUFMAN, B. N., YOUNG, W. J. (1962) A chromosome abnormality with fragment in a paramongol child. *Bull. Johns Hopk. Hosp.* **111**, 221

MILES, C. P., LUZZATTI, L., STOREY, S. D., PETERSON, C. D. (1962) A male pseudoherma-
phrodite with a probable XO/XxY mosaicism. *Lancet*, **2**, 455
MILLER, J. Q., PICARD, E. H., ALKAN, M. K., WARNER, S., GERALD, P. S. (1963) A
specific congenital brain defect (arhinencephaly) in 13–15 trisomy. *New Engl. J.
Med.* **268**, 120
MILLER, O. J., BREG, W. R., SCHMICKEL, R. D., TRETTER, W. (1961) A family with an
XXXXY male, a leukæmic male, and two 21-trisomic mongoloid females. *Lancet*,
2, 78
MITTWOCH, U. (1952) The chromosome complement in a mongolian imbecile. *Ann.
Eugen., Lond.* **17**, 37
MOORE, K. L. (1959) Sex reversal in newborn babies. *Lancet*, **1**, 217
MORRIS, J. M. (1953) Syndrome of testicular feminization in male pseudohermaphrodites.
Amer. J. Obstet. Gynec. **65**, 1192
MULDAL, S., OCKEY, C. H. (1962) Deletion of Y chromosome in a family with muscular
dystrophy and hypospadias. *Brit. med. J.* **1**, 291
NAIK, S. N., SHAH, P. N. (1962) Sex chromatin anomalies in newborn babies in India.
Science, **136**, 1116
NAKAGOME, Y., HIBI, I., KONOSHITA, K., NAGAO, T., AIKAWA, M. (1963) Incidence of
Turner's syndrome in Japanese dwarfed girls. *Lancet*, **2**, 412
NATTRASS, F. J. (1957) Primary diseases of muscle, in *Modern Trends in Neurology*,
2nd series, ed. D. Williams, Butterworth, London
NILSSON, I. M., BERGMAN, S., RIETALU, J., WALDENSTRÖM, J. (1959) Hæmophilia A
in a "girl" with male sex chromatin pattern. *Lancet*, **2**, 264
NOWELL, P. C. (1960) Phytohemagglutinin: an initiator of mitosis in cultures of normal
human leukocytes. *Cancer Res.* **20**, 462
OIKAWA, K., BLIZZARD, R. M. (1961) Chromosomal studies of patients with congenital
anomalies simulating those of gonadal aplasia. *New Engl. J. Med.* **264**, 1009
PALMER, C. G. (1963) Chromosome studies in patients with supravalvular aortic stenosis.
Lancet, **2**, 788
PATAU, K., SMITH, D. W., THERMAN, E., INHORN, S. L., WAGNER, H. P. (1960) Multiple
congenital anomaly caused by an extra autosome. *Lancet*, **1**, 790
PATAU, K., THERMAN, E., SMITH, D. W., INHORN, S. L., PICKEN, B. F. (1961) Partial-
trisomy syndromes I. Sturge-Weber's disease. *Amer. J. hum. Genet.* **13**, 287
PEARSON, H. A., GRELLO, F. W., CONE, T. E. (1963) Leukemia in identical twins.
New Engl. J. Med. **268**, 1151
PENROSE, L. S. (1939) Maternal age, order of birth and developmental abnormalities.
J. ment. Sci. **85**, 1141
PENROSE, L. S. (1951) Maternal age in familial mongolism. *J. ment. Sci.* **97**, 738
PENROSE, L. S., ELLIS, J. R., DELHANTY, J. D. A. (1960) Chromosomal translocations
in mongolism and in normal relatives. *Lancet*, **2**, 409
PENROSE, L. S., DELHANTY, J. (1961) Triploid cell cultures from a macerated fœtus.
Lancet, **1**, 1261
PENROSE, L. S. (1962) Paternal age in mongolism. *Lancet*, **1**, 1101
PENROSE, L. S. (1963) *The Biology of Mental Defect.* Sidgwick and Jackson, London
PFEIFFER, R. A., SCHELLONG, G., KOSENOW, W. (1962) Chromosomenanomalien in den
Blutzellen eines Kindes mit multiplen Abartungen. *Klin. Wschr.* **40**, 1058
PITT, D. B. (1962) A family study of Fallot's tetrad. *Austr. Ann. Med.* **11**, 179
PITT, D., FERGUSON, J., BAIKIE, A. G. (1964) Normal and abnormal sibs with a familial
chromosomal translocation. *Austr. Ann. Med.* **13**, 178
POLANI, P. E., BRIGGS, J. H., FORD, C. E., CLARKE, C. M., BERG, J. M. (1960) A mongol
girl with 46 chromosomes. *Lancet*, **1**, 721
POLANI, P. E. (1963) Cytogenetics of Down's syndrome (mongolism). *Pediat. Clin. N.
Amer.* **10**, 423
REISMAN, L. E., TRUJILLO, J. M. (1963) Chronic granulocytic leukemia in childhood.
J. Pediat. **62**, 710
ROSENFIELD, R. L., BREIBART, S., ISAACS, H., KLEVIT, H. D., MELLMAN, W. J. (1962)
Trisomy of chromosomes 13–15 and 17–18: its association with infantile arterio-
sclerosis. *Amer. J. med. Sci.* **244**, 763
SANDBERG, A. A., KOEPF, G. F., CROSSWHITE, L. H., HAUSCHKA, T. S. (1960) The
chromosomal constitution of human marrow in various developmental and blood
disorders. *Amer. J. hum. Genet.* **12**, 231
SCHUSTER, J., MOTULSKY, A. G. (1962) Exceptional sex-chromatin pattern in male
pseudohermaphroditism with XX/XY/XO mosaicism. *Lancet*, **1**, 1074
SERGOVICH, F. R., SOLTAN, H. C., CARR, D. H. (1962) A 13–15/21 translocation chromosome in carrier father and mongol son. *Canad. med. Ass. J.* **87**, 852
SHAH, P. N., NAIK, S. N., MAHAJAN, D. K., DAVE, M. J., PAYMASTER, J. C. (1961) A new

variant of human intersex with discussion of the developmental aspects. *Brit. med. J.* **2**, 474

SHAW, M. W., GERSHOWITZ, H. (1962) A search for autosomal linkage in a trisomic population: blood group frequencies in mongols. *Amer. J. hum. Genet.* **14**, 317

SMITH, D. W., THERMAN, E., PATAU, K., INHORN, S. L. (1962a) Mosaicism in mother of two mongoloids. *Amer. J. Dis. Child.* **104**, 534

SMITH, D. W., MARDEN, P. M., McDONALD, M. J., SPECKHARD, M. (1962b) Lower incidence of sex chromatin in buccal smears of newborn females. *Pediatrics*, **30**, 707

SMITH, D. W. (1963) The No. 18 trisomy and D₁ trisomy syndromes. *Pediat. Clin. N. Amer.* **10**, 389

SMITH, D. W., PATAU, K., THERMAN, E., INHORN, S. L., DE MARS, R. I. (1963) The D₁ trisomy syndrome. *J. Pediat.* **62**, 326

SOHVAL, A. R., CASSELMAN, W. G. B. (1961) Alteration in size of nuclear sex-chromatin mass (Barr body) induced by antibiotics. *Lancet*, **2**, 1386

SOHVAL, A. R. (1963) "Mixed" gonadal dysgenesis: a variety of hermaphroditism. *Amer. J. hum. Genet.* **15**, 155

SOHVAL, A. R. (1964) Hermaphroditism with "atypical" or "mixed" gonadal dysgenesis: relationship to gonadal dysgenesis. *Amer. J. Med.* **36**, 281

STALDER, G. R., BÜHLER, E. M., WEBER, J. R. (1963) Possible trisomy in chromosome group 6–12. *Lancet*, **1**, 1379

STERN, C. (1960) *Principles of Human Genetics.* 2nd Ed., Freeman, San Francisco.

STEWART, J. S. S. (1959) Testicular feminization and colour-blindness. *Lancet*, **2**, 592

SWANSON, C. P. (1958) *Cytology and Cytogenetics.* Macmillan, London

TAYLOR, A. I. (1963) Sex chromatin in the newborn. *Lancet*, **1**, 912

THERMAN, E., PATAU, K., SMITH, D. W., DE MARS, R. I. (1961) The D trisomy syndrome and XO gonadal dysgenesis in two sisters. *Amer. J. hum. Genet.* **13**, 193

TJIO, J. H., PUCK, T. T., ROBINSON, A. (1960) The human chromosomal satellites in normal persons and in two patients with Marfan's syndrome. *Proc. nat. Acad. Sci., Wash.* **46**, 532

TJIO, J. H., WHANG, J. (1962) Chromosome preparations of bone marrow cells without prior in vitro culture or in vivo colchicine administration. *Stain Technol.* **37**, 17

TOUGH, I. M., BUCKTON, K. E., BAIKIE, A. G., BROWN, W. M. C. (1960) X-ray-induced chromosome damage in man. *Lancet*, **2**, 849

TOUGH, I. M., BROWN, W. M. C., BAIKIE, A. G., BUCKTON, K. E., HARNDEN, D. G., JACOBS, P. A., KING, M. J., McBRIDE, J. A. (1961) Cytogenetic studies in chronic myeloid leukæmia and acute leukæmia associated with mongolism. *Lancet*, **1**, 411

TOWNES, P. L., KREUTNER, K. A., KREUTNER, A., MANNING, J. (1963) Observations on the pathology of the trisomy 17–18 syndrome. *J. Pediat.* **62**, 703

TURNER, B., JENNINGS, A. N. (1961) Trisomy for chromosome 22. *Lancet*, **2**, 49

TURNER, B., JENNINGS, A. N., DEN DULK, G. M., STAPLETON, T. (1962) A self-perpetuating ring chromosome. *Med. J. Austr.* **2**, 56

TURNER, B., DEN DULK, G. M., WATKINS, G. (1964) 17–18 trisomy and 21 trisomy in siblings. *J. Pediat.* **64**, 60

UCHIDA, I. A., CURTIS, E. J. (1961) A possible association between maternal radiation and mongolism. *Lancet*, **2**, 848

UCHIDA, I. A., LEWIS, A. J., BOWMAN, J. M., WANG, H. C. (1962a) A case of double trisomy: trisomy No. 18 and triplo-X. *J. Pediat.* **60**, 498

UCHIDA, I. A., PATAU, K., SMITH, D. W. (1962b) Dermal patterns of 18 and D₁ trisomics. *Amer. J. hum. Genet.* **14**, 345

UCHIDA, I. A., SOLTAN, H. C. (1963) Evaluation of dermatoglyphics in medical genetics. *Pediat. Clin. N. Amer.* **10**, 409

VALENCIA, J. I., DE LOZZIO, C. B., DE CORIAT, L. F. (1963) Heterosomic mosaicism in a mongoloid child. *Lancet*, **2**, 488

VAN WIJCK, J. A. M., TIJDINK, G. A. J., STOLTE, L. A. M. (1962) Anomalies of the Y chromosome. *Lancet*, **1**, 218

WAARDENBURG, P. J. (1932) Das menschiche Auge und seine Erbanlagen. *Bibliogr. genet.* **7**, 44

WALKER, N. F. (1957) The use of dermal configurations in the diagnosis of mongolism. *J. Pediat.* **50**, 19

WALTON, J. N. (1956) The inheritance of muscular dystrophy. *Ann. hum. Genet., Lond.* **21**, 40

WALTON, J. N. (1957) The amyotonia congenita syndrome. *Proc. roy. Soc. Med.* **50**, 301

WARKANY, J., CHU, E. H. Y., KAUDER, E. (1962a) Male pseudohermaphroditism and chromosomal mosaicism. *Amer. J. Dis. Child.* **104**, 172

WARKANY, J., RUBINSTEIN, J. H., SOUKUP, S. W., CURLESS, M. C. (1962b) Mental retardation, absence of patellæ, other malformations with chromosomal mosaicism. *J. Pediat.* **61**, 803

WAXMAN, S. H., GARTLER, S. M., KELLEY, V. C. (1962a) Apparent masculinization of the female fetus diagnosed as true hermaphroditism by chromosomal studies. *J. Pediat.* **60**, 540

WEINSTEIN, E. D., WARKANY, J. (1963) Maternal mosaicism and Down's syndrome (mongolism). *J. Pediat.* **63**, 599

WEISS, L., DIGEORGE, A. M., BAIRD, H. W. (1962) Four infants with the trisomy 18 syndrome and one with trisomy 18 mosaicism. *Amer. J. dis. Child.* **104**, 533

WHITE, M. J. D. (1961) *The Chromosomes*, 5th Ed., Methuen, London

WILKINS, L. (1960) Abnormalities of sex differentiation. Classification, diagnosis, selection of rearing and treatment. *Pediatrics*, **26**, 846

WILLEMSE, C. H., VAN BRINK, J. M., LOS, P. L. (1962) XY/XO mosaicism. *Lancet*, **1**, 488

WRIGHT, S. W., DAY, R. W., MOSIER, H. D., KOONS, A., MUELLER, H. (1963) Klinefelter's syndrome, Down's syndrome (mongolism) and twinning in the same sibship. *Pediatrics*, **62**, 217

CHAPTER 8

DISORDERS OF GROWTH

Douglas Hubble

Physiological Control of Growth

Skeletal growth is accompanied by the coincidental growth of other organs and systems; if in measurement we concentrate on the linear growth of the skeleton we do so for ease of examination and we do not forget that there is a growth of other organs and systems—such as the skull, the brain and the sexual organs—which is quite dissociated from linear growth. There is one aspect of development—skeletal maturation—which requires special consideration when linear growth is being considered.

The two processes of *chondroplasia*, growth of cartilage, and *osteogenesis*, epiphyseal development and increase in bone structure, are normally synchronous, but they are under different hormonal and metabolic controls, so that in disease processes the comparison and contrast between the maturation of the skeleton (osteogenesis) and linear growth (chondroplasia) provide us with important diagnostic clues. One of the earliest recognitions of this dissociation was provided by Park (1954) who suggested that in childhood illness the well-known Harris lines in the long bones were attributable to the fact that the linear growth of bone was arrested while the accretion of new bone continued.

In animals thyroxine is concerned with *skeletal maturation* and growth hormone with *linear growth*. In man the evidence from a study of disease processes is that these two hormones are synergistic for both processes, thyroxine being required predominantly for skeletal maturation and growth hormone for linear growth but, in the absence of either hormone, neither process proceeds at the normal rate (Talbot *et al.* 1952). The androgens accelerate both processes, but they advance skeletal maturation (a frequent clinical observation) at a greater rate than linear growth, so that fusion of the bones is advanced and ultimate height is reduced. Skeletal maturation also goes faster than linear growth if an excess of thyroxine is administered (as also in thyrotoxicosis) and we may expect that the reverse would occur in the presence of an excess of growth hormone, so that ultimate stature would be increased. This pathological condition rarely occurs in childhood, but when human growth hormone is readily available for treatment we may expect clinical confirmation of these facts to be obtained. Even in the fœtus the dissociation between the control of linear growth and skeletal maturation is apparent. In fœtal cretinism epiphyseal development is grossly retarded while linear growth proceeds normally. Thyroxine is in fœtal life the essential hormone for normal skeletal maturation, and an excess of androgen, as in congenital virilising adrenal hyperplasia, does not advance epiphyseal development. Other examples of the dissociation between the processes of osteogenesis and chondroplasia will be referred to below.

Fœtal and Postnatal Growth

The astonishing rate of fœtal growth and the agents which control it are subjects about which we know little but in which increasing attention to nature's experiments is teaching us something. The effects of placental insufficiency, hypoxia, toxic agents and twinning on the retardation of fœtal growth demand much more study. The uterine environment appears to be all-important and the optimal conditions for growth normally present in the *milieu exterieur* of the fœtus appear to be sufficient to overcome, at least in some degree, any factors causing growth resistance or retardation which the fœtus carries, as in cretinism, mongolism, Turner's syndrome, and congenital hypopituitary dwarfism. The hormonal equipment of the fœtus, if we may accept the evidence of cretinism, appears to make little contribution to this optimal growth. The cause for this astonishing growth appears to lie in the capacity of the fœtus for mitotic division and cellular multiplication when given optimal nutrition (Seckel 1960). We can assume that this cellular gargantuanism carries over into the postnatal period but in gradually diminishing degree. In the first year of life the baby increases its birth length by an average of 50%, in the second year there is 16% of linear growth and in the third year 10%. During these first years the baby's innate growth capacity diminishes and its own hormonal apparatus takes over the regulation of linear growth. For example, in congenital hypopituitary dwarfism the slowing of growth is seldom recognised until the third year of age, though when adequate records are available there is some evidence of slowing of growth during the first and second years of life.

If the child suffers from some condition in the first year or two of life which interferes with his obtaining the full benefit from this period of exceptionally rapid growth, it may be that the later correction of such a condition does not allow him to achieve his full growth potential. This, although not proven, is suggested by the follow-up of some patients with cœliac disease and hypothyroidism referred to below. If this is so, then it suggests that the regulation of growth during these early years is set by a genetic time clock which does not allow this period of exceptionally rapid growth to be achieved later. The phenomenon of the compensatory growth spurt (catch up growth) has only a limited effect when disease has supervened in the first year of life.

The operation of the genetic time clock, and the dissociated control of linear growth and skeletal maturation, is again exemplified in patients with hypopituitarism or with eunuchoidism. Linear growth usually slows down at the predestined age despite the retarded skeletal maturation and the failure of bone fusion. The eunuchoid giant is a rare specimen.

The Compensatory Growth Spurt (Catch-up Growth)

During a period of illness, malnutrition, or hormonal lack the linear growth of bone may be retarded, and when the underlying condition is corrected a period of accelerated growth occurs. Accelerated growth over very short periods may be three times, and even four times, the average rate for the age, and this rapid rate is best seen in hypothyroid children in the first few months of thyroxine treatment. The maximal growth which can be achieved over longer periods when such causes of growth retardation are corrected is about twice the average rate. If this is a recovery phase from disease or malnutrition, then the rate gradually slows down until, in a varying time, the previous rate of growth is reached, and the child's growth then advances along its predetermined curve (Prader *et al.* 1963).

The Adolescent Growth Spurt

This is a well documented accleration of growth occurring in both sexes. The hormonal factors associated with it are not defined—in girls they are assumed to be the adrenal androgens and œstrogen, in boys adrenal and testicular androgens. As can be seen dramatically in children suffering from precocious puberty, skeletal maturation advances at a greater rate than linear growth, so that it is reasonable to assume that the androgens and the œstrogens (p. 212) play a major role in the growth spurt. It may well be that other hormones—growth hormone, gonadotrophins, thyrotrophin, thyroxine, insulin—are all directly concerned in this process, which may be the result of a generalised anterior pituitary hyperplasia, but exact definition is lacking.

The Control and Rate of Skeletal Maturation

Epiphyseal development. This appears to depend primarily on thyroxine and to a lesser extent on the growth hormone, while the androgens, and to a lesser extent œstrogen, notably advance it. It is considerably retarded in hypothyroidism, less so in congenital hypopituitary dwarfism, and greatly accelerated in thyrotoxicosis and congenital virilising adrenal hyperplasia. It is also retarded in states of malnutrition, such as cœliac disease and kwashiorkor, but advanced in overnutrition (obesity). It might be assumed that this delayed maturation in malnutrition is the result of protein deficiency, but the possibility that a secondary hormonal deficiency is also concerned has to be remembered.

There are some curious facts about the rate of skeletal maturation that are not easy to explain. When treatment by a protein anabolic drug is stopped, the stimulus to skeletal maturation cannot be finally assessed until 6 to 12 months afterwards. In some patients there is also a continuing stimulus to linear growth, but this is less invariable and less prolonged (Hubble and Macmillan 1962). When the treatment of congenital virilising adrenal hyperplasia is begun, suppression of the abnormal steroids rapidly results in retardation of linear growth, but the rate of skeletal maturation may be maintained for as long as a year.

The site of this continuing androgenic stimulus in both these conditions must lie in the epiphyses, though how this effect is sustained is not clear. The anabolic agent may be stored in the liver or in the peripheral tissues.

The Convention of Height Age

Most pædiatricians learnt the useful conventions of height age, weight age and skeletal age at the hands of Lawson Wilkins. Tanner has criticised the validity of height and weight age on the grounds that they are not an accurate index of maturity; as for example, the child of 6 years who has a height age of 4 years may be of constitutionally short stature, may be a late maturer, or may have some pathological cause for growth retardation. He makes a similar criticism of the intelligence quotient. He writes in one place of the "idea of 'height age' and 'weight age' previously used in pædiatric medicine" (Tanner 1961). It would be a mistake for the clinician to give way too easily to the understandable requirements of the anthropometrist. These conventions have considerable value for us still.

Pædiatricians have always recognised that the interpretation of these conventions requires a consideration of the three possibilities stated above. The patients in whom we are considering the performance of investigations on account of growth retardation usually fall well below the 3rd centile for height, and where the height is at the 3rd centile or above the convention of height age is not useful. Pædiatricians find the charts prepared by J. M. Tanner and R. H. Whitehouse (University of London, Institute of Child Health, for The Hospital for Sick Children, Great Ormond Street, London) of great value in the diagnosis of constitutional short stature or of retarded maturity, but they also find that the convention of height age provides them with an acceptable picture of the degree of retardation, and of the response to treatment, in pathological conditions. Moreover, a consideration of height age, weight age and bone age when taken together may provide some useful diagnostic clues. Many examples will occur in the further discussions. One illustration may be given here. Talbot (Talbot et al. 1952) many years ago pointed out that where the height age was retarded, and the weight age still more retarded, malnutrition should be considered as a possible contributory factor in the dwarfism. These reasons for the retention of these conventions appear to me to be adequate and they will be used in the following pages.

Diagnosis in the Clinic

History taking. In the clinic this will include the approximate heights and weights of parents and siblings; the birth history of the patient, including his length and weight; his subsequent growth and development; his appetite and nutrition; his bowel habit; his infections and diseases; his personality, his intelligence and his academic performance.

The *examination* of the patient requires the accurate record of his height and weight which must be plotted on the relevant charts; the measurement of skull circumference; the search for systemic disease—heart, lungs and nervous system; the enlargement of abdominal organs—liver, spleen and kidneys; the search for abnormalities of the face, skull, skeleton and skin—such as eye, ear malformations, underdeveloped mandible, neck-webbing, cubitus valgus, defective extension of the elbow and pronation of the forearm, incurved fifth digit and so on; subcutaneous fat deposit, sexual maturation; and the assessment of intelligence and personality.

The required *investigations* include the examination of the urine; the hæmoglobin estimation; the radiographic assessment of skeletal maturation and the nature of skeletal abnormalities clinically observed; and such further investigations as are indicated by the history and examination.

This examination usually allows a presumptive diagnosis to be made, at least in the terms of the admittedly imprecise clinical classifications set out below. It must define those patients for whom further investigation is required.

Further Investigations When Required

1. When malabsorption is suspected

(a) Sweat for sodium chloride content
(b) Estimate of steatorrhœa
(c) Xylose absorption test
(d) Barium meal and follow through
(e) Duodeno-jejunal biopsy
(f) Fæces for intestinal parasites, especially *Giardia lamblia*

2. In all girls with short stature

(a) Buccal mucosal smear
(b) If the cells are chromatin negative, a chromosomal study

3. Endocrine investigations

(a) *Skull radiography* (pituitary and hypothalamic disease)
(b) *Pituitary disease*

    (1) Growth hormone assay, where available
    (2) Insulin sensitivity test
    (3) Metapirone test

(c) *Thyroid function*

    (1) Serum protein bound iodine
    (2) Blood cholesterol
    (3) ^{132}I or ^{131}I uptake
    (4) Thyroid antibodies, etc.
    (5) Enzymatic studies (perchlorate discharge and labelled MIT) in goitre with or without hypothyroidism

(d) *Adreno-cortical function*

    (1) Water-load test
    (2) Urinary 17-OHCS and 17-KS before and after ACTH
    (3) Fraction 2/3 ratio (Morris) in urine ⎫ congenital
                                         ⎬ virilising
                                          adrenocortical
    (4) Pregnanetriol in urine ⎭ hyperplasia

(e) *Sex hormones*

    (1) Gonadotrophins in urine
    (2) Prostatic secretion ⎫ boys
          Examination of semen ⎭
    (3) Vaginal smear ⎫ girls
          Œstrogens in urine ⎭

Disturbances of Growth

These will be now considered under the two classifications of A. *Tall Stature* and B. *Short Stature*.

A. Tall Stature

A.1. Constitutional

A.2. Overnutrition

A.3. Hormonal

(a) Precocious puberty
(b) Precocious sexuality
(c) Gigantism and acromegaly

A.4. Arachnodactyly (differentiation from 3(c))

A.1. Constitutional Tall Stature

The only diagnostic line to be obtained in these patients is the family history of tall stature in sibs, parents, grandparents and aunts and uncles. At best this provides no more than an uncertain guide to diagnosis. The assessment of skeletal maturation is of prognostic importance, and reference to the tables of Bayer and Bayley (1959) will provide a prediction of reasonable accuracy.

In differential diagnosis, gigantism, acromegaly and arachnodactyly have to be considered (see below). Treatment is considered later.

A.2. Tall Stature Accompanied by Overnutrition (Obesity)

Obesity is the index of overnutrition, and obese children are advanced in height (Wolff 1955 and see also Chapter 9, p. 227). Their ultimate height is not greater than expected and it may be less, since the early advance in height is accompanied by an earlier puberty in these children (Lloyd and Wolff 1961). Overnutrition may have done no more than bring forward the time of the adolescent growth spurt. An advance in skeletal maturation parallels and may exceed the advancement of height. When obese children are dieted the height velocity is slowed.

The advancement in height in obese children is not so rapid as that which accompanies the treatment by thyroxine of hypothyroid children, nor as the growth rate of children exposed to an excess of androgen. We assume that the nutritional excess causes the growth potential of the child to be fulfilled, having regard to the child's endocrine and metabolic status at the time. The amount of nutrients which cannot be absorbed in the processes accompanying growth are deviated to the fat depots. The large children born of diabetic mothers have been shown not only to be heavier than average but also a little longer than average. This condition is thought to be due to overnutrition associated with hyperinsulinism and hyperplasia of the β-cells of the pancreas (Baird and Farquhar, 1962 and see also Chapter 6, pp. 125, 133).

It is legitimate to assume that if an obese child has a height velocity below expectation, then some factor leading to growth retardation is present —such as the lack of thyroxine in hypothyroid children who are occasionally obese. Or some actual factor of growth resistance, as may be observed in obese children suffering from Turner's syndrome or mongolism, and in children suffering from the Laurence-Moon-Biedl syndrome, or the less well-defined Prader-Willi syndrome comprising muscular hypotonia in early childhood, short stature, mental retardation and hypogenitalism (see below). Some of these points are illustrated in the following four cases.

Case 1. Retarded growth despite obesity—hypothyroidism

K. C. Aged 10½ years. She had grown very little in the previous 2 years but her weight had been increasing for 5 years or so despite a poor appetite. Height 45½ inches. Weight 82 lb. (height age 8 years, weight age 12 years). Skeletal age 5 years. Serum protein-bound iodine 3·5 μg./100 ml.

Case 2. Retarded growth despite obesity—hypopituitarism presenting with hypoglycæmia

T. J. This boy was admitted twice to hospital during his fourth year with hypoglycæmic convulsions. His height was 33 inches, height age 1¾ years, his weight was 23 lb., weight age 1¼ years. His skeletal age was 1–1½ years. Following this period of hypoglycæmia he became obese in his fifth year and put on 15 lb. He is now 11 years of age, with a height age of 7 years. In his seventh year he was fully investigated and the only endocrine abnormality discovered was increased insulin sensitivity with hypoglycæmic unresponsiveness. Re-investigated at 11 years his insulin sensitivity had disappeared and once again thyroid and adrenocortical function were normal. He remained obese with a weight age of 13 years. The obesity, present for 6 years, had not encouraged an accelerated growth rate.

Case 3. Retarded growth despite obesity—Prader-Willi syndrome

K.P. This boy had shown mental and growth retardation since childhood. The history suggested muscular hypotonia in his early years. At the age of 13½ years his height was 47 inches and his weight 111 lb. (height age 7 years, weight age 13 years). The genitalia were tiny, with the testes undescended. At the age of 17 years the genitalia were still small although the testes were in the scrotum. The reduction of his weight had produced no acceleration of the rate of growth.

Case 4. Retarded growth despite obesity—Turner's syndrome

V. L. Aged 16½ years. This girl was diagnosed a few months ago as suffering from Turner's syndrome (chromosomal constitution—XO). She has no secondary sex characters. During the last two years she has become obese. Her weight is 131 lb. but her height is only 52½ inches (height age—9 years).

In 1956 Prader, Labhart, Willi and Fanconi described a syndrome mainly characterised by mental deficiency, obesity, abnormally short stature, muscular hypotonia and undescended testes. In 1961 Prader and Willi reported a total of 14 cases and added diabetes mellitus (in patients over the age of 12 years) to their description of the syndrome. Laurance (1961) has reported six cases. The syndrome affects girls as well as boys. In girls the differential diagnosis is from Turner's syndrome, and may be difficult in the Turner girls with a normal buccal mucosal smear (see Case 13, p. 201 and also Chapter 7, p. 176).

The pathogenesis of the short stature in these four conditions is discussed below—but the point is made here that overnutrition (obesity) will not overcome retarded growth in these disorders.

A.3(*a*). Precocious Puberty

Children who suffer from precocious puberty will not only show advancement in secondary sexual characters, but also an acceleration of linear growth and skeletal maturation. This advancement in height and skeletal maturation is occasionally a useful confirmation of precocious puberty.

Case 5. Regression of the precocious puberty

D. L. At the age of 5 years this girl had vaginal hæmorrhage for only one month, accompanied by slight breast enlargement and fine pigmented pubic hairs. There was some elevation of urinary gonadotrophins and 17-hydroxy-corticosteroids. All signs of puberty regressed in the following year but her height which had been on the 75th centile at the time of her menstruation advanced to the 90th centile in this time. It had receded to the 75th centile two years later.

In precocious puberty there is a longer period for the effects of puberty to operate on the skeleton than in normal puberty so that the child's ultimate height will be reduced, since during this period skeletal maturation runs faster than linear growth (height age advancing more rapidly than skeletal age).

Case 6. Constitutional precocious puberty in a boy

D. H. Aged $6\frac{1}{4}$ years. This boy's precocious puberty appeared to have commenced in infancy. His height was $51\frac{1}{2}$ inches and his height age $8\frac{1}{2}$ years. His skeletal age was 14 years, certainly more than two years advancement in each year. His height had advanced less than two years in each year. His ultimate height will not be more than 58 inches.

A.3(*b*). Precocious Sexuality

Children suffering from precocious sexuality who show advancement of linear growth are usually suffering from congenital virilising adrenal hyperplasia, of the prenatal type diagnosed late or the postnatal type; or much more rarely from adrenocortical, testicular or ovarian tumour. They show similar rates of advancement of linear growth and skeletal maturation as do the children with precocious puberty.

Case 7. Precocious sexuality due to an adrenal adenoma

A. C. At the age of $8\frac{1}{2}$ years an adenoma of the left adrenal cortex was diagnosed. He had begun to develop signs of precocious sexuality at the age of 5 years. His height at diagnosis was 56 inches (height age 11 years) and in the $3\frac{1}{2}$ years from the demonstrable onset of his disease he had grown 15 inches, approximately twice his expected gain in height. His skeletal age was 13–14 years, so that if his skeletal age was chronological at the onset of his disease, the rate of skeletal maturation had proceeded at more than twice the normal rate.

Although we may attempt to assess these changes in linear growth and skeletal maturation by the duration of the disease and the amount of circulating androgens present, there is one factor which cannot be assessed and that is the individual variation in the response of osteogenesis and chondroplasia to these agents.

Case 8. Congenital virilising adrenal hyperplasia

P. H. The diagnosis was made at the age of $2\frac{1}{2}$ years. Urinary ketosteroids were 8 mg./24 hours, the 17-hydroxycorticosteroids 34 mg./24 hours, and pregnanetriol 7·3 mg./24 hours. His height was 41 inches (height age $4\frac{1}{2}$ years) and his skeletal age was 9–10 years. On the assumption that his skeletal age was not advanced at birth, skeletal maturation had advanced nearly four years for each year of life.

In antenatal life the effect of an excess of androgens on linear growth is much less marked than it becomes later. The average birth length of six full term children suffering from congenital virilising hyperplasia of whom I have records was $20\frac{1}{2}$ inches. Mellman *et al.* (1959) state, and this is my experience also, that skeletal maturation in the fœtus is not advanced in congenital virilising hyperplasia. The assumption from these facts is that fœtal growth is maximal when optimal nutrition is assured in intra uterine life, and that the circulation of additional growth stimulants has no, or little, effect. If the essential stimulus to skeletal maturation, thyroxine, is in adequate supply, the addition of androgen will produce no further advancement in epiphyseal development.

A.3(c). Gigantism and Acromegaly. A.4. Arachnodactyly

These causes of tall stature may be considered together. When there is evidence of a pituitary tumour and the signs of gigantism or acromegaly are present, there is no difficulty in diagnosis. If hyperpituitarism occurs before the epiphyses are closed it is stated that gigantism occurs; it is then presumed that the excess of growth hormone results in enhanced linear growth. If this occurs after epiphyseal fusion has taken place then increased deposition of bone results with the characteristic signs of acromegaly. In fact, the skeletal distinction between gigantism and acromegaly is not so clear cut. In the rare cases of an eosinophilic adenoma of the pituitary developing in childhood or adolescence, acromegalic changes may be seen in the bones although the predominant feature is gigantism. Growth hormone is primarily concerned with chondroplasia but it also has an effect on osteogenesis.

If however there is no enlargement of the sella turcica and no evidence of hyperpituitarism, despite the presence of gigantism, then diagnosis becomes more difficult.

Case 9. Gigantism due to presumed excess of growth hormone

J. J. Male, aged $13\frac{1}{2}$ years. Height 81 inches. Span 80 inches. Lower segment 45 inches. The increased rate of growth started at the age of 8 years. He was pubertal. Skeletal maturation was chronological. There was no enlargement of the sella turcica and no impairment of visual fields. Endocrine assays were within normal limits except that the assay of serum growth hormone (Read's method) was 144 μg./100 ml. (D. MacMillan)—the highest level obtained in a large series of estimations.

In such patients the differential diagnosis is from Marfan's syndrome—arachnodactyly. This latter disease is congenital, and often familial, and is frequently accompanied by other anomalies—skeletal, ocular and cardiac—all of which were absent in this patient. However the diagnosis in sporadic cases when none of these other abnormalities may be present is not easy.

Case 10. *Arachnodactyly—forme fruste*

B. M. Aged 13¾ years. This boy was long at birth particularly in the arms. When first seen his height was 69½ inches, the lower segment being 6½ inches longer than the upper segment. The metacarpal index was 9·6 (see below). The span was 77 inches—7½ inches in excess of height. There were none of the other features of arachnodactyly.

The essential differences between these two boys were the apparent congenital origin in Case 10, and the much greater height of Case 9. In such patients a diagnosis can often not be firmly made, and the possibility of constitutional tall stature must also be considered. The eldest brother of Case 9 was 75 inches tall but without any disproportionate growth of limbs.

It has been suggested by Sinclair *et al.* (1960) that a metacarpal index $\left(\dfrac{\text{length}}{\text{width}}\right)$ greater than 8·4 is abnormal, and if the patients lower segment is greater than the upper segment by more than 2 inches the diagnosis of Marfan's syndrome should be considered. Case 9 (J.J.) however, had a metacarpal index of 10 and his lower segment exceeded his upper segment by 8 inches. These measurements then do not distinguish Marfan's syndrome in its incomplete forms from hyperpituitary gigantism. Important in diagnosis in Case 9 was the fact that J.J.'s growth rate did not accelerate until he was 8 years old, while increased length of limb in Case 10 was recognised in early life.

B. Short Stature

B.1. Familial and congenital dwarfism

(*a*) Hereditary short stature

(*b*) Syndromes

(*c*) Chromosomal disorders—mongolism and Turner's syndrome

B.2. Intra-uterine growth retardation

B.3. Malnutrition

(*a*) Specific protein deficiency

(*b*) Malabsorption

B.4. Hormonal causes

(*a*) Growth hormone deficiency

(*b*) Thyroxine deficiency

(*c*) Corticosteroid excess

(*d*) Androgen and œstrogen action

B.5. Factors disturbing cellular nutrition

(*a*) Hypoxia

(*b*) Renal disease

(*c*) Hepatic disease

Familial and Congenital Dwarfism

B.1(*a*). Hereditary Short Stature

In considering the differential diagnosis of short stature in the clinic it is necessary to make an assessment of the family growth patterns. The inadequacy of this assessment is well recognised. Nonetheless, such evidence as can be obtained from the measurement of sibs and parents should not be ignored. It is not uncommon for the diagnosis of hereditary short stature to be made in the clinic in patients attending on account of retarded growth. The degree of retardation may well be greater than has occurred in near relatives.

Usually in these children the skeletal maturation is within average limits (3rd to 97th centile), but sometimes epiphyseal development is severely retarded in children who appear to be of short stature by inheritance. This might be comfortably regarded as indicating plenty of growth potential in reserve, but it is doubtful whether such a conclusion is justifiable. Bayer and Bayley (1959) in their tables for height prediction have prepared additional tables for children with anomalous growth whose skeletal ages are one or more years retarded or accelerated for their chronological ages.

B.1(b). Three Congenital and Familial Syndromes with Short Stature

Vitamin D resistant rickets. This disease is inherited as a dominant and in some families the trait may be sex linked so that the heterozygous females have the disease more mildly than do males with an unopposed X chromosome. The dwarfism which accompanies the rickets may be due to the disturbance of phosphorus metabolism. The hypophosphatæmia which occurs is difficult to correct by calciferol without the production of hypercalcæmia, and the persistence of short stature may be due to defects of bone growth consequent on mild chronic hypophosphatæmia even in treated patients. (Winters et al. 1958, Steendijk 1962). However, the possibility of another genetic cause for the short stature has been raised.

Pseudohypoparathyroidism. This disorder is congenital, and sometimes familial (MacGregor and Whitehead 1954). It is characterised by stunted growth, mental retardation, characteristic facies and bone abnormalities. The short stature is a genetic defect unrelated to the disturbance of phosphorus metabolism.

Laurence-Moon-Biedl syndrome. This is a congenital and sometimes familial disorder characterised by retinitis pigmentosa, polydactyly, diabetes insipidus, obesity and short stature. The mechanism of the obesity is undetermined and the syndrome provides an example of short stature accompanied by obesity (p. 195).

B.1(c). Chromosomal Disorders Causing Growth Retardation

Mongolism. Mongolism is now attributable to a chromosomal disorder causing a trisomy of the autosome 21. One of the most invariable features of mongolism is retarded growth. Dutton (1959) examined forty-two adult male mongols whose age was greater than 19 years. The arithmetic mean of their height was 59 inches, and only one attained a height of 64 inches. If the average male adult stature is 68 inches—the height of mongols is 9 inches below this or approximately an average reduction of 13%. Dutton reported that the skeletal maturation of mongols is within average limits but other authors have recently stated that moderate degrees of skeletal retardation occur in mongolism (Ravick *et al.* 1964). Reference has already been made to the possibility that in fœtuses suffering from an innate growth resistance this retardation may to some extent be overcome in intra-uterine life. There are no statistics concerning the birth length of mongols. However, Smith and McKeown (1955) showed that the prenatal growth retardation of mongol children is not extreme, since their mean birth weight was 2900 gms. (6 lb. 6 oz.) with a mean duration of gestation of 269 days. This represents a calculated reduction in average birth weight of less than 9%.

Turner's syndrome. This is a sex chromosome anomaly occurring in girls usually with the karyotype XO (see Chapter 7, p. 175). The mean height of 49 patients aged 17 years and older suffering from Turner's syndrome is 55 inches. If the mean height of normal adult women is 64 inches this represents a reduction of mean height of more than 15%. If the same degree of growth retardation was shown by the fœtus, this would be represented by a reduction of 3 inches below a 20 inch mean. The birth length in 21 patients, all full term, recorded by Lemli and Smith (1963) showed a mean of 18·6 inches— a reduction of about 7%. A tentative conclusion which may be drawn from these figures is that while there is some intra-uterine growth retardation in Turner's syndrome it is of a lesser degree than is shown later in extra-uterine life.

Cases 11 *and* 12. *Identical twins, the one suffering from Turner's syndrome and the other normal* (Dr B. D. Bower)
Identical twins, the one suffering from Turner's syndrome (45 chromosomes— XO) and the other with a normal chromosomal constitution, were prematurely born. The normal child weighed 4 lb. 1 oz. at birth and the child with Turner's syndrome weighed 3 lb. 12 oz. The birth length of each twin was $17\frac{1}{2}$ inches. At 14 weeks of age the length of the normal baby was $24\frac{1}{2}$ inches and the length of the baby with Turner's syndrome was $22\frac{1}{2}$ inches.

The growth resistance of the bones in Turner's syndrome is to some extent overcome by uterine nutrition.

Although it is usually stated that linear growth in patients with Turner's syndrome is not accelerated by the use of protein anabolic drugs, it can in fact be so stimulated, though the advancement in height is paralleled, or outdistanced, by the acceleration of skeletal maturation (Hubble and Mac-Millan 1962). Blizzard (1963) states that linear growth in Turner's syndrome may be stimulated by the use of human growth hormone.

Case 13. *Variant of Turner's syndrome: X chromosomal abnormality with dwarfism, mental retardation, obesity and failure of sexual development*
J. A. Now aged $19\frac{1}{2}$ years. She was first seen at the age of 15 years on account of short stature. Her height was then 50 inches (height age 7 years) and her weight was 74 lb. (weight age 10 years). There was moderate obesity which increased in the subsequent 4 years so that she reached the 50th centile for weight at $17\frac{1}{2}$ years with a height of 54 inches (height age $10\frac{1}{4}$ years). There was no sexual development at 15 years or since. The serum protein-bound iodine was below normal levels (3·1 and 3·9 μg./100 ml.) but she had none of the signs of hypothyroidism. The IQ was 80.

The presenting signs were then dwarfism, obesity, mental retardation and delayed sexual development. The differential diagnosis included Turner's syndrome, hypopituitarism with mild hypothyroidism, and the Prader-Willi syndrome. A variant of Turner's syndrome appeared to be the most probable diagnosis, but the buccal mucosal smear on repeated occasions showed chromatin positive nuclei. The suspicion of some form of congenital hypogonadism was confirmed by a rising output of urinary gonadotrophins (despite the lack of sexual characters) which, although giving varying levels over the years, rose as high as 50 mg. IRP-HMG/24 hrs. in 1960, when she was 16. Chromosomal analysis (Dr J. H. Edwards) done in 1963 showed a normal number of chromosomes, with no mosaicism either in bone marrow cells or in lymphocytes. There was however present an unusually long "short arm" in an X (presumed) chromosome. This undescribed abnormality has been seen by Dr Edwards in another patient (Dr W. H. Cant and the author). Laparotomy (Mr Henry Roberts) showed a very small uterus (1 cm. by 1 cm.) with minute round ligaments and fallopian tubes. There was a white streak at the gonadal ridge.

There are two conclusions to be drawn from this patient, the one practical and the other theoretical. The first is that the presence of chromatin positive nuclei does not exclude some variants of the Turner syndrome. The second, that the somatic manifestations of the Turner syndrome—especially dwarfism—cannot be adequately explained by the death of an X chromosome. Any hypothesis would now have to include the inactivation of an X chromosome by the presence of an abnormal short arm.

B.2. Intra-uterine Growth Retardation (Dysmaturity)

It is now sixty years since writers like Gilford, Hansemann and Ballantyne recognised that the fœtus might grow defectively in the uterus, *despite a fœtal life of normal duration*. These authors bestowed on these infants such descriptions as fœtal ateleiosis, nanosomia primordialis and fœtal microsomia. Modern authors like Seckel (1960) (bird-headed dwarfs) and Russell (1954) (intrauterine dwarfism) have sought to characterise new syndromes while adding little to our knowledge of ætiology, and making but small additions to the natural history of these disorders.

Recently there has arisen a widespread feeling that what is now required are large-scale prospective studies of these children in order to answer certain fundamental questions. What are the intra-uterine factors which have caused this dysmaturity? What is the prognosis for these children as regards development? Why should some of them be mentally retarded, and others not? Why should some have skeletal abnormalities, and others not? How important are nutritional and endocrine factors in retarding postnatal development? Are placental abnormalities of causative importance, or are the placentas small and abnormal for the same reasons as the fœtuses they nourish?

The introduction of the term intra-uterine growth retardation (Warkany *et al.* 1961) is, in fact, an attempt to approach the problem from the point of view of a prospective enquiry, meanwhile describing as completely as possible the clinical features and relevant genetic and environmental conditions. Many of the syndromes of which growth retardation is a prominent sign are well characterised, many others are ill defined. All these many conditions are of great importance and interest, and their present clinical descriptions will have an enhanced importance when their ætiological factors are understood.

B.3. Malnutrition and Growth

The advancement of the rate of linear growth, and of ultimate height, in this century has been attributed to improved nutrition, though since it is seen in all classes of society, both rich and poor, other causes have been sought for it (Tanner 1962). That malnutrition is a cause of retarded growth has been a common observation, both in animal and human biology, for many a day. Malthus wrote in 1798, "Indeed, it seems difficult to suppose that a labourer's wife who has six children and who is sometimes in absolute want of bread, should be able always to give them the food and attention necessary to support life. The sons and daughters of peasants will not be found such rosy cherubs in real life as they are described to be in romances. It cannot fail to be remarked by those who live much in the country, that the sons of labourers are very apt to be stunted in their growth, and are a long while arriving at maturity. Boys that you would guess to be fourteen or fifteen, are when inquiring, frequently found to be eighteen or nineteen. And the lads who drive plough, which must certainly be a healthy exercise, are very rarely seen with any appearance of calves to their legs; a circumstance, which can only be attributed to a want either of proper, or of sufficient nourishment."

Inadequate growth due to the inadequate provision of calories is now very uncommon in children of school age. In hospital practice it is still quite commonly seen in younger children. Ignorance, neglect and poverty are the usual determining environmental factors. In mentally retarded children a failure to provide adequate calories for those without clamant appetites is an additional cause for growth retardation.

A failure of appetite due to emotional inhibition, food resistance, or physical disease is still a common cause of growth retardation. The mechanism by which appetite is depressed in brain damaged children is unexplained, though reduced activity and lowered basal metabolism are no doubt contributory causes. A vicious circle is soon established, small children have both small appetites and small stomachs, and a reduced demand soon results in a diminished supply. Depression in children appears to have an effect on growth rates which is not due to diminshed intake of food (Widdowson 1951, Acheson 1959, Patton and Gardner 1962). Whether this inhibition is mediated via the hypothalamus to the anterior pituitary, with depression of growth hormone output is unknown. Illness also results directly in retardation of growth and this result is more apparent in boys than in girls, and appears to affect chondroplasia more than osteogenesis. This is the explanation given for the appearance of Harris lines in the radiographs of growing bones.

The dwarfism of diabetes insipidus, both cerebral and renal, has been attributed to inadequate caloric intake (Hillman et al. 1958, Vest et al. 1963). It is suggested that these patients recognise that the more they eat, the more urine they have to void (to excrete their solute load) and therefore the intake of food is, consciously or unconsciously, reduced. While the failure of appetite in these children is not in doubt, it seems possible that the frequent filling of the stomach with large quantities of fluid may depress the appetite by a peripheral mechanism.

Although the mechanisms causing malnutrition and growth retardation

are not always easy to unravel, their results can be studied in protein deprivation—the disease known as kwashiorkor occurring in children living in
tropical countries, and in the disorders of malabsorption, cœliac disease and
fibrocystic disease of the pancreas, common in temperate climates.

B.3(a). Specific Protein Deficiency

Kwashiorkor. This disease is prevalent in African children during the
post-weaning phase, 85% of the cases (Trowell, 1954) occurring between the
7th and 36th months of life. Although this disease may be regarded basically
as one of specific protein malnutrition, there is no doubt that other factors
are concerned—such as total caloric malnutrition, infection and malabsorption (see Chapter 10, pp. 235, 251). Whatever the exact ætiology, retardation
of growth is one of the cardinal signs and this is accompanied by retardation
of skeletal maturation (Jones and Dean 1956).

Other disorders resulting in protein deficiency. Bridge and Holt (1945)
attributed the growth retardation of children with *glycogen storage disease*
to the non-availability of carbohydrate for ordinary metabolic processes,
with a resultant switch to protein utilisation; this is essentially the same
reason (although a different mechanism is involved) for growth failure that
occurs in the presence of increased cortisone production or administration—
gluconeogenesis.

Collis *et al.* (1963) reported that children suffering from *cystinuria* were
2·5 cm. shorter than the mean normal height for children of the same age and
sex, while children suffering from *Hartnup disease* were 5·0 cm. shorter than
the mean normal height for children of the same age and sex. This short
stature they attributed to a defective transport of amino-acids across the
small intestine and to the loss of essential amino-acids in the urine.

B.3(b). Malabsorption

The common causes of malabsorption in childhood are cœliac disease and
fibrocystic disease of the pancreas. In malabsorption there is not only a
total caloric deficiency but also malabsorption of protein and specific
nutrients, such as calcium, phosphorus, B_{12} and folic acid. All these deficiencies may have an adverse effect on linear growth rates. Chronic malnutrition
may result, too, in depression of the activity of the anterior pituitary with
further interference with linear growth.

Cœliac disease. In cœliac disease there is the further possibility that the
absorption of a toxic substance (? a glutamine-containing peptide) may have
a directly harmful influence on growth; and also that there may not only be
impaired absorption of protein, but also a further loss of protein through the
damaged mucosa of the small intestine. It would be difficult to decide
which of these many causes is chiefly responsible for growth retardation;
certainly protein deficiency and total caloric inadequacy are important.

Retardation of linear growth is an important diagnostic sign in cœliac
disease; and an improved rate of growth following the institution of a
gluten-free diet is a reliable index of correct diagnosis and successful treatment (Sheldon 1959). In 13 patients of mine with cœliac disease there was
one group of 9 patients whose average age at diagnosis was 3 years 4 months

and in whom the degree of retardation of skeletal maturation was greater than the retardation of linear growth. This was demonstrated by the height age/chronological age ratio which was 0·74, while the bone age/chronological age ratio was 0·56. Of the four cases whose average age at diagnosis was greater than 3 years 4 months, the bone age/chronological age ratio was 0·43. The longer the duration of the untreated disease, the greater was the degree of skeletal retardation. In a second group of 7 cases in whom the average age at diagnosis was $2\frac{1}{2}$ years, the height age was more retarded than the bone age, the height age/chronological age ratio being 0·58 and the bone age/chronological age ratio being 0·72. The earlier the onset and the more severe the disease in the first two years of life, the greater will be the impairment of linear growth and the more reduced will be the height age/chronological age ratio. It is in this group too that the patients are seen in whom it may be inferred that a pathological cause operating against growth in the first year or two of life may result in a permanent impairment of height (see page 191).

Fibrocystic disease of the pancreas. Although malabsorption is an important contributory cause of the growth retardation which occurs in fibrocystic disease of the pancreas, in a majority of patients there is a severe complicating pulmonary lesion. To the factors causing retarded growth in malabsorption syndromes must be added that of recurring pulmonary infection. There is retardation of skeletal maturation as well as of linear growth in severe cases.

Other diseases causing malabsorption. There are several examples of such disorders in childhood although any one of them occurs but rarely. They have been reviewed by Anderson et al. (1961). Sobel et al. (1962) have studied growth retardation in chronic regional ileitis in childhood.

B.4. Hormonal Causes

Anterior pituitary hormones and growth. The two hormones secreted by the anterior pituitary which have a direct effect in promoting growth are the growth hormone, and thyrotrophin acting on its target organ, the thyroid gland. The sex hormones operating in the adolescent period and throughout puberty are important growth promoting agents. The effect of corticotrophin, acting through the adrenal cortex on protein, fat and carbohydrate metabolism, must have important consequences for cellular nutrition and therefore for growth, but in the absence of disease the adrenocortical hormones play a largely undetermined though essential part in the processes of growth.

The essential requirements in the diagnosis and treatment of an endocrine deficiency are a biological or biochemical assay of the circulating hormones, and substitution therapy, whether derived from animal sources or from synthetic production of the hormone. In regard to the diagnosis of growth hormone deficiency the readily available assay is still awaited; and the failure of animal-derived growth hormone to cause growth promotion in man makes therapy still a distant prospect for all who need it. For the diagnosis of growth hormone deficiency we cannot rely, as in other endocrine disorders, on the failure of a target organ. Growth hormone deficiency can only declare itself in the failure of growth, and of this failure the causes are legion.

While growth hormone assays are not generally available it appears probable that they soon may be. Read's assay often gave results which were clinically meaningful (Macmillan 1961) but the assay was interfered with by non-specific protein inhibitors. The use of the sulphation factor as a bioassay for growth hormone has been found accurate by some workers (Aarskog 1963, Nadler *et al.* 1963). Most promising is the isotope dilution method, or some variant of it (Greenwood *et al.* 1964). The amounts of growth hormone circulating in the plasma are very small and there is considerable diurnal variation.

There will never be any large amount of human growth hormone available for therapy, so that treatment must await its synthesis.

B.4(*a*). Growth Hormone Deficiency

There are two types of pituitary disorder which produce a deficiency of growth hormone production—the one without a demonstrable organic lesion, the other in which there is evidence of a lesion.

The first type is called *congenital hypopituitary dwarfism;* the second *organic hypopituitarism.*

Congenital hypopituitary dwarfism. The author has previously stated the diagnostic criteria of this variety of short stature as: 1, the gradual onset of growth retardation in the second and third year of life; 2, immaturity of facies; 3, a height age which is more retarded than the retarded skeletal age; 4, height well below the 3rd centile after the 4th year of life; 5, the eventual failure, partial or complete, of sexual development; 6, hypercholesterolæmia; 7, increased insulin sensitivity; and 8, a late failure of other endocrine glands.

In the absence of a reliable assay for growth hormone, it will be seen that this is at best a presumptive diagnosis, which is clinically confirmed only when there is partial or complete failure of sexual development. While the diagnostic position has not improved in recent years, the ætiology of the condition has been to some extent clarified by the recognition that even in those patients who presented the clinical picture of congenital hypopituitary dwarfism, and whose disease was presumed to be therefore of an idiopathic nature (without known pathogenesis), there were some patients in whom an ætiological factor could be suspected. In some this has been a history suggestive of perinatal brain damage; in others, the presence of skeletal abnormalities suggests a developmental abnormality, comparable to primordial dwarfism in which the pituitary gland appears also to have been involved.

In the first group the presence of hypoglycæmia convulsions, or the evidence of the partial failure of other endocrine functions in early life, may suggest such an ætiology. While in other patients suffering from an obvious cerebral defect accompanied by dwarfism, evidence of some failure of pituitary function may be obtained, such as an increased insulin sensitivity. Such ætiological assumptions can only be clarified by the wide application of an accurate growth hormone assay.

The author feels convinced that there will remain, even when these patients with secondary hypopituitarism are better understood, a group of patients for whom the diagnosis of congenital hypopituitary dwarfism will be required. It is assumed that in these patients the pituitary is unable to synthesise growth hormone, and that in later life there is a failure, partial or complete, to synthesise the sex hormones. The disorder is much more common in boys than in girls—10 to 1 in Lawson Wilkins' series (Martin and Wilkins 1958), while I have had 18 boys and 4 girls under my care in the last twenty years in whom I have considered the appearances sufficiently classical to make the diagnosis.

Case 14. *Congenital hypopituitary dwarfism*

T. B. This boy is now $20\frac{1}{2}$ years of age. He has been studied for 15 years. His height is now 54 inches and his epiphyses are fused. Both the external genitalia and the prostate are small. Although the output of gonadotrophins remained at a prepubertal level until his 20th year <5 mg. IRP-HMG/24 hrs., in the last year it has risen to 50 mg. IRP-HMG/24 hrs. There is no evidence of thyroid or adrenocortical failure, although the plasma cortisol level of 3·0 µg./100 ml. plasma is below the normal adult range (5–15 µg./100 ml.). The total serum lipid is 980 mg./100 ml. and the total cholesterol 324 mg./100 ml., while the serum protein-bound iodine has always been within the average range.

The failure of growth is not noticed as a rule until the second or third year of life, and while this is related to the fact that growth before this is not dependent on the growth hormone, yet other authors have suggested that some unnoticed retardation of growth occurs before this (Aarskog 1963). This has been my experience too, when height records are available for the first two years.

Case 15

R.E. Now aged $6\frac{1}{2}$ years. Height $38\frac{3}{4}$ inches (height age $3\frac{1}{2}$ years). When he was first investigated at the age of $2\frac{1}{2}$ years his height was $28\frac{1}{4}$ inches (height age 10 months). The clinical appearances and the investigations were consistent with the diagnosis of congenital hypopituitary dwarfism. Corticotrophin and adrenocortical functions were normal, thyroid function may have been a little depressed. This boy must have had growth retardation occurring during the first and second years of life.

The presence of hypercholesterolæmia in some of these patients deserves a comment. It was first described by me in 1957 but it was assumed by Martin and Wilkins (1958) to be related to hypothyroidism. The senior author, however, agreed with me later (Wilkins, personal communication) that this did in fact occur in congenital hypopituitary dwarfism without evidence of hypothyroidism. It occurred in 11 out of 17 of my patients, and in 8 out of these 11 patients the serum protein-bound iodine was normal. It was reported as present in 14 out of 19 cases of Martin and Wilkins (1958) and in only 6 of these patients was the protein-bound iodine below 4·0 µg. per 100 ml. The cause of the hypercholesterolæmia is unknown, it may be related to a deficiency of growth hormone. In one of my patients it appeared to be associated with a delay in the clearing of lipid from the serum after a fatty meal.

Congenital hypopituitary dwarfism with hyperlipæmia

Case 16. *Congenital hypopituitary dwarfism with hyperlipæmia*

C.H. Aged $4\frac{1}{2}$ years. This girl's height is 33 inches (height age 2 years). She has the features of congenital hypopituitary dwarfism. The fasting total lipids were 870 and the cholesterol 281 mg./100 ml. After a fatty meal the serum was not cleared in eight hours (normal clearance occurs in 4–5 hours).

Two groups of patients are of special interest: 1, those in whom the presentation is with hypoglycæmic convulsions; 2, those in whom the presenting disorder is hypothyroidism. I have seen two patients in each group.

With hypoglycæmic convulsions

Case 17.

T. R. Now aged 6 years. Her height is now $33\frac{1}{2}$ inches (height age 2 years). She had severe hypoglycæmic convulsions in the second year of life. Her length was 24 inches at 2 years (height age 4 months). She had suffered perinatal brain damage. Some depression of both thyroid and adrenocortical function was probable.

Case 2

T.J. (p. 196). Now aged 11 years. His height is $48\frac{1}{4}$ inches (height age $7\frac{1}{4}$ years). His height at the age of 4 years was 33 inches (height age $1\frac{3}{4}$ years). He had several hypoglycæmic convulsions during the fourth year of life, and following these became very obese. Despite his obesity he showed no acceleration of growth rate.

In one of these patients there was evidence of perinatal brain damage, and, as I have said, this ætiology should always be suspected. It may be as suggested by Nadler *et al.* (1963) that this syndrome depends on an extreme deficiency of growth hormone.

In children who present with a clear picture of hypothyroidism but in whom adequate dried thyroid or thyroxine therapy produces the relief of all the symptoms of hypothyroidism, *with the exception of the expected growth response*, a deficiency of growth hormone may be suspected, in addition to a failure of thyrotrophin production.

With hypothyroidism

Case 18

J. W. Now aged $11\frac{1}{2}$ years. Patient of Dr Thursby Pelham. He was diagnosed as suffering from hypothyroidism by unimpeachable criteria at the age of $5\frac{1}{2}$ years. His height was then $34\frac{1}{2}$ inches. In the intervening 6 years, despite thyroid therapy, his height has advanced only 9 inches ($1\frac{1}{2}$ inches a year), and his height age is 6 years. The skeletal maturation is at the same level. The growth hormone level (Read's assay, 1960) was 35 μg./l. (normal range 200–350 μg./l.).

Case 19

J. B. Now aged $7\frac{1}{4}$ years. Patient of Dr D. MacCarthy. This girl was diagnosed by adequate criteria to be suffering from hypothyroidism in the first year of life. At $1\frac{1}{4}$ years her height was 23 inches and now 6 years later with adequate thyroxine therapy it is no more than 36 inches— a height age of 3 years. Her skeletal maturation is less retarded than linear growth but still behind her chronological age. The growth hormone level was 10 μg./l.

Organic hypopituitarism. Although these patients present rarely in childhood the causes of their hypopituitarism are numerous. In the patients seen by me the causes have included trauma with intra-sellar calcification, presumed craniopharyngioma with intra-sellar calcification, surgery for neoplasm, supra-sellar calcification associated both with tuberculous meningitis and with craniopharyngioma, chromophobe adenoma, encephalitis, Hand-Schüller-Christian syndrome, and eosinophilic granuloma. The diagnosis is usually not difficult and the growth retardation is usually the least of these children's troubles. The benign prognosis of intra-sellar calcification—whether due to trauma or due to a presumed craniopharyngioma—is worthy of comment. Here the condition appears to be stationary through long years of observation, but the prognosis of supra-sellar calcification due to craniopharyngioma is much less benign. The hypopituitarism due to the supra-sellar calcified lesion of tuberculous meningitis is permanent, but the lesion does not advance.

B.4(*b*). Thyroxine Deficiency

Cretinism is associated with an average birth length. This was shown by Andersen (1960) who recorded the birth length of 22 cretins—with a range of 48 to 56 cm. and an average of 51·7 cm. (20·4 inches). Maternal thyroxine passes over the placenta slowly and in small amounts (Grumbach and Werner 1956) but in insufficient quantity to promote normal cerebral and skeletal maturation in fœtal cretins. It is apparently not required for normal linear growth. Evidence of growth retardation soon appears after birth. Since a child's average growth is nearly one inch a month in the first six months, measurement of length is a valuable clinical enquiry when the diagnosis is considered. The serum protein-bound iodine is the essential investigation. When children present with hypothyroidism in the first or second decade of life the complaint is nearly always of growth failure. Other symptoms of hypothyroidism are present when enquired for, and other signs are present when looked for, but retardation of growth is the common observation to have been made by the parents. It is frequently surprising how a child's academic performance has been maintained despite the insidious onset of hypothyroidism. Skeletal maturation will also be retarded, and the essential diagnostic investigation is again the serum protein-bound iodine, which will always be lower than 4·0 μg./100 ml. in older children and below 4·5 μg./*l*. in infants. The advancement of skeletal maturation proceeds very rapidly with treatment and the acceleration of linear growth proceeds at a slower rate. When these children have missed the first two years of maximal growth it is doubtful whether they ever achieve their intended height potential.

Case 20

K.C. Now aged 15½ years. This girl was diagnosed as suffering from hypothyroidism at the age of 10 years. Her height was 45½ inches (height age 6 years), and the skeletal age advanced 5–6 years in the 5 years of treatment but her height response was much slower, taking 5 years to reach the 3rd centile.

Case 21

A. V. Now aged 10½ years. This girl was diagnosed as suffering from hypothyroidism at the age of 5¼ years. Her height was 36½ inches (height age 2 years) and the skeletal age was 1½ years. On thyroid therapy the skeletal age became chronological in 2 years (6 years advancement) but the height did not reach the 10th centile for 3 years. Her height has travelled along the 10th centile since.

B.4(*c*). Corticosteroid Excess

The hormones of the adrenal cortex—hydrocortisone, cortisone and its synthetic analogues—are well known to cause both retardation of linear growth and of skeletal maturation. The pathogenesis of these changes is uncertain. The obvious explanation is that of gluconeogenesis. If protein is converted to carbohydrate then less is available for bone growth and for skeletal maturation.

Case 22

R. K. This boy, aged $8\frac{1}{2}$ years, was $43\frac{1}{2}$ inches tall at the time of the operation of bilateral adrenalectomy for Cushing's syndrome. During the subsequent year his height advanced to 49 inches and the skeletal maturation advanced by four years.

The effect of exogenous cortisone on linear growth is described on p. 213.

B.4(d). Androgens and Œstrogens

Hormones which accelerate skeletal maturation faster than they advance linear growth will eventually retard growth. This has long been recognised as occurring in untreated congenital virilising adrenal hyperplasia. Œstrogens have been claimed to have this same dissociated action and they have therefore been used to promote epiphyseal closure in girls who are growing very tall (see below).

B.5. Factors Disturbing Cellular Nutrition
B.5(a). Tissue Hypoxia

Anæmia. Retardation of growth accompanies *chronic anæmia* from any cause. In some types of anæmia there may be associated factors contributing to growth retardation. In nutritional anæmia there may be a deficiency of other nutrients in addition to iron; also recurrent infection is common. In sickle-cell anæmia, recurring illness associated with thromboses may retard growth. In hæmolytic anæmia, steroid therapy may complicate growth patterns. In spherocytic anæmia, growth retardation has been described, remedied by splenectomy, and in this disease complicating factors are unusual and hypoxæmia may be the only cause of retarded growth.

Congenital cardiac disease. Campbell and Reynolds (1949) found some correlation between the severity of cyanosis and the degree of growth retardation in congenital heart disease. Mehrizi and Drash (1962) have recently reviewed their experience of growth patterns in congenital cardiac disorders. Growth retardation had occurred in the majority of their patients. It was greater in degree in cyanotic than in acyanotic lesions; and was least demonstrable in patients with coarctation of the aorta. Umansky and Hauck (1962) report that of 444 patients with patent ductus arteriosus, more than three times the expected number fell at or below the 10th centile for height, while 20% of the patients showed marked acceleration of linear growth post-operatively. Patients with pure pulmonary stenosis showed the greatest acceleration of growth rates after operation. Another possible mechanism involved in defective growth in congenital cardiac disease is diminished peripheral blood flow. An associated factor may be the frequent respiratory infections occurring in some types of lesion.

B.5(b). Renal Disease

Chronic renal disease produces growth retardation, and when the renal disease can be corrected the child returns to his normal growth pattern.

The important factors in causing growth retardation are chronic acidosis and anorexia (West and Smith 1956). The acidosis presumably acts by causing a harmful change in the cellular milieu and by retarding cell multiplication.

Retardation of growth occurs in aminoacidurias (see above). This has been attributed to loss of aminoacids in the urine, but, as in the Fanconi-de Toni-Debré syndrome, chronic renal acidosis may constitute an additional factor.

B.5(c). Hepatic Disease

Although there is no doubt that growth retardation occurs in chronic hepatitis, Sherlock (1963) drew attention to the fact that in adolescent girls with chronic liver disease acceleration of growth rates and pubertal changes occur. This appeared inexplicable until clinical evidence was produced (see below) that œstrogen is indeed a growth-promoting agent in adolescent girls. The interference with the conjugation of œstrogen in the liver has been regarded as the cause of gynæcomastia occurring in men and boys suffering from chronic liver disease, and the same mechanism must be invoked for the exaggerated adolescent growth spurt in girls.

The retardation of growth in glycogen storage disease is explained by the increased utilisation of protein (in the absence of glycogen) for daily metabolic needs (Bridge and Holt 1945, Hubble 1957) and a similar explanation is required for the dwarfism of the Mauriac syndrome occurring in inadequately treated diabetic children. The features of the Mauriac syndrome are dwarfism and hepatomegaly; the liver enlargement is caused by the deposit of glycogen and fat, and the syndrome is completely corrected by the provision of long-acting insulins, which prevent long periods of hyperglycæmia and nonmobilisation of glycogen (Hubble 1957). The mechanism of growth retardation is presumably the same as that occurring in glycogen storage disease, in Cushing's syndrome and in the therapeutic use of cortisone, i.e. the nonavailability of protein for linear growth.

The Effect of Drugs on Stature

Protein anabolic drugs. "Can a man by taking thought add a cubit to his stature?" The modern answer is that the growth rate of children can be accelerated, but that, except in the special cases where some specific replacement therapy can be used as in the treatment of hypothyroidism, there is as yet no certainty that the protein anabolic drugs will achieve an increase of ultimate height. All these drugs are weak androgens and therefore they accelerate skeletal maturation, and the estimate of the positive advantage gained by their use depends on the measurement of height gain, on the degree of skeletal advancement and on the prediction of ultimate height. The second and third of these criteria are both liable to error, for various reasons, and most cautious observers have not yet been persuaded out of their sceptical approach to such therapy (Bongiovanni 1961, Hubble and Macmillan 1962). Even the sceptics agree that, despite these uncertainties, it is often justifiable to treat the late maturing boy with these agents, providing that the courses of treatment are interrupted, and providing that 6–12 months is allowed to elapse before treatment is resumed. The reason for this interruption is that skeletal maturation continues at an increased rate even after treatment is stopped. The cause of this is unknown. The same observation can be made in congenital virilising hyperplasia. Once corticotrophin is suppressed and the hyperplasia is checked, retardation of the rate of growth occurs promptly, but acceleration of skeletal maturation proceeds unchecked for any period up to a year.

Growth hormone. The use of human growth hormone is not subject to this limitation—epiphyseal maturation is not disproportionately accelerated. This is true replacement therapy in hypopituitarism, and growth in the first 4 months of treatment may be accelerated to six or seven times the rate observed during the pre-treatment period. In some hypopituitary dwarfs the hormone has been effective for more than 5 years and the children continue to grow at two to three times the pre-treatment rate. Each child requires 6–10 mg. weekly, and Blizzard (1963) calculates that the full use of the pituitaries from every possible autopsy would permit treatment of 4000 children in the United States—and presumably more than 1000 children in this country. So far in Great Britain the Medical Research Council has only liberated small amounts for research purposes.

Œstrogen and arrest of height. Hormones have been used to retard growth in children suffering from gigantism or in those with a tall inheritance whose predicted height is thought to be excessive. Most parents would wish their daughters to be less than 6 feet tall, while most parents will accept without distress a height for their sons of from 6 feet 4 inches to 6 feet 6 inches. Advice is therefore more often sought concerning the possibility of checking the too rapid growth of girls.

The treatment of gigantism or excessively tall stature, when considered desirable, depends on the use of œstrogen in girls and methyl testosterone in boys. Both these preparations have the effect of advancing skeletal maturation and thus promoting earlier closure of the epiphyses. If these drugs are used their side-effects must be accepted. Both will depress the production of sex-hormones from the anterior pituitary, and therefore interfere with the development of the gonads. However, the evidence provided by the use of contraceptive preparations suggests that these effects are reversible. Girls treated with œstrogen will develop uterine bleeding and breast enlargement. These side effects require careful consideration before therapy is undertaken.

Bayley and his colleagues (1962), in a careful study, suggested that œstrogen therapy did not suppress growth when statistically adequate groups were treated. The value of their exemplary inquiry appears to have been spoilt by the fact that their girl patients were too old before treatment was begun. Whitelaw and Foster (1962) emphasised that treatment should be started before the age of 12 as the growth potential remaining after this age was too small to allow therapy to be successful. The five girls treated by these authors were between the ages of 8½ years and 11. Three of their patients were followed for 3 years, and two for 2 years. The average advancement of skeletal maturation was 2½ years in one year of treatment. The interesting fact which has emerged from all such observations is that, at least in most subjects, œstrogen is a stimulant to growth. Whitelaw and Foster's patients averaged 11·3 cm. (4½ inches) of growth in the first year of treatment. A more recent report by these authors arrives at a similar conclusion (Whitelaw, Foster and Graham 1963). Œstrogen has not been regarded as playing any part in the prepubertal growth spurt in girls (Tanner 1962), but this further clinical evidence makes it probable that it is indeed one of the hormones responsible.

In summary, it may be said that while such treatment is rarely necessary in boys, it may occasionally be used in girls, but then always before the age of 12.

Steroids and growth retardation. Blodgett et al. (1956) reported that doses of cortisone above 50 mg./sq.m. of body surface per day would retard growth in a majority of children and Van Metre and his colleagues (1960) have observed that cortisone in comparable doses produced less growth inhibition than did prednisone.

In the treatment of chronic asthma by long continued steroid therapy Falliers and his colleagues (1963) found that linear growth rates were satisfactory when no more than 50 mg. of cortisone, 5 mg. prednisone and 0·37 mg. betamethasone were used per square m. of body surface per day— approximately therefore in ratios of 135 (cortisone) to 13·5 (prednisone) to 1 (betamethasone). The potency of steroids has usually been first assessed in terms of anti-inflammatory activity in rheumatoid arthritis, when weight for weight the methasones have been reported to be 30–50 times, and prednisone and prednisolone 4–5 times, as effective as cortisone. The evidence provided by these authors, and by Van Metre et al., is that the growth retarding effect of the methasones is 100 times and prednisone 10 times that of cortisone, weight for weight. The therapist treating diseases such as asthma, nephrosis and adrenocortical hyperplasia should bear these facts in mind, even though his primary objective is always to obtain the maximal therapeutic effect with the smallest possible dose. It seems probable that the effect on growth is associated with the steroid's anti-anabolic action on protein deposition. Experiments in rats suggest that cortisone inhibits growth by amino-acid deprivation, produced by a uniform increase in amino-acid transport or metabolism by all cells (Szentivanyi et al. 1961).

Intractable asthma will itself produce growth retardation, and a growth spurt has actually been observed in such children when steroid therapy improves their clinical condition (Falliers et al. 1963). Another fact which should always be remembered in hormonal therapy is that there is a considerable variation in individual response, and this variation is well seen in the growth-retarding effects of steroid therapy (see also Chapter 12, p. 299).

REFERENCES

AARSKOG, D. (1963) Human growth hormone in dwarfism since birth. *Amer. J. Dis. Child.* **105**, 368

ACHESON, R. M. (1959) The environment and the growth of children. *Irish J. med. Sci.* **11**, 11

ANDERSEN, H. J. (1960) Studies of hypothyroidism in childrem. *Acta pœdiat., Suppl.* 125

ANDERSON, C. M., TOWNLEY, R. R. W., FREEMAN, M., JOHANSEN, P. (1961) Unusual causes of steatorrhœa in infancy and childhood. *Med. J. Aust.* **2**, 617

BAIRD, J. D., FARQUHAR, J. W. (1962) Insulin secreting capacity in infants of normal and diabetic women. *Lancet*, **1**, 71

BAYER, L. M., BAYLEY, N. (1959) *Growth Diagnosis*. Univ. Chicago Press

BAYLEY, N., GORDAN, G. S., BAYER, L. M., GOLDBERG, M. B., STORMENT, A. (1962) Attempt to suppress growth in girls by œstrogen treatment: statistical evaluation. *J. clin. Endocr.* **22**, 1127

BLIZZARD, R. M. (1963) The past, present and future of pituitary growth hormone. *Amer. J. Dis. Child.* **106**, 439

BLODGETT, F. M., BURGIN, L., IEZZONI, D., GRIBETZ, D., TALBOT, N. B. (1956) Effects of prolonged cortisone therapy on the stature, growth, skeletal maturation and metabolic status of children. *New Engl. J. Med.* **254**, 636

BONGIOVANNI, A. M. (1961) Anabolic drugs to promote growth. *Pediatrics*, **27**, 519

BRIDGE, E. M., HOLT, L. E. JR. (1945) Glycogen storage disease: observation on the pathologic physiology of two cases of the hepatic form of the disease. *J. Pediat.* **27**, 299

CAMPBELL, M., REYNOLDS, G. (1949) Physical and mental development of children with congenital heart disease. *Arch. Dis. Childh.* **24**, 294

COLLIS, J. E., LEVI, A. J., MILNE, M. D. (1963) Stature and nutrition in cystinuria and Hartnup disease. *Brit. med. J.* **1**, 590

DUTTON, G. (1959) The physical development of mongols. *Arch. Dis. Childh.* **34**, 56

FALLIERS, C. J., TAN, L. S., SZENTIVANYI, J., JORGENSEN, J. R., BUKANTZ, S. C. (1963) Childhood asthma and steroid therapy as influences on growth. *Amer. J. Dis. Child.* **105**, 127

GREENWOOD, F. C., HUNTER, W. M., MARRIAN, V. J. (1964) Growth hormone levels in children and adolescents. *Brit. med. J.* **1**, 25

GRUMBACH, M. S., WERNER, S. C. (1956) Transfer of thyroid hormone across the human placenta at term. *J. clin. Endocr.* **16**, 1392

HILLMAN, D. A., NEYZI, O., PORTER, P., CUSHMAN, A., TALBOT, N. B. (1958) Renal (vasopressin resistant) diabetes insipidus: definition of the effects of a homeostatic limitation in capacity to conserve water on the physical and emotional development of a child. *Pediatrics*, **21**, 430

HUBBLE, D. V., MACMILLAN, D. R. (1962) A study of growth promotion in children. *Arch. Dis. Childh.* **37**, 518

HUBBLE, D. V. (1957) Hormonal influence on growth. *Brit. med. J.* **1**, 601

JONES, P. R. M., DEAN, R. F. A. (1956) The effects of kwashiorkor on the development of the bones of the hand. *J. trop. Pediat.* **2**, 51

LAURANCE, B. (1961) Proc. 32nd Annual Meeting Brit. Pædiat. Assoc., *Arch. Dis. Childh.* **36**, 690

LEMLI, L., SMITH, D. W. (1963) The XO syndrome. *J. Pediat.* **63**, 577

LLOYD, J. K., WOLFF, O. H., WHELEN, W. S. (1961) Obesity in childhood—a long term study of the height and weight. *Brit. med. J.* **2**, 145

MACGREGOR, M. E., WHITEHEAD, T. P. (1954) Pseudoparathyroidism: a description of three cases and a critical appraisal of earlier accounts of the disease. *Arch. Dis. Childh.* **29**, 398

MACMILLAN, D. R. (1961) Proc. 32nd Annual Meeting Brit. Pædiat. Assoc., *Arch. Dis. Childh.* **36**, 690

MALTHUS, T. R. (1798) *First Essay on Population*. Johnson, London

MARTIN, M., WILKINS, L. (1958) Pituitary dwarfism. *J. clin. Endocr.* **18**, 679

MEHRIZI, A., DRASH, A. (1962) Growth disturbance in congenital heart disease. *J. Pediat.* **61**, 418

MELLMAN, W. J., BONGIOVANNI, A. M., HOPE, J. W. (1959) The diagnostic usefulness of skeletal maturation in an endocrine clinic. *Pediatrics*, **23**, 530

NADLER, H. L., NEWMANN, L. L., GERSHBERG, H. (1963) Hypoglycæmia, growth retardation and probable isolated growth hormone deficiency in a one year old child. *J. Pediat.* **63**, 977

PARK, E. A. (1954) Bone growth in health and disease. *Arch. Dis. Childh.* **29**, 269

PATTON, R. G., GARDNER, L. I. (1962) Influence of family environment on growth: The syndrome of maternal deprivation. *Pediatrics*, **30**, 957.

PRADER, A., LABHART, A., WILLI, H. (1956) Ein Syndrom von Adipositas, Kleinwuchs, Kryptorchismus und Oligophrenie nach myatonieartigem Zustand im Neugeborenenalter. *Schweiz. med. Wschr.* **86**, 1260

PRADER, A., WILLI, H. (1961) Das Syndrom von Imbezillität, Adipositas, Muskelhypotonie, Hypogenitalismus, Hypogonadismus und Diabetes mellitus mit "Myatonie"—Anamnese. *IInd Internat. Congr. Mental Deficiency*, Vienna

PRADER, A., TANNER, J. M., VON HARNACH, G. A. (1963) Catch-up growth following illness or starvation. *J. Pediat.* **62**, 646

RAVICK, L., RAPOPORT, I., SEEFELDT, U. (1964) Bone development in Down's disease. *Amer. J. Dis. Child.* **107**, 7

READ, C. H. (1960) The immunologic assay of human growth hormone. *Clin. Endocr.* **1**, 598

RUSSELL, A. (1954) Syndrome of "intra-uterine" dwarfism recognisable at birth with cranio-facial dysostos, disproportionately short arms and other anomalies (five examples). *Proc. roy. Soc. Med.* **47**, 1040

SECKEL, H. P. G. (1960) Concepts relating the pituitary growth hormone to somatic growth of the normal child. *Amer. J. Dis. Child.* **99**, 349

SECKEL, H. P. G. (1960) *Bird Headed Dwarfs.* Thomas, Springfield, Ill.

SHELDON, W. S. (1959) Celiac disease. *Pediatrics*, **23**, 132

SHERLOCK, S. (1963) *Diseases of the Liver and Biliary System.* 3rd Ed., Blackwell, Oxford,

SINCLAIR, R. J. G., KITCHEN, A. H., TURNER, R. W. D. (1960) The Marfan Syndrome. *Quart. J. Med.* **29**, 19

SMITH, A., McKEOWN, T. (1955) Pre-natal growth of mongoloid defectives. *Arch. Dis. Childh.* **30**, 247

SOBEL, E. H., SILVERMAN, F. N., MARSHALL LEE, F. JNR. (1962) Chronic regional enteritis and growth retardation. *Amer. J. Dis. Child.* **103**, 569

STEENDIJK, R. (1962) Studies on growth in refractory rickets. *J. Pediat.* **60**, 340

SZENTIVANYI, A., RADORICK, J., TALMAGE, D. W. (1961) The effects of cortisone on the incorporation of S35 labelled amino acids into serum and tissue protein. *Fed. Proc.* **20**, 379

TALBOT, N. B., SOBEL, E. H., McARTHUR, J. W., CRAWFORD, J. D. (1952) *Functional Endocrinology.* Harvard Univ. Press

TANNER, J. M. (1961) *Education and Physical Growth.* Univ. Lond. Press, p. 46

TANNER, J. M. (1962) *Growth at Adolescence.* Blackwell, Oxford

TROWELL, H. C., DAVIES, J. N. P., DEAN, R. F. A. (1954) *Kwashiorkor.* Arnold, London

UMANSKY, R., HAUCK, A. J. (1962) Factors in the growth of children with patent ductus arteriosus. *Pediatrics*, **30**, 540

VAN METRE, T. E. JNR., NIERMANN, W. A., ROSEN, L. J. (1960) A comparison of the growth suppressive effect of cortisone, prednisone, and other adrenal cortical hormones. *J. Allergy*, **31**, 531

VEST, M., TALBOT, N. B., CRAWFORD, J. D. (1963) Dwarfism and hydronephrosis in diabetes insipidus. *Amer. J. Dis. Child.* **105**, 175

WARKANY, J., MONROE, B. B., SUTHERLAND, B. S. (1961) Intrauterine growth retardation. *Amer. J. Dis. Child.* **102**, 249

WEST, C. D., SMITH, W. C. (1956) An attempt to elucidate the cause of growth retardation in renal disease. *Amer. J. Dis. Child.* **91**, 460

WHITELAW, J. M., FOSTER, T. N. (1962) Treatment of excessive height in girls. *J. Pediat.* **61**, 566

WHITELAW, M. J., FOSTER, T. N., GRAHAM, W. H. (1963) Estradiol valenate: its effects in anabolism and skeletal age in the prepubertal girl. *J. clin. Endocr.* **23**, 1125

WIDDOWSON, E. M. (1951) Mental contentment and physical growth. *Lancet*, **2**, 152

WINTERS, R. W., GRAHAM, J. B., WILLIAMS, T. F., McFALLS, V. W., BURNETT, C. H. (1958) A genetic study of familial hypophosphataemia and vitamin D resistant rickets. *Medicine, Baltimore*, **37**, 97

WOLFF, O. H. (1955) Obesity in childhood. *Quart. J. Med.* **24**, 109

CHAPTER 9

OBESITY IN CHILDHOOD

O. H. WOLFF

OBESITY is the most frequent nutritional disturbance in rich countries. Many fat children become fat adults. Obesity presents a challenge to the pædiatrician because he is concerned with the health of the child as well as with prevention of adult morbidity and mortality which are increased by obesity.

Recognition

Obesity may be defined as the condition in which there is an excess of adipose tissue distributed more or less evenly over the body. The diagnosis is usually and reliably made by looking at and weighing the child. Children whose weight exceeds the mean weight for height and sex by 20% or more are obese, provided they are not œdematous. Many children whose weight exceeds the mean by only 10–20% are also too fat. Quaade (1955) and Börjeson (1962) regarded a weight which exceeds the mean by more than 2 standard deviations as excessive.

More direct estimates of body fat can be obtained by determination of total body water or by underwater weighing to determine the density of the body (Behnke, Feen and Welham 1942). These methods are valuable research tools but are too complicated for clinical practice. On the other hand, measurement of the thickness of skin folds including subcutaneous fat with a skin caliper is a simple method which deserves wider use (Hammond 1955). Heald and colleagues (1963) from a study of various measures of body fat and hydration in adolescent boys concluded that this technique using the Harpenden caliper provides a practical and accurate estimate of adiposity, and Fletcher (1962) found in adults that total body fat can be estimated from fat fold measurements.

Incidence

In Wakefield, Yorkshire, in 1960 as many as 2·7% of school children were found to be overweight (Chief Medical Officer of the Ministry of Education 1962). In the United States the incidence is even higher; Johnson, Burke and Mayer (1956a) classed 10% of a cross section of Boston school children as overweight. Börjeson (1962) in a survey of Stockholm school children noted peak incidences for the girls at the ages of 9·6 and 14·5 years, and for the boys at 11·7 and 14·5 years. The overall incidence was higher among children from the poorer social classes and was approximately the same for boys and girls. No systematic study of the incidence of obesity in children below school age appears to have been made.

Ætiology

The ætiology of childhood obesity is rarely simple and the search for a single responsible factor is almost always in vain. It is often impossible to separate cause from effect. Thus physical inactivity may be a cause of obesity—obesity may make a child inactive. An emotional disturbance may be a cause of obesity—obesity may make a child unhappy. Overnutrition has important metabolic effects, but the possibility that a primary metabolic deviation may be a cause of overnutrition cannot be excluded, though the evidence for such a sequence of events is not convincing.

Genetic factors. Edwards (1963) explained on theoretical grounds the difficulty, if not impossibility, of assessing the extent to which genetic factors play a part in the causation of common diseases. His observations apply to the ætiology of obesity. Genetic factors are undoubtedly important, but it is impossible to differentiate the effect of environment, which begins to act immediately after conception, from that of the numerous genes which must be involved in determining the food intake, physical activity, metabolic processes and growth potential of the individual.

Börjeson (1962) studied the incidence of obesity in the sibs of over-weight children and found it to be higher than in the sibs of the control group. Dizygotic twins showed no greater similarity in bodyweight than did other sibs. However, amongst the few monozygotic twins the incidence of obesity was higher than amongst others sibs. Edwards stressed the limitations of twin studies as a method for determining qualitatively the genetic basis of common disease. Similarly the birth weight of the infant destined to become obese cannot be used as a measure of the importance of genetic factors, because it will reflect not only the infant's genetic make up but also the intra-uterine environment, which in turn will depend on the mother's genetic make up and her environment. Thus in man there can be no answer to the question of the relative importance of heredity and environment in the ætiology of childhood obesity.

Appetite regulation and the hypothalamus. Anand (1961) reviewed our state of knowledge of the mechanisms that regulate food intake. The hypothalamus plays a central part in facilitating or inhibiting the various spinal and brain stem reflex mechanisms concerned in this regulation. In its turn the hypothalamus is under the influence of impulses from the frontal and temporal lobes. The aim of the appetite-regulating mechanism is to maintain normal body weight or, in other words, to adapt calorie intake to expenditure, taking into account calories needed for growth.

The hypothalamus is acted upon and responds to a number of peripheral stimuli. Mayer (1953) postulated the existence of a glucostatic regulating mechanism dependent on glucose utilisation as reflected by arterio-venous or capillary-venous glucose differences. This cannot be the only mechanism, however, because Quaade (1962) showed that hunger can be felt at a time when marked capillary-venous glucose differences exist. Kennedy (1953) suggested that the hypothalamic satiety mechanism is concerned with the prevention of an overall surplus of energy intake over expenditure which would cause excessive deposition of fat. He proposed that "lipostasis" could be achieved through sensitivity of the hypothalamus to the concentration of unspecified circulating metabolites which might depend on the amount of fat in the depots. Sensations received from the gastrointestinal tract are also important in the regulation of food intake.

Most of the experimental work on the place of the hypothalamus in maintaining normal body weight has been done on animals. In the human gross disturbances of the hypothalamus, such as occur with a craniopharyngioma, tuberculoma, or as a sequel of an attack of meningitis or encephalitis, are rare causes of obesity and are usually associated with other localising signs and symptoms. With a perfectly functioning appetite-regulating mechanism obesity will not occur, but an otherwise normal mechanism may fail for a variety of reasons. Like other regulating mechanisms, it functions best over a certain range of physiological activity. Thus when energy expenditure is below a certain level, such as in extreme physical inactivity or in hypothyroidism or conceivably in primary abnormalities of intermediary metabolism, it is more likely to fail than when energy expenditure is normal. Similarly emotional disturbances resulting in abnormal stimuli from the cerebrum may upset normal hypothalamic regulating mechanisms.

The hypothalamus may also influence fat deposition and mobilisation through the sympathetic nervous system, which innervates adipose tissue (Barnett 1962). Confalonieri, Mazzucchelli and Schlechter (1961) showed that in the rat denervation of adipose tissue depresses all metabolic activities, but lipid mobilisation is affected more than synthesis and deposition, with a consequent net increase in fat. Hypothalamic damage may also lead to obesity by reducing physical activity (Kennedy 1963).

Diet and physical activity. After Newburgh (1942) had shown that in most cases of obesity there is no gross disturbance of endocrine or alimentary function or of intermediary metabolism, it was widely assumed that overeating, i.e. gluttony, is the main cause. More recently interest has been revived in the energy output of obese people and particularly in their physical activity.

Diet. Johnson, Burke and Mayer (1956b) found the calorie intake of obese adolescent girls to be no higher, and in most cases lower than that of the non-obese controls. Peckos (1953) studied the calorie intake of children in relation to their physique and found that the stout endomorph had a lower mean intake than the slender ectomorph, the mesomorph having an intermediate intake. From our observations of children admitted to hospital for weight reduction we can confirm that many overweight children have a very low energy expenditure. An example is that of a 12 year old girl who weighed 82 kg. when she was admitted to hospital. She was given a 300 cal. diet during the next 129 days and lost 21 kg., an average weight loss of 0·16 kg. per day. She was therefore in negative calorie balance to the extent of approximately 1300 calories per day (1 kg. of human fat being equivalent to approximately 8250 cal.). On a diet of 1700 cal. this girl would not have lost weight. On an average daily calorie intake for her age of 2500 cal. (Burke *et al.* 1959), she would have continued to gain excessive weight. If overeating means eating more than other children of the same age and sex, it appears to be uncommon, and many fat children have been unjustly accused of gorging themselves.

It is not possible to generalise about the proportion of calories these children obtain from carbohydrate, fat or protein. There is a tendency for overweight children, particularly those from poorer families, to eat an excess of carbohydrates. Foods such as chocolate, ice-cream, biscuits, cakes and sugary drinks make up a disproportionate part of their diet and protein may even be deficient. Yudkin (1963) stressed the undesirability of such a diet rich in refined and processed carbohydrate foods and Kemp (1963) coined the term "carbohydrate addiction." Not all obese children eat this type of diet; the adolescent girls studied by Johnson, Burke and Mayer (1956b) ate no more carbohydrate than the controls.

It is equally impossible to generalise about the periodicity of eating in overweight children. Some eat at frequent intervals and take much carbohydrate containing food between the conventional meals; others have just one or two meals a day; yet others take the three or four conventional meals. The periodicity of food intake cannot be ignored in a consideration of calorie equilibrium and intermediary metabolism. Cohn (1961) observed that the carcasses of rats fed twice daily by stomach tube contained almost twice as much body fat as those of animals freely eating the same amount of food. "Gorging" as opposed to "nibbling" may predispose to the deposition of body fat in the human as it does in the rat, because all animals have a very limited capacity for storing calories in any form other than fat (Gwinup et al. 1963).

Physical activity. The study of this aspect of energy equilibrium is held back by the lack of simple techniques to measure ordinary everyday physical activity. It is now recognised that food intake and physical activity must always be considered together. Mayer and colleagues (1954) showed in the rat that over the range of moderate physical activity calorie intake decreases with decreasing physical activity, so that weight remains constant. When, however, physical activity is further reduced, calorie intake increases and the animal gains weight. Passmore (1958) made the same observation in the dog and Kennedy (1963) stressed the importance of decreased activity as a factor in the production of hypothalamic obesity in rats. Using a treadmill he found that a normal rat would run abut 20 km. a day, but after destruction of the ventro-medial nuclei of the hypothalamus activity decreased almost to zero and simultaneously the animal's weight increased. From their study of obese girls Johnson, Burke and Mayer (1956b) concluded that marked inactivity accounted for a positive calorie balance in the face of a calorie intake which was no greater and often smaller than in the controls. In another study of schoolchildren these authors (1956a) found that there was a tendency to gain excess weight in late autumn, winter and early spring. They suggested that this was due to the reduced activity during these seasons compared with summer. Stunkard (1958) used a mechanical pedometer for the measurement of physical activity as reflected in the mileage walked; this instrument is cheap and simple to use and deserves wider application in the study of physical activity. Even when obese children take part in sports they tend to be less active than the non-obese. Mayer (1963), using cinematography, showed that obese girls when playing tennis were stationary on the court for 80% of the time.

In a consideration of the energy expended by obese children account must be taken not only of the amount of physical exercise they take but also of the small movements that occur to a greater or lesser extent when people stand, sit or even lie and which are not recorded by the pedometer. Widdowson (1962) stressed the very great individual variation in calorie requirements and suggested that, whereas when a person is having his oxygen consumption measured he is expected to lie, sit and stand still, under more natural circumstances these accompanying movements may use up much energy. Rose and Williams (1961) found that fidgeting increased oxygen consumption by 80%. Anybody dealing with children knows that many cannot keep still for a moment during the waking hours and some are even restless in their sleep. In contrast the immobility of many obese children is remarkable. When a fat child is admitted to hospital for weight reduction, home treatment having failed, it is usually easier to persuade him not to eat more than the prescribed diet than to encourage him to become more active.

Enforced inactivity is of special importance in the causation of obesity in the child who is confined to bed for long periods, in the child with cerebral palsy other than the athetoid variety, primary muscle disease or other hypotonic states and in some mentally retarded children. Once a child has become overweight the accumulation of fat will further interfere with activity and the child feels too embarrassed to engage in sports. At this stage, not uncommonly, the doctor plays his part in the completion of a vicious circle by forbidding the child to take part in strenuous exercise.

Psychological considerations. Emotional factors can play a part in the causation of obesity by influencing not only food intake but also physical activity and possibly metabolic processes. Bruch (1943) in her studies of obesity in New York children found in many of the families a disturbed parent child relationship: the mother's feelings towards the child, often an only one, are ambivalent; she rejects him and at the same time overprotects and overfeeds him; the child becomes overdependent on his mother and comes to identify food with love. The child's physical inactivity may serve mother's need of offering services to a passively accepting child and the child is appreciated for the rôle which he fulfils in the emotional life of his parents, usually his mother. Quaade (1955) from a study of obesity in Danish children was unable to confirm Bruch's hypothesis but nevertheless concluded that less specific psychological factors are of importance in determining a child's attitude to food.

Probably several psychological mechanisms play a part in the causation of obesity (Apley and MacKeith 1962). Most parents regard a good weight gain in their child as evidence of health and proper parental care. It is difficult for them to recognise when the gain is becoming excessive. The modern pædiatrician teaches that it is impossible to overfeed a healthy infant. Do we play our part in the causation of obesity? The warning that overfeeding may be dangerous is not out of place at any time after the first 4–6 months of life. Overprotection and overfeeding often go together, but it is probably incorrect to assume that overfeeding is invariably the result of an ambivalent mother-child relationship. For some mothers, particularly from poorer homes, the giving of plenty of food to their children is simply and understandably their way of expressing concern and sincere affection. Other mothers are insecure and need to keep their child closely attached to themselves; they use food especially sweets, ice-cream, etc., to maintain this close relationship and often at the same time complain that the child will not eat a proper meal. Apley and MacKeith coin the term "persistent umbilical cord syndrome." Such mothers often also prevent their children from taking part in sports.

From the child's point of view overeating may result from a need for oral gratification as a substitute for other forms of emotional satisfaction or as a means of gaining parental approval. An uncontrolled craving for food may then develop (Trethowan 1963).

The attitude of the doctor who looks after the overweight child is also of interest. Recently pædiatricians have become more concerned with the emotional problems of their patients and their families and have developed certain skills in dealing with the less severe disturbances without the help of a child psychiatrist. However, when dealing with the overweight child we tend to be less patient, less interested in the emotional background and more ready to suggest that the mother is overfeeding the child or that the child is greedy. Yet many overweight children eat less than do non-obese children of the same age. Further, when the dietary advice is not followed by weight loss we are too ready to assume, sometimes rightly sometimes wrongly, that the prescribed diet has not been followed and accordingly reprimand mother and child. If by the next visit weight loss has still not occurred the family may be labelled unco-operative and it is hinted that there is little more we can do for them. We tend to become irritable with our patients and their parents when deep-seated emotional problems prevent them from accepting our well-intentioned advice. The doctor's unconscious feelings about the significance of food presumably play a part in determining his attitude towards the obese child and his family.

The importance of emotional factors varies greatly from child to child and can only be assessed for the individual child by careful history taking, mother and child being interviewed separately and the doctor ridding himself, as far as possible, of preconceived ideas.

It is often difficult or impossible to differentiate between psychological causes of obesity and the effects of the obesity on the psyche. Most overweight children are teased about their appearance and withdraw from the company of other children into an even more inactive existence. They become too embarrassed to engage in active pursuits. Again a vicious circle is set up.

Metabolic Aspects

Though great variations exist in the diet and physical activity of overweight children, nevertheless in the individual child obesity can only result from a calorie intake in excess of that child's requirements. It is probably immaterial whether the excess is taken mainly as carbohydrate, fat or protein. If the excess consists of carbohydrate, only a small proportion can be stored as glycogen (the liver of a child weighing 30 kg. cannot store more than about 100 g. of glycogen), the remainder will be converted into fat and stored in the fat depots; to this process there is no limit. If the excess consists of fat, it will again be stored in the fat depots. If the excess consists of protein, part will be used to form new body protein, i.e. it will stimulate growth; but the child's growth potential is limited by factors other than nutritional, and the remainder of the protein will be converted into carbohydrate and fat and then be stored to a limited extent as glycogen and mainly as depot fat. Even when protein intake is not in excess, a high total calorie intake will spare protein for increased anabolism, i.e. for accelerated growth. Thus the outstanding consequence of overnutrition is increased deposition of depot fat derived from dietary fat and from conversion of protein and carbohydrate into fat.

Certain metabolic changes result from overnutrition. Whether primary metabolic disturbances also play an important or frequent rôle in the causation of obesity is not yet clear. In a consideration of this possibility it is essential to bear in mind the concept of nutritional individuality (Widdowson 1962). In normal individuals, who maintain a steady body weight, there exists a wide variation in calorie intake from one person to another. Widdowson found that of twenty or more normal boys in every yearly age group from 1 to 18 there was without exception one who ate enough food to provide twice as many calories as the food of another. Big children did not necessarily take the most calories and the calorie intake per kg. body weight varied nearly as much as the total calorie intake. If we understood the factors responsible for this great variability among individuals of normal weight, we might find it easier to explain why some children become obese on a calorie intake which would not be excessive for another child of the same age and sex. Why are the energy requirements of some obese children so low? The basal metabolic rate of most overweight children is normal when related to surface area, and increased in relation to chronological and height age (Mossberg 1948). Their expenditure of calories for a given amount of muscular work is increased because body movements involve greater physical exertion than they do in normal children. The importance of differences in physical activity has already been mentioned. The efficiency with which food is absorbed from the intestine also varies from individual to individual. Long-term balance studies of overweight and normal children are needed to show whether overweight children tend to absorb food more efficiently. However, as the normal child absorbs as much as 95% of ingested calories it is *a priori* unlikely that increased absorption could play more than a minor role in determining the low calorie requirements of many overweight children. The specific dynamic action of food has to the author's knowledge not been determined in a series of overweight children, but Strang, McClugage and Evans (1931) found it to be no lower in the obese adult than in the non-obese.

Adipose Tissue and Intermediary Metabolism

Adipose tissue. In biochemical terms obesity may be defined as the condition in which the rate of synthesis and laying down of fat in adipose tissue greatly exceeds that of its mobilisation from that tissue. A knowledge of the nature and functions of adipose tissue is therefore essential for an understanding of obesity (Kekwick 1960).

Composition. Wishnofsky (1952) assumed an average fat content of human fatty tissue of 87% and calculated that the calorie equivalent of 1 kg. is approximately 8250 kcal. Whether variations occur in the gross composition of human fatty tissue is not yet established. Morse and Soeldner (1963) observed a mean water fraction of adipose tissue of 15%, with no difference between obese and non-obese subjects. On the other hand, Pawan and Clode (1960) and Thomas (1962) found adipose tissue from obese subjects to contain rather less water. According to Thomas, biopsy specimens from non-obese subjects have the following composition: fat 82·8%, water 13·5%, protein 2·6%; and from obese subjects: fat 88·2%, water 9·6%, protein 2%. He concluded that the total amount of cellular tissue is also increased in the obese subject because with a 2–3 fold increase in total body fat the percentage of protein in adipose tissue was only slightly less than in the non-obese. Similarly Peckham, Entenman and Carroll (1962) concluded from a study of the influence of a high calorie diet on the composition of adipose tissue in the rat that adipose tissue retains the capacity for forming new cells for at least the first 34 weeks of the animal's life. When the overfed rats were placed on an ordinary diet, they reverted to normal weight and normal body composition. However, a basic difference persisted between these rats and the controls: when the high calorie diet was reintroduced, the rats which had previously been overweight showed a weight increase 40% greater than the control animals fed the same high calorie diet. The authors suggested that the greater weight gain may be related to the greater number of adipose tissue cells in the rats that had once been obese. Perhaps some similar mechanism explains at least in part the strong liability in the human for obesity to relapse after successful weight reduction.

Insulating effect of subcutaneous adipose tissue. Quaade (1963) measured skin and deep subcutaneous temperatures in normal, lean and obese subjects and observed that during exposure to cold the deep subcutaneous temperature fell much less in the obese than in the other subjects. In neutral room temperature the obese group had lower skin temperatures and higher deep subcutaneous temperatures than the other groups. Such effective subcutaneous insulation probably limits the obese person's calorie expenditure and may be one reason why obesity often persists in the absence of gross overeating.

Metabolic activity of adipose tissue. The lipid stored in adipose tissue is almost entirely triglyceride (glycerol esterified with three fatty acids). Much of the body's requirement for energy is supplied by adipose tissue in the form of free fatty acids, which have an extremely rapid turnover rate. Adipose tissue is thus a highly active tissue from which fatty acids are constantly being released and in which fatty acid synthesis into triglyceride takes place. It is also the major source of stored energy. Fatty acids required for synthesis of triglyceride reach adipose tissue from chylomicron triglyceride derived from ingested fat, from low-density lipoproteins and from the fatty acid-albumin complexes in which free fatty acids are carried in the blood. Fatty acids are also synthesised within the adipose tissue cells from glucose via acetyl coenzyme A (Fig.). Insulin is required for this process. Glucose and insulin are also needed to provide glycerol phosphate (Fig.), which is essential for the synthesis of triglyceride, adipose tissue being unable to utilise again for triglyceride synthesis the glycerol which has been formed by lipolysis of

triglyceride (Vaughan and Korn 1962). Finally, glucose metabolism is needed
to supply the energy for the synthesis of triglycerides.

Release of fatty acids from adipose tissue is enhanced by growth hormone,
ACTH, cortisol, thyroid-stimulating hormone, adrenaline and nor-adrenaline
(Winegrad 1962, Masoro 1962). Certain other lipid mobilising factors,
probably of pituitary origin, have been identified by Seifter and Baeder
(1957), Chalmers, Pawan and Kekwick (1960) and Rudman and colleagues
(1960), and their possible physiological rôles were discussed by Rudman

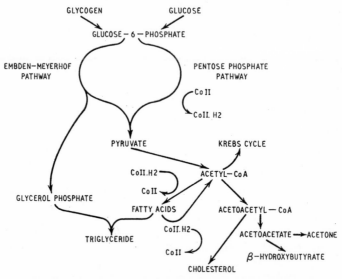

Inter-relationships between carbohydrate and fat metabolism.
(Only intermediates referred to in the text are included.)
CoII = nicotinamide adenine dinucleotide phosphate (NADP)
CoII . H$_2$ = reduced NADP = NADP H$_2$

(1963). Theoretically a deficiency of any of these factors could cause obesity
provided triglyceride synthesis was not simultaneously depressed. Evidence
in support of such a hypothesis is at present lacking.

Obesity and carbohydrate metabolism. When much triglyceride is being
formed requirements for insulin are great and Rabinowitz and Zierler (1961)
confirmed that hyperinsulinism occurs as an adaptive phenomenon in
obesity. Conceivably this secondary hyperinsulinism will further stimulate
appetite and complete a vicious circle. Primary hyperinsulinism is a rare
cause of obesity in children. After a period of adaptive hyperinsulinism
exhaustion of the β-cells of the islets of Langerhans may occur, and Weill and
Bernfeld (1957) found impaired glucose tolerance in one-third of the obese
children they investigated; after weight reduction glucose tolerance became
normal in two-thirds of the originally abnormal patients. Not many fat
children show the classical picture of diabetes mellitus, presumably because
it takes some years of adaptive hyperinsulinism before exhaustion of the
β-cells occurs.

Recently Vallance-Owen and Lilley (1961) suggested another mechanism to explain the coexistence of obesity and diabetes: they identified an insulin antagonist in the plasma of diabetic and "prediabetic" adults, which antagonises the action of insulin on glucose uptake by rat diaphragm, but not that on glucose uptake by adipose tissue. Compensatory hyperinsulinism then leads to increased synthesis of fatty acids and deposition of triglycerides. The high levels of insulin necessary to overcome the action of the antagonist on muscle might then lead to obesity before the diabetic disturbance of carbohydrate metabolism would become obvious. It is not known whether this insulin antagonist occurs with greater frequency in obese than non-obese children. Randle, Garland, Hales and Newsholme (1963) also suggested that obesity may be a feature of early diabetes rather than a cause and postulated the following sequence of events: in early diabetes, in spite of normal or raised plasma concentration of insulin, the rate of triglyceride breakdown in muscle and adipose tissue is increased in the fasting state and the resulting high plasma concentration of free fatty acids impairs sensitivity to insulin. After intake of food or glucose plasma concentration of insulin rises still higher, and as a result lipolysis is inhibited in adipose tissue but not in muscle and the concentration of free fatty acids falls. Under the continuing influence of high concentrations of insulin and glucose, synthesis of fatty acids and deposition of triglyceride takes place in adipose tissue at an abnormally high rate. Muscle glycerides however continue to be broken down at an excessive rate and the liberated free fatty acids lead to further insensitivity to insulin.

Ketosis. Kekwick, Pawan and Chalmers (1959) found obese adults to be less susceptible to fasting ketosis than non-obese subjects, and Passmore (1961) suggested that this relative resistance to fasting ketosis might be due to an increased supply of reduced coenzyme II ($CoII.H_2$) derived from an unusually active use of the pentose phosphate pathway (Fig.) for carbohydrate metabolism; $CoII.H_2$ would then accelerate fatty acid synthesis from acetyl-CoA rather than condensation of acetyl-CoA to form acetoacetyl-CoA and the three ketone bodies. Passmore postulated that an increased use of the pentose phosphate pathway and decreased use of the Embden-Meyerhof pathway might be a primary metabolic deviation contributing to the onset of obesity. However, there is now some doubt whether lipogenesis in the fasting state is limited by the rate of formation of $CoII \cdot H_2$ via the pentose phosphate pathway (Masoro 1962). In our experience obese children differ in this respect from obese adults and start to excrete large quantities of ketone bodies in the urine within 24–48 hours of being placed on a 300 cal. diet; this excretion continues for as long as they are given this diet.

Cholesterol. Serum cholesterol levels do not appear to have been studied systematically in obese children. In young men Tanner (1951) found a small correlation between the amount of subcutaneous fat and the level of serum cholesterol. Increased cholesterol synthesis from acetoacetyl-CoA (Fig.) is likely in overnutrition when glycolysis occurs at an increased rate and yet Krebs cycle activity is not significantly increased, unless fatty acid synthesis from acetyl-CoA proceeds at such a rate that no excess acetoacetyl-CoA is formed. $CoII.H_2$ is required for synthesis of cholesterol from acetoacetyl-

CoA and it is possible, though not proven, that an increased use of the pentose phosphate pathway for glycolysis may supply the coenzyme and thus stimulate cholesterol synthesis. A diet rich in animal fat, such as some overweight children eat, would also raise serum levels of cholesterol; the responsible mechanism has not yet been elucidated.

Other studies of intermediary metabolism. Knorr, Liebrich and Baitsch (1961) found that in the fasting state obese children have higher blood levels of free fatty acids than do children of normal weight. Pawan (1959, 1961) noted the same in adults and also observed that when adults are given a 1000 cal. diet, providing 90% of calories as fat, the non-obese subjects within a few days developed hypoglycæmia as well as marked ketonæmia and a negative nitrogen balance; whereas the obese subjects showed essentially no change in blood sugar, blood ketones or nitrogen balance. Pawan suggested that under these circumstances net conversion of fat into carbohydrate might occur. We have observed that obese children can be maintained on a 300 cal. diet containing 30 g. carbohydrate, 28 g. protein and 7 g. fat for several months without developing hypoglycæmia, though ketonuria occurs and growth in height slows down. These findings suggest that the obese subject during periods of calorie deprivation can obtain almost all his energy requirements from breakdown of fat and depends only to a limited extent on glucose metabolism. This low rate of glucose oxidation in certain obese subjects has recently been confirmed by Gordon and colleagues (1962). Whether these metabolic peculiarities of the obese should be regarded as fundamental factors in the causation of obesity or as the body's adaptation to overnutrition is not clear. There is need for such studies of intermediary metabolism to be repeated after the patient has regained and is maintaining normal weight. Only then will it be possible to differentiate between cause and effect.

Adrenocortical Function

The influence of body size on cortisol production and urinary corticoid excretion is recognised. Mlynaryk and colleagues (1962) and Migeon, Green and Eckert (1963) found cortisol production to be increased in obese subjects of various ages. In obese children and adolescents Cohen (1958) found the urinary excretion of 17-ketogenic steroids to be elevated, whereas 17-ketosteroid excretion was usually at the upper limit of normal or only slightly raised. Weight reduction was invariably associated with a fall in both 17-ketosteroid and 17-ketogenic steroid excretion. Thus overactivity of the adrenal cortex must be regarded as one of the effects of overnutrition, though in its turn it may aggravate the obesity.

The mechanisms responsible for the hyperadrenocorticism are not clear. Cohen suggested that overnutrition leads to hyperpituitarism which in turn leads to increased adrenocortical activity. Migeon and colleagues proposed that the increased adrenocortical activity is the body's means of counteracting the effects of adaptive hyperinsulinism on blood glucose levels (Rabinowitz and Zierler 1962). The hyperadrenocorticism could also be regarded as an adaptive process by means of which the excess protein, which cannot be used for anabolism—i.e. growth—is converted into carbohydrate and fat.

Adrenocortical overactivity is at least partly responsible for the striæ which are so frequently found in obese adolescents. Simkin and Arce (1962) provided evidence that these striæ are produced not only by stretching of the skin by rapid excessive subcutaneous fat deposition, but also by weakening of the elastic fibres of the skin by an increased production of corticosteroid hormone. Adrenocortical overactivity may also be responsible for the moderate hypertension which is not uncommon in overweight adolescents and which subsides as weight is lost. (When measuring the blood pressure of an overweight child with a fat upper arm, a wide arm band must be used; otherwise a false high reading will be obtained.) Hyperadrenocorticism may also contribute to the impaired carbohydrate tolerance of the obese child.

Difficulties in the differential diagnosis of obesity with secondary hyperadrenocorticism from Cushing's syndrome are infrequent. Cushing's syndrome is rare in childhood; the height is usually below average whereas in "simple" obesity it is usually above average; hirsutism and osteoporosis are frequent in Cushing's syndrome and glucose tolerance is usually more impaired than it is in simple obesity. In the rare instances where difficulty arises tests of the pituitary-adrenal axis are helpful. Simkin and Arce (1962) and Migeon, Green and Eckert (1963) found that the pituitary-adrenal axis of obese subjects responds normally to corticosteroid suppression and ACTH stimulation tests, or that it may even show some hyper-responsiveness to ACTH. In Cushing's syndrome the response is abnormal.

Development of Obese Children

Birth weight. Most infants who subsequently become obese have a normal birth weight (Bruch 1939, Wolff 1955, Haase and Hosenfeld 1956), but Börjeson (1962) found that the children who became overweight before the age of 7 had a slightly higher mean birth weight than the control group.

Onset of obesity. Reliable information is scarce and can only come from prospective studies of height and weight of a large number of children and ideally extending from birth to the end of adolescence. Börjeson (1962) suggested that the onset of obesity frequently coincides with, and is due to, the natural "fat spurts" (Tanner 1962).

Height. Bruch (1939), Mossberg (1948) and Wolff (1955) found the average height of obese children to be greater than the standard. The increased height is regarded as one of the effects of overnutrition. Quaade (1955) however found obese Copenhagen school-children to be no taller than their non-obese classmates. A possible explanation for this discrepancy is that the nutrition and general health of Scandinavian children is so good that they already achieve their maximum growth potential and therefore overnutrition cannot result in a further increase in height. Compatible with this explanation is the finding of Börjeson (1962) that the average height of Scandinavian school children, which, like in many other countries, had shown a secular trend to increase (Broman, Dahlberg and Lichtenstein 1942), has not further increased during the last decade. The observation of Wolff (1955) that the obese children in his series, though taller than normal children of various social classes, were not significantly taller than children of the professional class may lend some support to this speculation.

Just as height gain can be accelerated by overnutrition, so it can be slowed
down by a reduction in food intake and Wolff (1955) showed that the obese
children who during treatment lost weight rapidly gained in height about
20% less than expected; but those who failed to lose weight continued to
gain in height 5–10% more than the standard. A close inverse relationship
was shown to exist between rate of weight loss and height gain.

The unusual coexistence of obesity and an unexpectedly low height suggests
the presence of a factor counteracting the growth stimulus of overnutrition;
in such circumstances a diagnosis of hypothyroidism or Cushing's syndrome
has to be considered (Wolff 1962) (see Chapter 8, p. 195).

Lloyd, Wolff and Whelen (1961) showed that after obese children have
passed through puberty their average height is no longer above standard.

Skeletal maturation is usually advanced in relation to chronological age
and more consistent with the child's height age (Mossberg 1948).

Puberty. In obese girls puberty occurs on average half to one year sooner
than in the general population (Mossberg 1948, Wolff 1955). Contrary to
previously held beliefs, it is now established that the average onset of puberty
in obese boys is not delayed (Quaade 1955, Mossberg 1948) and may even be
advanced (Wolff 1955). Quaade further showed that the size of the testes
does not differ between obese and non-obese boys and that cryptorchidism is
no more frequent amongst the obese than the non-obese.

In Fröhlich's syndrome, a rare condition due to a space occupying lesion in the
region of the sella turcica, usually a craniopharyngioma, symptoms and signs of
increasing intra-cranial pressure and localising signs such as visual field defects
dominate the clinical picture, in which sexual infantilism and obesity are relatively unimportant. The terms "Fröhlich's syndrome" or "dystrophia adiposo-
genitalis" no longer serve a purpose and cause avoidable confusion.

That overnutrition speeds up a child's development is clear, but the
mechanisms responsible are not. Stimulation of anterior pituitary function
probably plays a part. Increased height gain with skeletal maturation consistent with height age is likely to be the result of increased secretion of
growth hormone. Concentrations of this hormone have not yet been systematically determined in obese children. The increased adrenocortical activity
and the early onset of puberty are also consistent with anterior pituitary
overactivity. Conceivably the substrate excess which results from a calorie
intake greater than the individual's requirements may directly lead to
adaptive hyperinsulinism and to increased adrenocortical activity, and it
may even cause the cells of the growing child to increase their protein anabolic
activity irrespective of increased hormonal stimulation.

Prognosis, Complications and Associated Conditions

Long-term prospective studies (Haase and Hosenfeld 1956, Abraham and
Nordsieck 1960, Lloyd, Wolff, and Whelen 1961, Börjeson 1962) show that
childhood obesity has a poor prognosis. Approximately four-fifths of overweight children will grow into overweight adults. For grossly overweight
children the outlook is even worse, and with advancing years many of these
patients become even more overweight. Children who lose weight during the
initial period of treatment often relapse later. The importance of childhood

obesity as a precursor of obesity in adult life was confirmed by Mullins (1958), who found that about one-third of adults attending an out-patient department were over-weight and that in one-third of these the obesity dated from childhood. The influence of overweight on morbidity and mortality of adults is recognised (Marks 1960) and it has been shown that weight reduction brings improved health and longevity. Even in childhood obesity has serious consequences. Börjeson (1962) showed that the obese child's circulatory adjustment to physical exercise is less adequate than that of the non-obese and that he therefore has a lowered physical working capacity. The obesity can become so extreme as to interfere with normal cardio-respiratory mechanisms giving rise to the "Pickwickian syndrome," which is characterised by alveolar hypoventilation, arterial hypoxæmia, polycythæmia, right heart failure and somnolence (Ward and Kelsey 1962). The deaths of three children from this condition have been reported. Flat feet, knock knee and an increased lumbar lordosis are less serious complications.

When obesity is found in association with another condition there is too often a tendency to postulate the existence of a syndrome in which the hypothalamus is usually implicated. Wolff (1962) suggested that before doing so at least three other possibilities must be considered.

(i) Chance association: with a condition as common as obesity it is to be expected that occasionally a second quite unrelated abnormality will be present, e.g. cryptorchidism.

(ii) The associated condition giving rise to the obesity: any condition that interferes with movement, e.g. hypotonic states, will predispose to obesity. Any child with constitutional growth retardation is unable to respond to relative overnutrition with increased growth in height and will then become fat. Mentally retarded children as a group are of below average height and this mechanism may operate in them. They are also prone to be given too much to eat because their parents find it difficult to show them their love except in the form of food.

(iii) Obesity giving rise to the associated condition: this applies to the "Pickwickian syndrome."

In the Laurence-Moon-Biedl syndrome there is probably a congenital malformation of the hypothalamus associated with other congenital defects.

Treatment

Present treatment is unsatisfactory and the following remarks are, therefore, to be interpreted not as recommendations based on successful experience but as suggestions deserving a trial. That childhood obesity needs treatment both for its own sake as well as because it is a precursor of adult obesity is clear.

Preventive treatment. This may be the most fruitful approach. The dangers of obesity should be brought home to parents. Such education must come mainly from general practitioners and infant welfare and school medical officers and should concern itself not only with the family's eating habits but also with physical exercise. The concept of nutritional individuality needs stressing. What is too much for one child may be too little for another of the same age.

Curative treatment. Early treatment is more likely to be successful. It is unwise to suggest that the child will spontaneously lose his "puppy fat," though occasionally this does happen. If, as a result of advice given, the weight returns to normal a check should thereafter be kept on the weight because the tendency to relapse is great, particularly just before and during puberty. The adolescent is easily embarrassed by his or her appearance and may become deeply depressed. Treatment should therefore be started before puberty. Fat girls at puberty develop enormous breasts which even after weight has been lost are not transformed into their normal attractive shape but become empty and pendulous.

Diet. This is still the essential of treatment. Despite earlier suggestions, Fletcher, McCririck and Crooke (1961) showed that, given a certain calorie intake, the composition of the diet has no effect on the rate of weight loss. Most but not all children will lose weight on a 1000 kcal. diet containing about 100 g. carbohydrate, 60 g. protein and 40 g. fat. If on this diet weight is not lost, one cannot assume that the child has eaten more and the daily intake may have to be reduced further to 800 or even 600 kcal.

Appetite suppressants. These have a limited place. If the child is finding it difficult to follow the diet, amphetamine sulphate or dexamphetamine sulphate may be used for a short period; their effect often wears off after a month or two. These drugs are habit forming but addiction is rare in children. The more recent appetite suppressants such as methylamphetamine, phenmetrazine (Preludin), diethylproprion, phentermine and chlorphentamine have no advantages over amphetamine (*British Medical Journal* 1963, MacGregor 1963).

Psychological approach. If more attention were paid to emotional factors, results might improve. Apley and McKeith (1962) outline the psychological approach. This is important whether emotional disturbances play a rôle in the causation of the obesity or not. Any weight reducing regime in itself is a great strain for the child and to be told that his or her appearance is not desirable and needs changing is an insult to a child's personality. If the parents are also fat, the doctor may well encounter strong unconscious opposition from the child—and the parent—when he suggests that obesity is not desirable. Tact is needed in handling this delicate situation. For children who are emotionally very disturbed insistence on a strict reducing diet is dangerous and may even precipitate anorexia nervosa; in the early stages of their treatment an entirely psychological approach is indicated.

Physical activity. The children should be encouraged to become physically more active.

Hospitalisation. For the grossly overweight child the results of treatment at home are so unsatisfactory that inpatient treatment deserves a trial. The dietitian can then provide a 300 cal. diet containing approximately 30 g. protein and carbohydrate and 7 g. fat. The nurses and physiotherapists ensure increased physical activity and the child is given friendly encouragement and if necessary systematic psychotherapy. Under this regime, which has been tried for the past few years at the Birmingham Children's Hospital, a daily weight loss of $\frac{1}{4}$–$\frac{1}{2}$ kg. occurs. When normal or near normal weight has been achieved the calorie content of the diet is slowly increased and it is often found that even on a relatively low calorie intake, e.g. 1000 cal. per day, the rate of weight gain once more becomes excessive. It is too soon to report on the ultimate outcome of such a regime, but it is already clear that, as with all obese patients, continued supervision is essential if relapse is to be avoided.

Conclusion

The ætiology of childhood obesity is multifactorial; physical inactivity and psychological factors deserve more attention than they have received. Overnutrition has important psychological, endocrine and metabolic effects. With present forms of treatment the prognosis is poor. More research is needed into the endocrine and metabolic consequences of overnutrition and the possibility that primary metabolic deviations may play a rôle in the ætiology also requires further investigation.

REFERENCES

ABRAHAM, S., NORDSIECK, M. (1960) Relationship of excess weight in children and adults. *Publ. Hlth. Rep., Wash.* **75**, 263

ANAND, B. K. (1961) Nervous regulation of food intake. *Physiol. Rev.* **41**, 677

APLEY, J., MACKEITH, R. (1962) *The Child and his Symptoms, a Psychosomatic Approach.* Blackwell, Oxford

BARNETT, R. J. (1962) The morphology of adipose tissue with particular reference to its histochemistry and ultrastructure, in *Adipose Tissue as an Organ* (Kinsell, L. W. ed.). Thomas, Springfield

BEHNKE, A. R., FEEN, B. G., WELHAM, W. C. J. (1942) Specific gravity of healthy men. *J. Amer. med. Assoc.* **118**, 495

BÖRJESON, M. (1962) Overweight children. *Acta Pœdiat.* **51**, suppl. 132

British Medical Journal (1963) Today's drugs: drugs for obesity. *Brit. med. J.* **2**, 853

BROMAN, B., DAHLBERG, G., LICHTENSTEIN, A. (1942) Height and weight during growth. *Acta pœdiat.* **30**, 1

BRUCH, H. (1939) Obesity in childhood, 1. *Amer. J. Dis. Child.* **58**, 457

BRUCH, H. (1943) Psychiatric aspects of obesity in children. *Amer. J. Psychiat.* **99**, 752

BURKE, B. S., REED, R. B., VAN DER BERG, A. S., STUART, H. C. (1959) Calorie and protein intakes of children between 1 and 18 years of age. *Pediatrics*, **24**, 922

CHALMERS, T. M., PAWAN, G. L. S., KEKWICK, A. (1960) Fat-mobilising and ketogenic activity of urine extracts: relation to corticotrophin and growth hormone. *Lancet*, **2**, 6

CHIEF MEDICAL OFFICER OF THE MINISTRY OF EDUCATION (1962) Report on the health of the school child, 1960 and 1961

COHEN, H. (1958) 17-ketogenic steroid excretion in obese children before and after weight reduction. *Brit. med. J.* **1**, 686

COHN, C. (1961) Meal-eating, nibbling and metabolism. *J. Amer. diet. Ass.* **38**, 433

CONFALONIERI, C., MAZZUCCHELLI, M. V., SCHLECHTER, P. (1961) The nervous system and lipid metabolism of adipose tissue. *Metabolism*, **10**, 324

EDWARDS, J. (1963) The genetic basis of common disease. *Amer. J. Med.* **34**, 627

FLETCHER, R. F. (1962) The measurement of total body fat with skinfold calipers. *Clin. Sci.* **22**, 333

FLETCHER, R. F., McCRIRICK, M. Y., CROOKE, A. C. (1961) Reducing diets, weight loss of obese patients on diets of different composition. *Brit. J. Nutr.* **15**, 53

GORDON, E. S., GOLDBERG, E. M., BRANDABUR, J. J., GEE, J. B. L., RANKIN, J. (1962) Abnormal energy metabolism in obesity. *Trans. Ass. Amer. Physns*, **75**, 118

GWINUP, G., BYRON, R. C., ROUSH, W., KRUGER, F., HAMWI, G. J. (1963) Effect of nibbling versus gorging on glucose tolerance. *Lancet*, **2**, 165

HAASE, K. E., HOSENFELD, H. (1956) Zur Fettsucht im Kindesalter. *Z. Kinderheilk.* **78**, 1

HAMMOND, W. H. (1955) Measurement and interpretation of subcutaneous fat, with norms for children and young adult males. *Brit. J.; rev. soc. Med.* **9**, 201

HEALD, F. P., HUNT, E. E., SCHWARTZ, R., COOK, C. D., ELLIOTT, O., VAJDA, B. (1963) Measures of body fat and hydration in adolescent boys. *Pediatrics*, **31**, 226

JOHNSON, M. L., BURKE, B. S., MAYER, J. (1956a) The prevalence and incidence of obesity in a cross-section of elementary and secondary school children. *Amer. J. clin. Nutr.* **4**, 231

JOHNSON, M. L., BURKE, B. S., MAYER, J. (1956b) Relative importance of inactivity and overeating in the energy balance of obese high school girls. *Amer. J. clin. Nutr.* **4**, 437

KEKWICK, A. (1960) On adiposity. *Brit. med. J.* **2**, 407

KEKWICK, A., PAWAN, G. L. S., CHALMERS, T. M. (1959) Resistance to ketosis in obese subjects. *Lancet*, **2**, 1157

KEMP, R. (1963) Carbohydrate addiction. *Practitioner*, **190**, 358

KENNEDY, G. C. (1953) The rôle of depot fat in the hypothalamic control of food intake in the rat. *Proc. roy. Soc. B.* **140**, 578

KENNEDY, G. C. (1963) Metabolism and obesity. *Brit. med. J.* **1**, 1149

KNORR, D., LIEBRICH, K. G., BAITSCH, H. (1961) Über das Verhalten der freien Fettsäuren des Blutes im Kindesalter. *Klin. Wschr.* **39**, 1143

LLOYD, J. K., WOLFF, O. H., WHELEN, W. S. (1961) Childhood obesity: a long-term study of height and weight. *Lancet*, **2**, 145

MacGREGOR, A. G. (1963) Appetite suppressants. *Prescribers' J.* **3**, 25

MARKS, H. H. (1960) Influence of obesity on morbidity and mortality. *Bull. N.Y. Acad. Med.* **36**, 296

MASORO, E. J. (1962) Biochemical mechanisms related to the homeostatic regulation of lipogenesis in animals. *J. Lipid Res.* **3**, 149

MAYER, J. (1953) Genetic, traumatic and environmental factors in the etiology of obesity. *Physiol. Rev.* **33**, 472

MAYER, J. (1963) quoted by PASSMORE, R. VIth Internat. Nutr. Congr. *Lancet*, **2**, 457

MAYER, J., MARSHALL, N. B., VITALE, J. J., CHRISTENSEN, J. H., MASHAYEKHI, M. B., STARE, F. J. (1954) Exercise, food intake and bodyweight in normal rats and genetically obese adult mice. *Amer. J. Physiol.* **177**, 544

MIGEON, C. J., GREEN, O. C., ECKERT, J. P. (1963) Study of adrenocortical function in obesity. *Metabolism*, **12**, 718

MLYNARYK, P., GILLIES, R. R., MURPHY, B., PATTEE, C. J. (1962) Cortisol production rates in obesity. *J. clin. Endocr.* **22**, 587

MORSE, W. I., SOELDNER, J. S. (1963) The composition of adipose tissue and the non-adipose body of obese and non-obese man. *Metabolism*, **12**, 99

MOSSBERG, H. O. (1948) Obesity in children. *Acta pœdiat.* **35**, suppl. 66

MULLINS, A. G. (1958) The prognosis in juvenile obesity. *Arch. Dis. Childh.* **33**, 307

NEWBURGH, L. H. (1942) Obesity. *Arch. intern. Med.* **70**, 1033

PASSMORE, R. (1958) A note on the relation of appetite to exercise. *Lancet*, **1**, 29

PASSMORE, R. (1961) On ketosis. *Lancet*, **1**, 839

PAWAN, G. L. S. (1959) Some aspects of the metabolism of the obese. *Proc. nutr. Soc.* **18**, 155

PAWAN, G. L. S. (1961) Some metabolic aspects of human obesity. *Proc. Ass. clin. Bioch.* **1**, 148

PAWAN, G. L. S., CLODE, M. (1960) The gross chemical composition of adipose tissue in the lean and obese human subject. *Biochem. J.* **74**, 9p

PECKHAM, S. C., ENTENMAN, C., CARROLL, H. W. (1962) The influence of a hypercaloric diet on gross body and adipose tissue composition in the rat. *J. Nutr.* **77**, 187

PECKOS, S. P. (1953) Caloric intake in relation to physique in children. *Science*, **117**, 631

QUAADE, F. (1955) *Obese Children*. Danish Science Press, Copenhagen

QUAADE, F. (1962) On the "glucostatic" theory of appetite regulation. *Amer. J. med. Sci.* **243**, 427

QUAADE, F. (1963) Insulation in leanness and obesity. *Lancet*, **2**, 429

RABINOWITZ, D., ZIERLER, K. L. (1961) Forearm metabolism in obesity and its response to intra-arterial insulin. *Lancet*, **2**, 690

RABINOWITZ, D., ZIERLER, K. L. (1962) Forearm metabolism in obesity. Characterisation of insulin resistance and evidence for adaptive hyperinsulinism. *J. clin. Invest.* **41**, 2173

RANDLE, P. J., GARLAND, P. B., HALES, C. N., NEWSHOLME, E. A. (1963) The glucose fatty-acid cycle. *Lancet*, **1**, 785

ROSE, G. A., WILLIAMS, R. T. (1961) Metabolic studies on small and large eaters. *Brit. J. Nutr.* **15**, 1

RUDMAN, D. (1963) The adipokinetic action of polypeptide and amine hormones upon the adipose tissue of various animal species. *J. Lipid Res.* **4**, 119

RUDMAN, D., DiGIOLAMO, M., KENDALL, F. E., WERTHEIM, A. R., SEIDMAN, F., REID, N. B., BERN, S. (1960) Further observations on the effect of pituitary gland extracts upon the serum lipids of the rabbit. *Endocrinology*, **67**, 784

SEIFTER, J., BAEDER, D. H. (1957) Lipid mobilizer (LM) from posterior pituitary of hogs. *Proc. Soc. exp. Biol., N.Y.* **95**, 318

SIMKIN, B., ARCE, R. (1962) Steroid excretion in obese patients with colored abdominal striae. *New Engl. J. Med.* **266**, 1031

STRANG, J. M., McCLUGAGE, H. B., EVANS, F. A. (1931) The nitrogen balance during dietary correction of obesity. *Amer. J. med. Sci.* **181**, 336

STUNKARD, A. (1958) Physical activity, emotions and human obesity. *Psychosom. Med.* **20**, 366

TANNER, J. M. (1951) The relation between serum cholesterol and physique in healthy young men. *J. Physiol.* **115**, 371

TANNER, J. M. (1962) *Growth at Adolescence.* 2nd Ed., Blackwell, Oxford

THOMAS, L. W. (1962) The chemical composition of adipose tissue of man and mice. *Quart. J. exp. Physiol.* **47**, 179

TRETHOWAN, W. H. (1963) Obesity, addiction and the amphetamines, in *Final Report on the Symposium on Obesity*, W. R. Warner, Eastleigh, p. 39

VALLANCE-OWEN, J., LILLEY, M. D. (1961) Insulin antagonism in the plasma of obese diabetics and prediabetics. *Lancet*, **1**, 806

VAUGHAN, M., KORN, E. D. (1962) Metabolic activity of adipose tissue, in *Adipose Tissue as an Organ* (Kinsell, L. W. ed.). Thomas, Springfield

WARD, W. A., KELSEY, W. M. (1962) The Pickwickian syndrome. *J. Pediat.* **61**, 745

WEILL, J., BERNFELD, J. (1957) L'épreuve d'hyperglycémie provoquée chez les enfants obèses. *Sem. Hôp.* (Paris), **33**, 1661

WIDDOWSON, E. M. (1962) Nutritional individuality. *Proc. Nutr. Soc.* **21**, 121

WINEGRAD, A. I. (1962) Endocrine effects on adipose tissue metabolism. *Vitam. and Horm.* **20**, 142

WISHNOFSKY, M. (1952) Caloric equivalents of gained and lost weight. *Metabolism*, **1**, 554

WOLFF, O. H. (1955) Obesity in childhood. *Quart. J. Med.* **24**, 109

WOLFF, O. H. (1962) Obesity in childhood and its effects. *Postgrad. med. J.* **38**, 629

YUDKIN, J. (1963) Nutrition and palatability. *Lancet*, **1**, 1335

CHAPTER 10

KWASHIORKOR

R. F. A. DEAN

THE recent literature on kwashiorkor is so large that some system of selection is essential if a chapter on the subject is to be kept to a moderate length. Here the selection has been made chiefly by the omission of all animal work except that on one specific point—the experimental production of protein-calorie malnutrition—and by reliance on the very fine monograph of Waterlow, Cravioto and Stephen (1960) for most of the work earlier than 1960. The monograph most adequately supplements and brings up to date the book written in Kampala by Trowell, Davies and Dean in 1954. The topics for detailed discussion have also been selected, the choice being based on familiarity with certain of the problems. On the other hand, it has been necessary to avoid too many generalisations, because of the undoubted existence of regional differences.

The problem of kwashiorkor must be one of the most important of the nutritional problems of childhood. For the physician interested in the scientific basis of medicine, it must also be one of the most fascinating.

Marasmus and Kwashiorkor

It is convenient to start with a comparative list of some of the features of marasmus and kwashiorkor (see Table). It is curious that although marasmus has been recognised and clearly defined for at least 60 years, we now know less about it than we do about kwashiorkor, which has a literary life half as long, if we accept what might be called conscious description. It is also extremely difficult to find anything in British medical writing of the last two centuries that provides even a possible description. Exceptions may be some of the accounts of Irish children stricken by the famines of 1845 to 1848 (Woodham-Smith 1962). Mention is made of extreme wasting, bony changes (. . . "the jawbone was so fragile and thin that a very slight pressure would force the tongue into the roof of the mouth"—it would be interesting to know what was meant by this remarkable statement), apathy (children's "unmeaning, vacant stare" . . . "every trace of childish gaiety had disappeared"): pallor of the skin, hirsutism (probably during partial recovery) and loss of hair. The appalling incidence of louse-borne and dysenteric infections probably caused much marasmus, but some children can hardly have escaped kwashiorkor. Perhaps they included those in Belmullet in Erris, "who had previously been emaciated, (and) now exhibited frightful swelling though most of them were too weak to stand." Kwashiorkor may well have been prevalent in Europe from time to time. In recent years it has been reported in Sicily (Russo 1961) and (as kwashiorkor-like, but apparently fully acceptable to the canon) in gypsy children in Hungary (Kerpel-Fronius 1960).

It would be pointless to attempt to make a complete list of all the countries, from Turkey (Wray 1961) to Haiti (Jelliffe and Jelliffe 1960), from Egypt (Mameesh *et al.* 1963) and the Sudan (Hassan 1960) to Malaya (Dean 1961*a*)

TABLE

A COMPARISON OF THE USUAL FEATURES OF ADVANCED
MARASMUS AND SEVERE KWASHIORKOR*

Feature	Advanced Marasmus	Severe Kwashiorkor
Period of development of illness	Often short	Usually very prolonged
Usual age . . .	Under 12 months	12 to 36 months
Weight loss . . .	Great	Variable
Hair	Unchanged	Colour, texture and amount changed
Skin colour . . .	Unchanged	Pale
Skin lesions . . .	Absent	Often present
Subcutaneous fat . .	Lost	Preserved
Œdema	Not visible	Often gross
Diarrhœa. . . .	Often causative and persistent	Not always present
Vomiting. . . .	Often present	Unusual
Appetite	Retained	Lost
Other psychological disturbances	Absent	Marked
Water retention . .	Slight	Marked
Salt retention . .	Slight	Marked
Urine concentration . .	Normal or high	Reduced despite oliguria
Urea concentration in urine	Not reduced	Reduced
Potassium depletion ⎱ Magnesium depletion⎰ .	Dependent on extent of diarrhœa	Great: independent of diarrhœa
Total serum proteins. .	Normal or high	Reduced
Serum albumin. . .	Normal	Reduced
Anæmia	Unusual	Constant
Megaloblastosis . .	None	Present in 10–15% of cases
Liver size . . .	Normal	Sometimes enlarged
Liver lipid . . .	Normal	Grossly increased
Pancreas	Unaltered	Acinar tissue deranged
Pancreatic enzymes . .	Unaltered	Grossly reduced

* See also Trowell *et al.* 1955.

and New Guinea (Kariks 1962), from which accounts of kwashiorkor are now available. In many it is so common that it is a major public health problem, even if its extent is still not fully recognised. In some countries there is always the danger that, given favourable circumstances, it will appear explosively in a susceptible area, as it did recently in the Congo (Lowenstein 1962).

Ætiology

A great deal of circumstantial evidence has for many years pointed to a deficiency of dietary protein, in the presence—at least in the early stages—of a comparatively large supply of calories, as being of major importance in the ætiology of kwashiorkor. We believe that kwashiorkor is a primary condition of malnutrition, although it may become evident only after an infection. Marasmus nearly always results from prolonged or repeated illnesses, such as tuberculosis and epidemic diarrhœa, and is almost invariably secondary to the illnesses: it also occurs, but rarely, as the starvation of an infant who has been kept alive by a diet that is meagre, but not wildly unbalanced. We have seen, for instance, a child 7 months old who weighed less than 3 kg., and who had existed, according to his mother's account, on two or perhaps three tins of a proprietary baby food, with hardly any additions, and similar cases are not difficult to find in Mexico and Central America, and undoubtedly in many other countries.

The detailed measurements of the values of diets on which kwashiorkor has been acquired are so few that a critic who demands absolute proof of the protein-calorie imbalance cannot be satisfied, but animal experiments of extraordinary interest (Follis 1961, Platt 1961, Ramalingaswami et al. 1961) have shown that at least some of the features of kwashiorkor, including œdema, loss of hair, retention of subcutaneous fat, changes in the amounts of serum albumin, γ-globulins, cholesterol, iron and iron-binding capacity, and fatty liver, can be produced in monkeys and pigs by diets that are short of protein and overbalanced by calories: and that a state resembling marasmus can be induced in pigs by a diet that is low in both protein and carbohydrate. These findings are described in a very informative publication of the National Academy of Sciences (1961) containing the papers read at a meeting in Washington in 1960.

The experimental production of protein-calorie malnutrition in children could never be justified, and the accurate observation of children in their homes, over a long period of decline, is almost as impossible. We can, however, record the recognition of some adjuvant factors in the ætiology that seem to be important. They include not only the infections that have already been mentioned, but social, economic and psychological conditions, including the misery and altered behaviour characteristic of "maternal deprivation" (Geber and Dean 1956, Farmer 1960, Burgess and Dean 1962, Dean 1963a). In other words, malnutrition is at last being treated as an ecological problem, by the introduction of an approach through the methods, still rather suspect and alien to many physicians who regard them as inexact and subjective, of the sociologist and cultural anthropologist. Some of the pioneering attempts in this field were arranged by the Nutrition section of the World Health Organisation, in Malaya and Indonesia. The results of the approach in general terms are to be seen in the wide range of reports such as those of Someswara Rao (1962) from South India and Bailey (1961) from Indonesia, and in the series of papers by Jelliffe and his co-workers from East Africa (Jelliffe and Jelliffe 1963), Panama (Jelliffe et al. 1961), Haiti (Jelliffe and Jelliffe 1960) and South Trinidad (Jelliffe et al. 1960). The approach can also be detected in some recent accounts of experimental work on kwashiorkor. For instance, Simson and Mann (1961) writing in South Africa, did not merely cover the results of the use of their mixtures of maize and various high-protein foods: they included details of the incidence of illegitimacy, the causes and duration of separation of child and mother, the weaning diet, the serum chemistry, and the appearance of "clinical dysentery" during treatment—a useful term for the diarrhœa that is probably a manifestation of carbohydrate intolerance. Important nutritional work is being carried out in South Africa, much of it described by Brock (1961) in the series *Recent Advances*. A consequence of that work may be unique; in South Africa kwashiorkor has been made a notifiable disease (Editorial 1962).

A possible biochemical explanation of the ætiology of kwashiorkor that will, it is hoped, prove later in this chapter to have at least some foundation of fact, may be usefully stated at this stage. The child whose diet in the year after weaning is deficient in protein, but provides a relative excess of calories, maintains his protein metabolism for a longer or shorter length of time, according to the quality of the imbalance in the diet, by a slowing of growth and the autophagy of his body proteins, especially those of his muscles. Eventually this process of adaptation fails, and the failure is first shown by a decline in the rate of growth, and by an alteration in the ratios of certain groups of the free amino acids in the plasma. The antecedent causes of the alteration are at present unknown. There is a generalised retardation of protein metabolism, but conditions probably favour the continued synthesis of inessential amino acids whilst essential ones are being lost, and are not being replaced. From these origins flow the multiplicity of clinical and biochemical signs that characterise the fully developed syndrome of kwashiorkor.

Early Diagnosis

The most useful aid to the diagnosis of protein-calorie malnutrition, whether œdema is visible or not, is also the simplest—weight for age. Accurate height and weight standards applicable to the community studied are obviously required, but are usually lacking. Height, or measurement of some part of the skeleton, may be a better index of poor growth than weight, but is much more difficult to determine accurately. The great retardation in bony development, in the time of appearance of epiphyses and the shaping of the bones, as well as in their size (Jones and Dean 1956, 1959), must occur long before any clinical sign is recognised, and could perhaps be made a fine diagnostic tool.

The circumstances in which early diagnosis of malnutrition is needed usually preclude the use of elaborate equipment, and much thought has been given to simple field methods. Schemes for the determination of the degree of muscle wasting have been proposed, but are not yet fully worked out (Expert Committee 1963, Jelliffe and Welbourn 1963). We have come to use the disproportion of head and body as an index for rapid assessment, having used it subconsciously for some time before recognising, from a study of a large number of photographs of our clinic children, that we were doing so. This, and another disproportion we have noticed, that between foot length and the diameter of the calf, might be reducible to exact terms and become useful aids to other methods.

On the biochemical side, the use of indices based on creatinine excretion in the urine has been explored (Expert Committee 1963, Arroyave 1961, 1963). The excretion may be less constant in small children than in adults, in whom it is regarded as a valuable guide to muscle mass, and appears to be of little diagnostic value in obvious cases of malnutrition (Arroyave *et al.* 1961, Waterlow 1963c), but creatinine/urea and creatinine/height ratios have been used in surveys of children believed to be ill nourished, although not, apparently, in conjunction with other methods that would substantiate the validity of the ratios. In Guatemala it was found that children aged from 3 to 6 years in families of low economic status had a creatinine/height ratio as low as that found in kwashiorkor, but studies of younger children in the families were not made (Arroyave and Wilson 1961). The ratio of urea nitrogen to total nitrogen in the urine has been advocated (Arroyave 1961, 1963, Expert Committee 1963), but may give a better picture of the recent nitrogen intake than of the nutritional state (Waterlow 1963c). The test must be used cautiously. Unlike adults, young children are unable to maintain their urea concentration perfectly when they are fasting.

It is possible that the free amino acids of the plasma may be more helpful. There are large falls in the concentration of most of the essential amino acids, with the result that *the ratio of inessential to essential amino acids* is increased before any other alterations of biochemistry so far known can be detected (see p. 239).

Whitehead (Dean and Whitehead 1963b, Whitehead 1964b, Whitehead and Dean 1964b) has introduced a test making use of this principle and employing blood taken by finger prick—one of the few procedures usually tolerated in the field—into heparinised capillary tubes. The plasma is separated by the centrifuge, and analysed at leisure. The estimation is by one-way paper chromatography, in which the group of branch-chain inessential amino acids (leucine, isoleucine and valine) is separated from another group that contains the essential amino acids glycine, serine, taurine and glutamine. The spots bearing the two groups are cut out and eluted, and the ratio is obtained from the extinction coefficients of the colours given by the groups, read at 509 mμ in a spectrophotometer, or in a simple colorimeter such as the E.E.L., with a green filter. A critical study of the method (to be published) has shown that the results are closely reproducible and that samples stored at $-5°C$. give the same results after 6 months as they did on the day the blood was taken. The method is not, of course, either so exact or so informative as full-scale column chromatography, but it yields a large part of the data that are needed, and is infinitely simpler and less costly than any other method.

We applied Whitehead's method to several hundred children and found that in cases of potential kwashiorkor the height of the ratio could be related to the incidence of the clinical signs. To our surprise, the ratio was also found to correlate well with the most important sign, weight deficit. The only data that are in any way comparable are given, but with scant detail, in an account by Albanese *et al.* (1958) of the correlation of total α-amino nitrogen in the serum with weight deficit. The amino nitrogen of the serum of Egyptian children suffering from kwashiorkor was investigated by Awwaad and Eisa (1959), but did not show any correlation with weight for age.

Whitehead's method has so far been used only in Uganda and in Ethiopia, but the results obtained in both countries have been in close agreement. If the correlation with weight deficit is proved, it will lend support to weight and height as indicators of minor degrees of growth failure. It must be remembered, however, that only sophisticated communities possess records of birth dates from which ages can be calculated with certainty. It is also necessary to point out that any test of the amino acid levels in the serum may be temporarily vitiated by a recent meal containing more than a few grams of milk protein. Fortunately for the test, many of the children who attend clinics and health centres in developing countries have fasted for several hours before their arrival.

Some observations on the difficulty of salt excretion in children recovering from kwashiorkor led us to investigate the possibility of using a salt load as a diagnostic aid in potential kwashiorkor (Dean 1963b). The results were the exact opposite of those expected: weight was usually lost, not gained.

The Biochemistry of Severe Kwashiorkor

Protein metabolism. The evidence that has so far been obtained favours the concept of a slowing of protein metabolism with the preservation of many of the enzyme systems that are needed for synthetic processes of all kinds (Waterlow 1962a). Catabolism of protein in the gut (Wetterfors et al. 1960) is not excessive (Purves and Hansen 1962b), but anabolism is reduced, as shown by the small turnover rate of albumin and γ-globulin (Cohen and Hansen 1962, Purves and Hansen 1962a) and the low concentration of urea.

Waterlow (1962a) has reviewed the work on intra-cellular enzyme systems and shown that the degree of preservation of most systems is more remarkable than the extent of the loss of the others. For such work, the choice of a reference substance is of great importance. In his own studies (Waterlow 1962b), he used deoxyribonucleic acid, which is genetically determined and believed to be impervious to deprivation. Others have used non-collagen nitrogen, but that may be more variable. Organs and tissues of the body are known to be affected by malnutrition in an order that may be ascribed to their relative importance for the preservation of life of the organism as a whole. The preservation of mitochondrial enzymes may be an example of this process.

It is in the realm of amino acid metabolism that recent progress has chiefly been made towards the explanation of the biochemical changes of kwashiorkor, and one of the most important findings has been the demonstration by Snyderman et al. (1963) that, in 65 cases collected in 9 different countries, the pattern of the serum amino acids was altered in a consistent way. They had to rely on many different observers for clinical descriptions of the children, and were not able to show a close relationship between the degree of abnormality of the amino acid pattern and the degree of severity of the kwashiorkor. We believe, however, that such a relationship does exist and can be demonstrated, at least in children in Uganda and Ethiopia. A similar pattern has been found by Westall et al. (1958) in Mexico, Vis (Vis et al. 1958; Vis 1963) in the Congo, Edozien et al. (1960) in Nigeria, and Arroyave et al. (1962) in Guatemala, and we also have found it (Whitehead and Dean, 1964a). The most striking feature is the great reduction in the amounts of the *essential* amino acids leucine, isoleucine and valine; lysine is exceptional in being less reduced. Of the *inessential* amino acids, tyrosine, arginine, citrulline and α-aminoisobutyric acid are well below normal, but the others are at normal levels, or even increased. Holt et al. (1963) found a striking lack of correlation with severity in some children, especially in two who died 24 hours after admission, but whose amino acids were only affected by a small amount. This observation agrees with one of our own. The amino acid imbalance ratio increases as the signs of potential kwashiorkor accumulate, but in severe cases, although the ratio is always high, there is no discernible correlation with severity as measured by other criteria.

The identification in urine of a metabolite of histidine, imidazole acrylic acid (urocanic acid), led us to investigate the metabolism of histidine (Whitehead and Arnstein 1961, Whitehead 1962, 1964a). In severe kwashiorkor, breakdown of histidine is incomplete and the imidazole acrylic acid (normally an intermediate that is converted to formiminoglutamic acid (FIGLU) and eventually to formic and glutamic acids) appears in the urine. The altered metabolism becomes more evident if a loading dose of histidine is given. Histidine itself and the imidazole derivative are then excreted in larger amounts. For some unexplained reason, the excretion continues for several days. The tissues do not seem to be avid for histidine, despite its essential nature and its importance as a major constituent of some proteins such as hæmoglobin, and the renal threshold presumably fails.

Phenylalanine is like histidine in having a ring structure, and like histidine has a deranged metabolism in kwashiorkor (Dean and Whitehead 1963a, Whitehead and Milburn 1962 and unpublished). Normally it is converted to tyrosine, but in kwashiorkor the conversion is reduced; presumably this is the reason why in the serum the phenylalanine is at a comparatively high level and the tyrosine at a low one. The full extent of the biochemical lesion cannot be seen until phenylalanine is added to the diet. Then, metabolites of this amino acid and of tyrosine appear in the urine abnormally or in abnormal amounts.

The metabolism of the third important cyclic amino acid, tryptophan, is not notably deranged, although the urine contains a slight excess of indoles (Crawford 1963). It is quite clear that the utilisation of all the biologically active amino acids must be studied. A useful starting point for further work might be a study of the branch-chain amino acids, although very little is known about their functions, or of lysine, which seems to be little affected.

There have been several reports of *aminoaciduria* in kwashiorkor, and one of the earliest (Vis *et al.* 1958) showed, in a diagram, a large amount of histidine in the urine of untreated children. This histidine was not, however, thought worthy of special comment; the excessive excretions chiefly noted were those of taurine and α-aminoisobutyric acid. It now seems that although the α-amino nitrogen in the urine is increased in the acute stage, before treatment, the total amount is fairly small. Much larger amounts are excreted in the early days of treatment, and are probably due to a combination of overflow and failure of utilisation, rather than to dysfunction of the renal tubules (Schendel and Hansen 1962). Berman and Kench (1963) have pointed out that even in the acute stage, when conservation would seem to be imperative, essential amino acids are being lost in the urine. They found, as Edozien and Phillips (1961) had already noticed, that the ratio of bound to free amino acids was higher than normal, but that the excretion of free histidine was also raised, and they thought that the hydroxyproline and proline excretion showed that collagen degradation was proceeding despite the general depletion of body protein.

Protein complexes. It has recently become possible to assemble a group of data that exemplify a failure of protein binding in severe kwashiorkor. The serum levels of copper and iron, and the iron-binding capacity are all low. The amount of combined cholesterol in the serum is small (Schwartz and Dean 1957), although the amount free does not change, and Leonard and Mac-William (1964) have observed that the amount of protein-bound cortisol is much less at the beginning of treatment than at the end. There are probably many other instances awaiting discovery.

The copper-bearing α_2-globulin (cæruloplasmin), the iron-bearing β-globulin (ferritin), the hæmoglobin-bearing β-globulins (haptoglobins), all of which are at low levels in acute kwashiorkor (Lahey *et al.* 1958, Annual Report 1961–62, MacWilliam 1964) form parts of the larger fractions, such as α_2- and β-globulins, that are usually estimated *in toto*, and are then found to be reduced (Dean 1960). It is very unlikely that all the parts of a single fraction are affected equally, and a more refined method of analysis than is at present available might show some interesting inconsistency. Immunophoretic methods, as used by Peetoom (1962), are potentially suitable, but are not yet quantitative.

Partition of urinary nitrogen. The origin of our work on histidine was an attempt to explain the presence in the urine of a large amount of nitrogen in forms that we could not identify (Whitehead and Matthew 1960, Dean 1961b). The amount was 25% of the total in severe cases and 19% in those less severe. We had noticed the small percentage of urea nitrogen, sometimes down to 30, and with a mean of 75 instead of the usual 87–93, and wanted to know the percentages of the other constituents. Our findings, and those of Edozien and Phillips (1961) in Nigeria and workers in India (Annual Report 1961–62) can usefully be compared. There were extraordinary differences between the results from Nigeria and those from the other two countries, for which regional variation was presumably responsible. Except for the low urea, the only really notable abnormalities found in Uganda and India were the raised α-amino nitrogen and ammonia. In Nigeria, the urea was very low indeed, the α-amino nitrogen very much raised, the ammonia raised as in India, and uric acid slightly raised. We and the Indian workers found that 20% of the nitrogen was in unknown forms, but in Nigeria all the nitrogen was accounted for. Waterlow (1963a) has commented on some of these differences. He found in malnourished Jamaican infants an increase in the absolute amount of nitrogen residual to that of urea and ammonia, but did not give figures for the percentages represented by each of the seven items that we estimated. The average amount of his residual nitrogen was almost the same as that found by Macy in healthy children. The urea nitrogen in the urine bore a constant relationship to the total nitrogen, though there may have been some undisclosed qualitative abnormalities. He though that, as in Nigeria, all the nitrogen could be accounted for.

In a few Guatemalan cases of kwashiorkor, Arroyave and Wilson (1961) noted that the creatinine excretion was within the probable normal range on the day of admission but rose sharply by the seventh day of treatment. The rise could not have been due to increased muscle mass, and the results therefore confirmed that the measurement of creatinine was misleading, or at least difficult to interpret, in the acute stages. Expressing their results in mg. creatinine excreted for each cm. height, Arroyave and Wilson obtained figures that were low, even at the end of periods of treatment of between 21 and 69 days, compared with those obtained by Stearns from children in the United States. The concentration of serum creatinine was very small at the start of treatment and remained so.

We have found (unpublished work) that the creatine/creatinine ratio in the urine was from 0·1 to 0·4 in the untreated child, and rose gradually during treatment to 1·0 to 1·3. The synthesis of creatine is a function of the liver and involves arginine, glycine and methionine. The synthesis may be limited, in the acute stage of kwashiorkor, by the shortage of methionine.

In a paper recently published, Vasantgadkar et al. (1963) described a re-examination of the urine in kwashiorkor. They confirmed the presence of unidentified nitrogen in the early stages of treatment, but said that it did not disappear completely, even in the last stages, especially if the protein in the diet was of plant origin. Increases in ammonia and amino acid nitrogen, and uric acid and purine derivatives, were again found, but there was no increase in the output of histidine, and imidazole acrylic acid was not detected. They found a positive correlation between the level of the serum albumin and that of the urinary urea, and suggested that the ratio of the two substances might be a measure of severity.

Carbohydrate metabolism and diarrhœa in kwashiorkor. In comparison with the attention lavished on proteins, there has been a sad neglect of carbo-hydrates. If the explanation of the imbalance of serum amino acids is correct (p. 237), the deviation in favour of the synthesis of inessential amino acids must usually be encouraged by calories derived from carbo-hydrate—there is very seldom much fat in diets that lead to kwashiorkor. Again, there is the fact that carbohydrates are liable to cause diarrhœa, while the combination of severe diarrhœa with kwashiorkor is often fatal.

There is no doubt that the child acutely ill with kwashiorkor is intolerant of lactose. This was shown in 1952 (Dean 1952) and has been re-affirmed in Egypt more recently (Badr El-Din and Aboul Wafa 1961). The Egyptian workers have studied the galactose tolerance, because in the gut lactose is hydrolysed to galactose, and that is changed to glucose in the liver. After an oral dose of galactose, the serum level rose higher in one hour than in healthy children, and rose again in the second hour when it should fall. Even after an over-night fast, the children with kwashiorkor had a small amount of galactose in their blood, whereas normal children had none. Further study is required, but the strongly acid, bright yellow and frequent stools that are characteristic of the start of treatment with dried skimmed milk may be an indication of conditions in the gut that are against the hydrolysis of lactose. The loose stools can hardly be very favourable to absorption, although they obviously do not depress it very extensively. Recovery proceeds rapidly in many cases, in spite of them.

Bowie et al. (1963) writing from Cape Town, have suggested that the intolerance may extend to disaccharides other than lactose. Children who had received feeds of skimmed milk were given instead a carbohydrate-free diet: the mean daily stool weight changed from 534 g. to 170 g. and the improvement was obvious within 24–48 hours. In our own children, the beneficial results of lowering the lactose intake are usually visible in about 6 hours, and disaccharides other than lactose do not have such a marked effect on the stools.

One of the Egyptian children was thought to have died of hypoglycæmia: the blood sugar was only 5 mg./100 ml. Similar suggestions had been made before, but the only extensive work on hypoglycæmia is that of Wayburne and his colleagues (Kahn and Wayburne 1961, Wayburne 1963) in Johannesburg. After an 8-hour fast on the second night after admission to hospital, children with kwashiorkor had an average blood glucose of 51 mg./100 ml. compared with 76 mg./100 ml. in a control group. Hypoglycæmia was believed to be a common cause of death. In 32 out of 33 children who died, the blood sugar was less than 10 mg./100 ml. There were no convulsions or sweating, and even twitching was rare. In children whose blood sugar was from 20 to 30 mg./100 ml., liver biopsy within a few minutes of death showed the complete absence of glycogen. The authors made the interesting observation that the attacks of hypoglycæmia were always preceded by partial or complete failure to take food, and that out-patients arriving after a long journey, as well as in-patients, were affected. They thought a fast of more than 4 hours was dangerous. We came to the same conclusion some years ago and instituted frequent feeds, containing plenty of sugar (sucrose), and even continuous drip feeding for the worst cases. We now seldom have the sudden deaths that may be due to hypoglycæmia, but we cannot claim that our work has been systematic. The Johannesburg authors commented that despite the better understanding of the condition and the intravenous injection of 50% glucose, nearly all the children died. Our own experience is the same. We have revived about a dozen moribund children by glucose injections, and some of them have survived for as long as 24 hours; but all died except one, who happened to be having a blood transfusion when he collapsed, and was therefore swiftly treated. In Jamaica children have sometimes died whilst receiving 50% glucose solution into the inferior vena cava (McLean 1963). The reason for the hypoglycæmia remains unknown.

The whole subject of carbohydrate metabolism remains of great importance. No component of the diet is so likely to perpetuate diarrhœa during treatment as lactose. Vegetable oils are very well tolerated (Dean 1960, Waterlow 1961b, Dutra de Olivereira and Rolando 1963), and although some years ago we thought that butter fat was likely to produce loose stools and resolved not to use it, Indian workers (Annual Report 1961–62) have found that the fat, even if it provided nearly 40% of the total calories, caused neither diarrhœa nor fatty stools, while Bowie et al. (1963) used cream in the carbohydrate-free diets that were so successful in reducing the stool weights in their children. Our present standard diet (Dean and Swanne 1963) contains enough cotton seed oil to give more than 50% of the total calories.

Lipid metabolism. The fatty liver that is almost invariably part of the kwashiorkor syndrome, but is not found in marasmus (Macdonald 1960), may have various causes such as the synthesis of large amounts of triglyceride from excess dietary carbohydrate, the transport to the liver of non-esterified fatty acids released from fat depots, or an inability to transport fat from the liver because protein-fat combinations cannot be made (Macdonald 1962, Macdonald *et al.* 1963, and Lewis *et al.* (1963). The fatty liver is intense in severe cases in whom the appetite for carbohydrate has recently been poor, and some of the suggestions other than excess synthesis are perhaps more plausible. The liver and depot fat have much the same composition in kwashiorkor (Baker and Macdonald 1961), and non-esterified fatty acids in the plasma are at a higher level at the start of treatment than at the end. In the untreated child the liver fat and the fat in the blood have different iodine numbers, and during treatment changes occur that are consistent with the mobilisation of the liver fat (Schwartz 1958, Mey, Pretorius, Smit and du Toit 1961, Schendel and Hansen 1961). Treatment causes a considerable lipæmia, even if the diet is fat-free (Schwartz and Dean 1957), and the total fat may reach 2 g./100 ml. serum. The serum lipids are qualitatively affected by the dietary fat, vegetable oils causing smaller rises of cholesterol and the unsaturated fatty acids than the fat of milk (Matthew and Dean 1960, Mey, Smit, Labuschagne and Pretorius 1961).

There is, however, some evidence against the transport of depot fats to the liver. Although Macdonald *et al.* (1963) found that palmitic, palmitoleic and linoleic acids were roughly in the proportions of 7:1:1 in the liver, the proportions in the adipose tissue were 6:2:1. The proportions in both tissues remained the same throughout treatment. After ten days, the total lipid in the serum rose from 308 to 636 mg./100 ml., and glycerides from 90 to 203 mg. Phospholipid rose from 162 to 274 mg./100 ml., a finding that is not easy to understand. New formation seems to be a more likely explanation than phanerosis.

Further confirmation of the failure of transport of fat from the liver in the acute stage has come from Guatemala (Arroyave *et al.* 1963). A diet free of vitamin A or carotene, based on skimmed milk, caused an increase in the concentration of vitamin A in the serum, and the vitamin must obviously have been released by the tissues: the vitamin is transported by albumin and it was presumably the increase in this protein fraction that made the increase possible. The body's chief store of vitamin A is in the liver, and as the serum level rose, that of the liver fell.

Our own view is that the fatty liver is of secondary rather than primary importance. The presence of the fat does not seem to be associated with the depression of most of the functions of the liver, with the notable exception of albumin formation. The removal of bromsulphthalein from the blood is reduced (Kinnear and Pretorius 1962), but this does not necessarily imply that there is a fault in liver function. The removal depends on the capture of cysteine from glutathione, and a reduction in the available amount of this tripeptide would be limiting (Philp *et al.* 1961). The hypothesis needs support, but in its favour is the finding (Mody and Smith 1964) that the concentration of reduced glutathione in the red cells was lower than normal in severe kwashiorkor.

Signs of definite liver failure are unusual but are seen occasionally, and indicate a bad prognosis (McLean 1963). In severe cases glutamic pyruvate transaminase may be at high levels in the serum but at low levels in the liver tissue (McLean and Chan 1963). Such changes may be the result of increased permeability: they can occur without necrosis (Henly *et al.* 1963), which is not usually found in uncomplicated kwashiorkor.

The resemblance between the skin lesions of some cases of kwashiorkor to those produced experimentally by diets lacking essential fatty acids is sometimes striking. Naismith (1963), who believes that a deficiency may impair the utilisation of proteins, has found evidence suggesting that such a deficiency may exist in Nigerian children. He has pointed out that the children are weaned from breast milk (presumably at least 3·5% fat) in which 16% of the total fatty acids is the highly unsaturated linoleic acid, to a diet that contains only 1% fat. His work may help to explain the regional variation in the incidence and kind of skin lesions: but it is usually believed that the requirements of essential fatty acids are very small, and most diets, however limited, usually contain some items, such as groundnuts, that would in normal circumstances probably supply the requirements for the acids.

Mineral metabolism. Reference has already been made to changes in the intracellular electrolytes. The œdema of kwashiorkor is the retention of excess water with sodium and other electrolytes, and much of the excess is probably extracellular. When treatment succeeds in removing the œdema, there is a large excretion of salt in the urine. As the diuresis lessens, the salt excretion falls and may become almost unmeasurable, an anomalous condition that must indicate the "guarding" (in Darrow's parlance) of the serum sodium and may indicate a deficiency (Dean 1963b). There are interactions between sodium and potassium, and the addition of potassium to therapeutic diets probably helps to remove the excess sodium: there may even be a quantitative relationship between the intake of the one and the output of the other. Contrary to other groups, we have not found any consistent depression of the serum potassium, and we believe that if depression occurs, the cause may be diarrhœa that is not an integral part of kwashiorkor, although we recognise and have recently confirmed the depression of duodenal enzymes. Diarrhœa in our children is usually caused by sugar intolerance or by infection, and the drain of potassium seems to be the result of the loss of secretions that are known to be abundant in potassium. A fall in serum potassium should therefore be regarded as secondary, not primary, despite the fact that the body as a whole is short of potassium, as shown by the large retentions during treatment. In our cases, the serum concentration of sodium is usually unchanged, even in the acute stage of kwashiorkor. In Jamaica, where the serum sodium in healthy children is about 140 mEq./l., Smith and Waterlow (1960) and Smith (1963) found values over 121 mEq./l. in 98 out of 107 children with kwashiorkor, and values below 121 mEq. in the remaining 9. Only 12 of the 98 died in the first week, but 7 of the 9 died in that time. They thought that the reduced serum sodium was the result of dilution of the blood by excess water, and suggested that the extent of the dilution might be used as a rough indication of the amount of water being retained by the body. The amount was found to be related to the extent of pulmonary œdema, found clinically, and *post mortem* in children who died. Smith also pointed out that although children with kwashiorkor are over-loaded with sodium and cannot excrete it, some of them, who have been proved by muscle biopsy and by isotopic methods to be depleted of potassium, lose their ability to conserve that metal. The retention of the sodium and the loss of the potassium must be very much to their disadvantage. Even the acidification of the urine is impaired by potassium deficiency.

In the last few years the importance of magnesium has become obvious, largely through work by Montgomery (1960) in Jamaica. The discovery is belated, because the intracellular position of magnesium, its partnership with potassium, and its participation in enzyme reactions, have long been known. Muscle obtained by biopsy in the first days after admission from malnourished children contained 10 mEq. magnesium and 56 mEq. potassium/kg. wet weight. When the biopsy was repeated 5 to 9 weeks later, the respective values were 14 and 70 mEq.: the concentrations in healthy children are probably 16 to 20 mEq. magnesium/kg. wet weight and 89 to 92 mEq. potassium. In the children with kwashiorkor, at the beginning of treatment and later, and in the fatal cases, the serum magnesium was 1·73 mEq./l., with very small deviation; the level seems to be guarded even better than that of potassium, perhaps because absorption may continue even in the presence of diarrhœa. Montgomery gave figures for urinary excretion of magnesium that were low at first and confirmed the lack of the mineral, but the extent of the depletion was unknown. A large proportion of the total magnesium is normally in the skeleton, from which it may or may not be easily mobilised in states of malnutrition. This is one of the many points that will not be settled until the composition of whole corpses, and their component parts, is known in detail.

The work has been amplified by balance studies in Jamaica (Montgomery 1961) and South Africa (Linder et al. 1963). In nearly every case, the magnesium balance was positive, particularly when (in the South African children) extra magnesium was added to the diet. The positive balances continued throughout the periods of observation. The South African workers (who incidentally found a depression of serum magnesium below the normal range in 10 of 14 children) simultaneously with the magnesium balance estimated the balances of potassium, sodium, calcium, phosphorus and nitrogen. The retention of magnesium and potassium was greater than was expected from the nitrogen balance, and that of phosphorus was greater than was expected from the nitrogen and calcium balances. In both countries it was decided that urinary secretion of magnesium was a better guide to magnesium depletion than the serum concentration.

Magnesium deficiency affects many organs, including the heart (Hanna et al. 1960). In kwashiorkor, the ECG shows some marked changes. They were described in 1949 in Mexico (De la Torre et al. 1949), but were then believed to be related to a deficiency of vitamin B_1. The changes were described again in the Congo in 1957 (Schyns and Demæyer 1957) and in Cairo in 1960 (Awwaad et al. 1960), consisting of bradycardia, low voltage (specially in QRS), shortening of PR interval, and reduced or inverted T waves. Treatment reversed the changes, except for those of the PR interval. In the Congo, all the changes (most of which had been noticed in marasmic children by McCulloch in 1920) were thought to be more severe in the children who had the lowest levels of serum protein.

Findings in Cape Town (Smythe et al. 1962) were similar, but there were some important additions. The hearts were small; the cardiothoracic ratio was usually less than 0·5, and *post mortem* the hearts of two children who died at 16 and 24 months weighed only 23 and 32 g. In a few children, histological examination suggested myocardial œdema. During treatment, the T wave, previously inverted, became upright, as it did in the Congo and in Egypt. After one year the ECG was usually normal.

In the present context, the changes are of interest because they resemble those found in experimental magnesium deficiency (Wacker and Vallee 1958), as was recognised in a further South African study (Cronje and Pretorius 1963). Various therapeutic diets had little effect on the tracings, but improvement followed the addition of magnesium. In Kampala, where most of the changes described were also found, dramatic improvement followed the injection of magnesium sulphate in a few cases (Caddell 1963). Both sets of South African workers suggested that the changes in the heart might be a factor in the sudden death of children under treatment. In Jamaica, some moribund children have responded well to magnesium given intravenously.

Adrenal hormones. In malnourished Indian children, the cortex of the adrenals was uniformly degenerate (Chatterji and Sen Gupta 1960), and the changes were consistent with the finding in Chilean children (Monckeberg *et al.* 1956) of a generalised failure of cortical function, with no more than a brief response to ACTH. In South Africa, however, the histological appearance of the cortex was very variable, no constant change in function was found, and the response to ACTH was a little less at the start of treatment than at the end, but not grossly abnormal.

The South African workers (Lurie and Jackson 1962b) found that the output of 17-ketosteroids and 17-hydroxysteroids in the urine was the same at the beginning and end of treatment, and was unrelated to the presence or absence of œdema. Findings in our own laboratory have been similar. There was an excellent response to ACTH in the South African children, and the urinary output of the steroids rose steeply in one child who developed bronchitis during treatment. It was concluded that cortical function was not disturbed. On the days when ACTH was injected, the excretion of urinary creatinine was considerably enhanced: perhaps this finding is related in some way to the rapid increase in excretion that occurs at the start of treatment.

When aldosteronuria was investigated (Lurie and Jackson 1962a) the results were similar; there was no consistent relationship with the presence of œdema or its loss by diuresis, or with sodium retention. In two œdematous children, no aldosterone was detected until the diuresis began, and the excretion of the hormone did not rise when the sodium excretion fell, after the peak of the diuresis. It was thought possible that the usual relationship between œdematous conditions and the excretion of aldosterone did not obtain in kwashiorkor, and some evidence for this was mentioned by Smith (1963): 6 œdematous children had a lower mean aldosterone excretion than 5 who were not œdematous.

The recent work of Leonard and MacWilliam (1963) offers a probable explanation of some of the discrepancies. Cortisol exists in the serum in two forms, free and combined with protein. Of the combined portion, part is bound to transcortin, an α-globulin that has a very great affinity for cortisol but is saturated by low concentrations of the steroid, and the rest is bound to albumin which has a lesser affinity but a greater capacity. In acute kwashiorkor there is usually no change in the α_1-globulin and only a small fall in the α_2-globulin, but the albumin is greatly reduced. Leonard found that the total amount of cortisol excreted in 24-hour periods was the same at the beginning of treatment as at the end, but at the beginning 35% of the cortisol in the serum was in the free form, and at the end, only half as much—18%. The albumin level was fairly critical; if it was less than 1·7 g./100 ml. serum, there was a sharp increase in the proportion of cortisol that was free.

If other cortical steroids follow the same pattern, the apparent anomalies found by examination of the urine would be resolved. The total cortical production remains unchanged, but the amount of the serum proteins, especially the albumin, determines the amount of the total that is free, and therefore highly active. If there is, in effect, a hyperaldosteronism, this might be one of the factors responsible for a negative magnesium balance (Milne et al. 1957).

Growth hormone and thyroid activity. Some children who are recovering from severe malnutrition advance in every way except that they fail to gain weight satisfactorily. In Chile, a pituitary extract was given to 6 children by Monckeberg, Donoso, Oxman, Pak and Meneghello (1963). The response was thought to indicate a lack of pituitary hormone production in the malnourished child, that might be a protective adaptation.

The same authors (Monckeberg et al. 1956) had previously demonstrated in other children a low uptake of I^{131} and low levels of protein-bound iodine, proportional to the degree of malnutrition, but correctable by the administration of thyroid-stimulating hormone. In Jamaica, Stirling (1962a) found the thyroid gland of normal histological appearance.

Montgomery (1962b, 1962c) studied radio-iodine excretion and concluded that thyroid function was not responsible for initiating the large increase in oxygen consumption that had previously been shown to accompany the accelerated growth during recovery. The basic metabolic rate was approximately normal in terms of body solids and body weight, although it was reduced in terms of surface area, the parameter usually employed. For consistent increase of weight, calories in excess of the need calculated from the BMR need to be given, a detail of importance in therapy, the amount of gain being more closely related to the calorie intake than to the intake of protein (Waterlow 1961b).

The Anæmia of Kwashiorkor

In nearly all obvious cases of kwashiorkor there is a moderate degree of anæmia.

One of the most complete studies of the anæmia was that made in Kampala by Allen (1964). It followed a similar study in Kenya (Kondi et al. 1963), and the results were similar. In the Kampala children, the mean Hb level was 9·1 g./100 ml., the mean red cell count $3·61 \times 10^6/mm.^3$, and, as usually found elsewhere, the cells were normocytic and slightly hypochromic in most children.

Malaria and hookworm disease are very common in Kampala, and the presence of either one or the other was associated with a lowering of the Hb concentration by about 1 g./100 ml. A similar reduction was found in the most severe uncomplicated cases of kwashiorkor. A constant feature was a fall in the Hb concentration in the first ten days of treatment. The concentration reached about 8·5 g. and the fall was accompanied by a fall in hæmatocrit from 31·4 to 27·6, probably due to an increase in the blood volume. It is, of course, well known that the body water is greatly increased in kwashiorkor (Kerpel-Fronius 1960, Hansen et al. 1963), but the expansion of the volume in our children apparently represented a shift of some of the water from the extra-vascular compartment. It occurred at a time when œdema was being lost, and the fall in Hb correlated well with the rise in serum albumin. Other workers have measured the blood volume at the beginning and end of treatment and found a small but fairly consistent increase (Cronje et al. 1961). A few estimations have been made by the Evans Blue method in our unit, and they all showed an increase, usually of the order of 10 to 20% of the initial value, but the variations per kg. body weight were very large, as in the results of others (Smith 1960, Patel et al. 1960, Shah 1961). A striking feature of the blood in Kampala was a large rise in the number of platelets, the mean count rising from about 300,000/mm.[3] on admission to 638,000/mm.[3] ten days later. The eosinophil counts also rose steeply, and both rises occurred to the greatest extent in the children who, on admission to hospital, had the lowest total serum proteins.

In Kampala and in Kenya the bone marrow was inactive at first, and the ratio of erythroid precursors to myeloid was low. Treatment caused a brisk resumption of activity and occurred, in Kampala, even on diets that were very nearly vitamin-free. The Hb rose slowly, but the rise always stopped before the normal level for children of this age was reached, and was thought to be the result of "maturation arrest." If the anæmia tended to be microcytic, iron given by intramuscular injection, but not by mouth, was usually effective, as was already known (Trowell and Simpkiss 1957). The missing substance could not be identified: it appeared not to be vitamin C, folic acid or riboflavin. On a high-protein diet, rich in calories, the Hb rose slowly after the initial fall due to the dilution of the blood, and there was not a marked reticulocytosis at any time. The usual period of hospital treatment was about 17 days, and the mean Hb at the end of that time was 9·0 g. Most of the children returned for follow-up examination about a month later, and the mean concentration had then risen to 11·0 g. The platelet count had returned to about 300,000. As Vitale et al. (1963) have indicated, the most likely explanation of the typical anæmia of kwashiorkor is that it is an expression of the generalised failure of protein metabolism.

In Durban (Walt et al. 1962) and in Nairobi (Kondi et al. 1962), marrow erythroid aplasia or hypoplasia developed during treatment, usually two to three weeks after admission. There was some hypoplasia in the Kampala children, but only in those whose total serum proteins were less than 3·5 g./ 100 ml. In Durban, the marrow picture of all the children recovered spontaneously, riboflavin having no acceleratory effect. In Nairobi, where aplasia not merely hypoplasia was found, riboflavin seemed to have some value. In some cases prednisone also caused some improvement, and the suggestion was made that in the recovering child there might be a relative or absolute deficiency of corticosteroids that was relieved when the cortex was stimulated by the vitamin (Foy *et al.* 1961).

In various countries, including Uganda (Allen and Whitehead 1964), Kenya (Kondi *et al.* 1963), South Africa (Scragg and Rubidge 1960), Jamaica (Garrow *et al.* 1962), Colombia (Velez *et al.* 1963) and the Lebanon (Majaj, Dinning, Azzan and Darby 1963) there is a megaloblastic anæmia in 10 to 15% of the cases. The megaloblastosis is sometimes not seen on admission, but develops later. It seems that the condition is seldom due to a lack of vitamin B_{12}; the serum level of that vitamin is often high (Satoskar *et al.* 1962), but there may, of course, be a failure of utilisation. Folic acid will usually restore the bone marrow, as it did in Uganda, although Allen did not find a striking reticulocytosis. Very recently a response to vitamin E, given as α-tocopherol, has been found in the Lebanon (Majaj, Dinning, Azzan and Darby 1963, Majaj, Dinning and Darby 1963). In an illustrative example, a rise in Hb of about 6 g. occurred in the 25 days after the doses of the vitamin, and there was a reticulocytosis that reached 30% at its peak. The possibility arose that there might be inter-relations of the functions of vitamin E, vitamin B_{12} and folic acid. The serum level of vitamin E is sometimes very low in kwashiorkor (Trowell *et al.* 1954).

A phenomenon seen in Kampala could be explained by previous work on the amino acid histidine. It is well known that in many anæmias that appear to be due to folic acid deficiency, the urine contains formiminoglutamic acid (FIGLU). This substance is derived from a breakdown product of histidine, imidazole acrylic acid (urocanic acid). As already mentioned (p. 240), imidazole acrylic acid is excreted in severe cases of kwashiorkor, and it is thus not surprising that if there is an accompanying megaloblastosis, FIGLU cannot be found in the urine. When the metabolic block which prevents the breakdown of imidazole acrylic acid is removed by treatment with the usual high-protein diet, FIGLU appears in the urine and continues to be excreted until folic acid is given. The folic acid removes the second block, that in the metabolism of FIGLU, and that substance disappears in its turn. The results showed that when kwashiorkor and megaloblastic anæmia are present together, the FIGLU test (Luhby *et al.* 1959) may be misleading.

The binding of iron and copper in the serum has been mentioned in the discussion of protein metabolism. The serum levels of both metals are often reduced, and so is the total iron-binding capacity (Lahey *et al.* 1958, Edozien and Udeozo, 1960, Cronje *et al.* 1961, El Gholmy *et al.* 1962, Monckeberg, Vildosola, Figueroa, Oxman and Meneghello 1963). In Johannesburg, iron deficiency anæmia is frequent in kwashiorkor. In a study by Metz and Stein (1959) the mean Hb was 8·1 g. and the MCHC 28·6%. The bone marrow was rich in erythroid precursors. Reticulocytosis and a rise of Hb (in two children increases of over 6 g. were seen in 15 days) followed the intramuscular injection of iron. The diet was deficient in iron, the mean intake being assessed at less than 3 mg. daily, about half the allowance usually recommended. There may also have been defective absorption. In contrast to Kampala and other places, Johannesburg has neither malaria nor hookworm, and the part played by these parasites in iron-deficiency anæmias needs further study.

Infections in Association with Kwashiorkor

If adequate histories can be obtained for children admitted for the treatment of kwashiorkor, they nearly always contain references to episodes that may have been infective illnesses; and deterioration in general health is often said to have been noticed for the first time after such an episode (Scrimshaw *et al.* 1959, 1960).

Even in healthy children the common infections may cause a temporary decline in the secretion of digestive enzymes, and the anorexia that normally develops may be attributable, in part, to this cause. There is no good proof that malnourished children are especially liable to contract infections, but there is reason to believe that a period of anorexia may have severe consequences. In our wards we have seen that the effects of a short period of starvation may persist for many days, even in children whose condition had previously not given rise to any anxiety. We admit whenever possible children who are believed to be potential cases of kwashiorkor, so that we may study not only their biochemistry, but also the ease or difficulty with which they can be fed and their response to a good diet. For this work we sometimes use semi-solid diets that resemble the diet eaten at home. It is remarkable how often our diets are refused, despite the absence of any obvious psychological upset and the constant presence of the children's mothers, who also stay in hospital. In the face of this evidence the mothers often agree that they have had similar difficulty at home. Believing that the upset was due to the strange new circumstances, we have occasionally allowed the children to starve themselves, in the hope that they would soon be overcome by hunger: fluids, of course, are given liberally. In a few of the children, the general condition has suddenly worsened, and tube feeding has been necessary. We are now investigating the possibility that we may have allowed a dangerous hypoglycæmia to develop.

In children who were more or less well—they were recovering from kwashiorkor—Wilson *et al.* (1961) found that an attack of chicken-pox might cause a marked increase in the loss of nitrogen in the urine, and a negative nitrogen balance that began just after the exanthem. The adverse effect might last up to 2 weeks. The fever was not held to be responsible, but the food intake could not be maintained because of vomiting. That has not been our experience. We have found that the intake can be kept unaltered without any tendency to vomiting, if we use tube feeding, although there is considerable pyrexia and a complete lack of interest in food. Gandra and Scrimshaw (1961) also found in children who were not, presumably, malnourished—they were recovering from various infections in a private nursing home in Guatemala City—that a mild virus infection, induced by the injection of a yellow fever vaccine, caused an increase in urinary nitrogen that persisted for the whole 12-day period of observation.

The close link between infective diarrhœa and marasmus is undeniable: a link with kwashiorkor is less certain (Dean 1957). Common-sense favours malabsorption as the cause of diarrhœa, but in the absence of infection in the gut, malabsorption is not a striking feature of our cases, and Waterlow (1961b) has found that nitrogen absorption, even in the first days of treatment, may still be about 90% of the intake. We may cause malabsorption by such means as the feeding of lactose, but some experiments (unpublished) in which we measured the absorption of a test meal introduced into the duodenum showed little difference at the beginning and end of treatment.

Bacterial infections that we have observed in children recovering from kwashiorkor usually run an unremarkable course, and respond in a normal manner to antibiotics. The exceptions are usually lung infections, which are sometimes prolonged and fatal in spite of all we can do. The lungs of children with kwashiorkor have yet to be studied: nearly all our children have X-ray appearances that would be classed as abnormal in Europe, and an increase in pulmonary fluid has been noted elsewhere in malnourished children (Smith 1963). Many children are found to have patches of broncho-pneumonia *post mortem*, but seldom enough to be the certain cause of death.

In countries notorious for the malnutrition of the young children, measles has a very high mortality (Lowenstein 1963). The combination of measles and kwashiorkor almost deserves a chapter to itself: in our wards children usually become very ill, not from the complications of measles as in Europe, but from the infection itself, and many die. It is unlikely that different strains of virus are involved—the differences in response have been noticed in well-fed European and poorly-fed African children in the same hospital at the same time—and the nutrition of the host is probably the dominant factor.

There are several puzzling features in our children. We have had deaths from measles in children whose kwashiorkor was seemingly well under control, and whose blood chemistry had become almost normal. Further-more, in these children, as in nearly all of those we admit, the serum γ-globulins were at high (absolute) levels. Injected γ-globulin nevertheless gives very effective protection against measles: we have had no deaths in children who were given the injections within a few days of the exposure to infection.

Malnourished children in South Africa are thought to have poor resistance to infections. Isohæmagglutinin titres were not lower in malnourished children than in controls (Kahn *et al.* 1957). Similar results were obtained using Kahn lipid antigen (Bennett and Watson 1962) and typhoid and para-typhoid endotoxins (Pretorius and De Villiers 1962). In Mexico (Lowenstein 1963) the complementary activity of the serum of a few children was normal, although in another Mexican report (Olarte *et al.* 1956) there was retarded development of antibodies to diphtheria.

In South Africa (Becker *et al.* 1963) a remarkable association has been noticed between malnutrition and generalised herpes simplex. Nearly all the affected children die. These, and children who contract measles, might provide a profitable field for work on interferon, the substance produced by cells as a protection against "foreign" nucleic acids, especially those of viruses. It is possible that the production is hampered in a malnourished or deranged cell.

Treatment

The problem of treatment of kwashiorkor is to find means of restoring rapidly the processes by which the anabolism of protein can function at the optimal rate. Often an infection must be dealt with. More often the child is presented for treatment very severely ill from the late effects of an infection that may have run its course days or weeks earlier.

We give penicillin and streptomycin routinely for about a week, and substitute chloramphenicol for the penicillin if there is an infective diarrhœa (Dean and Swanne 1963). Urinary infections are rare, possibly because of this routine, and renal complications, known to be important in Jamaica (Stirling 1962b), are perhaps avoided by the use of the antibiotics.

In severe cases the diet must be liquid so that it can pass through a fine intragastric tube. It is nearly always impossible to spare the time and patience required to break the anorexia by hand feeding, and in most circumstances the only way to ensure that the child receives the stipulated amounts of his diet is to tube feed.

Some of the biochemical changes that are commonly regarded as part of kwashiorkor are probably the results of infection, or partly so. For instance, in South Africa diarrhœal disease brings most of the children to hospital, as the monthly incidence of cases shows clearly (Scragg and Rubidge 1960). Diarrhœas are also a major problem in Central America and Mexico, whereas in Uganda only a small proportion of the cases admitted for treatment have persistent diarrhœa that may be of infective origin. It is often extremely difficult to disentangle the effects of the infection from those of the underlying state of malnutrition, and it is certainly possible to simulate some of the effects by imperfect therapy. Thus it is common in our wards to find that a child who has only one or two stools on the day of admission and the day after, will have 5 or more each day in the succeeding week. We have thought since 1952 that the lactose in the dried skimmed milk incorporated in our diets is chiefly responsible, but so far measures such as reducing the amount of lactose, changing the proportions of lactose to that of other sugars in the diet, or providing a bland excipient such as sweet or cooked banana, have been no more than partially successful. The acid, bright yellow, frequent stools characteristic of lactose excess appear all too often. It may be difficult to provide cheaply carbohydrate-free diets of the kind that Bowie et al. (1963) found so effective. An inexpensive form of protein, as perfect as that of dried skimmed milk, is the chief necessity. Bowie et al. used egg, which we also have used with success. Most of the calories required could be obtained from a vegetable oil.

It has been claimed that loose stools are not of importance, because most children recover in spite of them (Venkatachalam and Srikantia 1961). Nevertheless, the number of deaths might be reduced and the period of treatment shortened, if the frequent stools could be avoided. An extensive trial of carbohydrate-free diets is clearly called for.

The mineral stores depleted by diarrhœa and vomiting require refilling. It is now known that in severe kwashiorkor the total losses of potassium and magnesium from the body are great, even if the serum concentrations are normal, and in some countries large quantities of both these minerals are being added to the diet. The sodium retained with the œdema fluid must be removed, and potassium seems to help in its removal (Hansen and Brock 1954). Sodium losses in the diuresis are sometimes excessive, and we add sodium chloride from the start of treatment, even in the presence of the most extreme œdema. The water retention and the weight increase temporarily, but the clinical appearance improves markedly: the improved appearance led us to add the salt in the face of the seemingly logical reasons for limiting or withholding it. The recent discovery in Jamaica, that a low serum sodium is a bad prognostic sign (Smith 1963) is relevant. We are now trying to combine a salt-poor diet in the first days of treatment, with a salt-rich diet starting as the excretion of sodium falls away. A day-to-day control of the salt output is necessary, and the added salt often produces a sharp rise in weight, with a visible increase in œdema, and a curious syndrome of rise of temperature and increase in the rate of respiration, which cannot be explained fully by a rise in the blood volume. The syndrome seems benign, but we would prefer to avoid it.

It is likely that in the first days of treatment, the overriding consideration is the removal of sodium, but very soon the depleted cells must need large quantities of all the electrolytes for their synthetic processes, and it may well be that a mixture such as that in dried skimmed milk—it is, presumably a balanced mixture, at least for the calf—is better than anything artificial we can devise. At the moment the optimum amounts of minerals needed are unknown.

It has been stated often that the addition of vitamins to therapeutic diets is valueless. It would be surprising if cure could proceed far on a vitamin-free diet, but which vitamins are most needed, and in what amounts, has yet to be determined. The signs accompanying kwashiorkor, such as angular stomatitis, cheilosis and changes of the tongue, that might be due to deficiencies of members of the B complex, clear up as the child's general condition improves, even when the total vitamin content of the diet is no more than that contained in a small amount of dried skimmed milk. Furthermore, the vitamin of which a shortage could most confidently be prophesied, vitamin B_{12}, has been found at a high concentration in the serum, even in severe cases in the acute stage (Satoskar et al. 1962, Satyanarayana 1963).

Anabolic steroids in our hands have been useless, and there have been some undesirable side effects: one boy gained 2 kg. weight and became visibly œdematous in about 10 days, and one girl's clitoris was considerably enlarged. Cortisone acetate, given by mouth, has also caused an increase in œdema in a few cases in Rhodesia (Piburn 1960).

We need to know how much protein should be given for the best results, but the problem is extremely complicated. It is necessary to take into account a large number of factors, including the form in which the protein is offered, the quantity and availability of the amino acids of the protein, the other nutrients in the diet with the protein, and the total caloric value of the diet.

One effect of recent work on serum amino acids has been to shake faith in the importance, in the development of kwashiorkor, of "limiting" amino acids in the diet; all the diets that are conducive to kwashiorkor cannot be deficient in the same amino acids, and the lack of total protein or of nitrogen, not of individual amino acids, is probably the chief cause of kwashiorkor. It is clear from many reports that plant proteins are not so rapidly effective in treatment as milk in promoting the synthesis of albumin, the removal of œdema, and the regain of weight (Dean 1952, Venkatachalam *et al.* 1956, Rao 1960, Scrimshaw *et al.* 1961).

The time may come when the complete exploration of the metabolism of amino acids in kwashiorkor, individually and in combination, will show the exact composition necessary for an ideal protein for treatment. Until more is known about the amino acid metabolism, it seems best to rely on the protein of cow's milk whenever possible. The complete protein might be even more effective than the calcium caseinate that is so often used: it has been said (Walt and Hathorn 1960) that skimmed lactic acid milk is so effective that the isolated protein need not be employed.

We have used mixtures of the caseinate, dried skimmed milk, cane sugar and cottonseed oil, and are at present using combinations that provide about 20 calories for each g. protein. Of the calories, more than half are derived from the oil. The results are fairly satisfactory in that only 15% of the worst cases die, many of these dying soon after admission. The essentially negative findings at most *post mortem* examinations show that the cause of death must be chemical.

Despite the contrary views of some, we favour high protein intakes. The synthesis of serum proteins, the loss of œdema and the gain in weight, all proceed faster the more protein there is in the diet, up to a level of about 7 g. protein/kg. body weight (Dean 1960). At higher levels there is sometimes an unsatisfactory rate of weight gain. Waterlow has reported success with diets containing less than 2 g. protein per kg., with a calorie : protein ratio as high as that in human milk (66:1). He and his colleagues (Garrow *et al.* 1962) and others (Dumm *et al.* 1963) now find about 4 g. protein and 150 calories/kg. satisfactory. Some years ago, we arranged a series of experiments in which different amounts of protein were given at first, and afterwards, the amounts were varied step-wise. Our criteria were weight loss, serum protein increase, and weight gain. Progress was very slow on 2·5 g. protein/kg. and only slightly faster on 3·0 g./kg: 4·0 to 5 g./kg. gave much better results (Dean 1961d). This work was not published in full because the weight gains proved to depend greatly on the minerals in the diet, and therefore on water retention.

Progress in such investigations is inevitably slow. Although exceptionally equipped, we cannot undertake the observation of more than 10 children at a time; at least 6 months' work is needed, and between 60 and 80 cases, for the assessment of any alteration in treatment.

The Late Effects of Treatment

Follow-up examination has usually shown that recovery from kwashiorkor appears to be complete (Garrow *et al.* 1962, Moodie 1961). We have found in Uganda that the impetus to growth given by a short period of intense hospital treatment lasts for about a year, but usually falls away before the height and weight for age have become entirely satisfactory (Dean 1961c, 1962a). Our studies (Geber and Dean 1956) of the mentality of children who had been treated for kwashiorkor led us to believe that no residue of the psychological disturbances remained, if the social circumstances were favourable to the child, but two recent investigations suggest we may have been over optimistic. Mexican workers (Cravioto and Robles 1963) have found that Gesell scores can be correlated with weight and height deficit for age in children aged 3 years and more, who were probably malnourished earlier. If physical recovery is incomplete, therefore, mental recovery might also be so. The result of a South African study (Stoch and Smythe 1963) is even more ominous, for the victims of kwashiorkor showed the mental stigmata throughout a period of observation that covered several years. If this is confirmed, the need for better treatment will be obvious: our success may be less complete than we believe.

Certainly, the electroencephalographic changes that are found in some of the severe cases of kwashiorkor (Nelson 1959, Nelson and Dean 1959) are known to persist for many months.

In conclusion, we offer a piece of speculation. If Selye (1958) is correct, permanent ill-effects may be produced by a combination of magnesium and potassium deficiencies with a relative excess of sodium (in some forms) and of certain steroids. Characteristically, hæmorrhages and necroses are succeeded by fibrosis, especially in the heart. In kwashiorkor it seems that all these contributory factors are present simultaneously. Mineral abnormalities of the same kinds, and at least one hormonal abnormality—excess active steroid (p. 248)—almost certainly co-exist. In Uganda there is not only a great deal of kwashiorkor, but in later life a great deal of disease, especially of a cardiac kind, that might arise on a basis of the sequence of necrosis and fibrosis: heart failure in pre-adolescent children, with severe changes in the left side of the heart; nutritional cardiopathies, such as endomyocardial fibrosis; pancreatic lithiasis; malabsorption syndromes; hepatic cirrhosis and primary carcinoma. Are these conditions legacies of kwashiorkor in early childhood? If so, why are most of these conditions rare in other countries that have much kwashiorkor? (Scrimshaw 1961). The answer may not be known for 20 years, or the length of time that must elapse before a sufficient number of groups of proven cases of kwashiorkor in various countries have been followed into adult life. At the moment, we do not even know how many live to become adult, let alone the extent of their permanent damage.

Prevention

The prevention of any disease must be much more important, even if less spectacular and less immediately satisfactory to the clinician, than the most remarkable cure. Here we cannot consider the alterations in social and economic circumstances, and the improvements in education, that seem to be inevitable if malnutrition is to be eradicated, and must limit discussion to the provision of foods that will adequately supplement the diet of the newly-weaned child.

The essence of the problem is to ensure that there is a daily intake of about 4 g. protein/kg. body weight, with an adequacy of calories. In some circumstances vitamin deficiencies must be corrected. In others, there may be shortages of minerals, but the plants that form the largest proportion of most poor diets nearly always provide plenty of potassium and magnesium at least. Whether these minerals are utilised is, of course, another problem. The importance of kwashiorkor would be greatly diminished if every child could be assured of a pint of milk a day, and it may not be going too far to say that the pint of milk, or its equivalent in some other form of animal origin, must be included in the diet if the potential for growth is to be fully realised. Several products, most of which have been used successfully for the treatment of kwashiorkor and can therefore be assumed to prevent it, are described in the National Academy of Sciences 1961 publication. The choice of the materials emphasised the need to use plant proteins, sometimes in accordance with the well-established principle of mixing the proteins so that they supplement each other's deficiencies, but no combination of the proteins has yet been proved to be as effective as milk protein over a long period for the restoration of the malnourished child to a state of apparent good health.

Compared with many other regions, East Africa is fortunate in its capacity for milk production, part of which has already been realised in the well-developed dairy industry of the Kenya Highlands. That industry could undoubtedly be developed further, and recent work has shown that in some parts of Uganda the prospects for the efficient production of milk are much better than was formerly believed. The Uganda Government has therefore decided to concentrate on the use of milk in their schemes for supplementing post-weaning diets. The ratio of protein to calories in dried skimmed milk is insufficient to ensure that the protein of the milk is used in the most economical way, and edible vegetable oil and sugar, both produced locally, are added to the dried milk in amounts sufficient to bring the protein : calorie ratio to that of full milk. The mixture is made by simple stirring: the oil distributes itself and does not settle out. In polyethylene packets that contain approximately the equivalent of a pint of milk (20 g. protein and 400 calories) it keeps for a year without special precautions. The mothers are advised to stir it into the child's food, but most of them prefer to reconstitute it into a liquid, a process that unfortunately introduces the hazard of dirty, or at least unboiled, water. The use of the packets in the treatment of kwashiorkor in thinly-staffed hospitals—a very simple dosage system is possible, on the principle of one packet for a small child and two packets for a large one—has proved successful, and a scheme for distribution to clinics and dispensaries throughout the country is being gradually brought into operation (Burgess and Burgess 1962, Dean 1962b).

The use of dried skimmed milk brings the disadvantage of loose stools, a universal finding that has not been given the attention it deserves. A practical method by which the loose stools could be prevented is urgently wanted; it would not only greatly improve home treatment, but might also obviate the expensive use of calcium caseinate for the hospital treatment of the most severe cases. (An Indian caseinate (Doraiswamy et al. 1961), relatively inexpensive to manufacture and capable of giving excellent results, is not yet in commercial production.) In much the same way, a method is needed for preventing the loose stools that are caused by dried yeast, and largely restrict the use of that food for its protein.

We have come to the conclusion that in many circumstances the most profitable course may be to discover the minimum proportion of milk (dried skimmed milk is the form most likely to be available) that must be added to diets of plant origin for the maximum effect; and others seem to be of like mind (Jayalakshmi and Mukundan 1961, Bhagavan *et al.* 1962, Sabry *et al.* 1963). In a small series of experiments (Clegg and Dean 1960, Dean 1961d), maximum nitrogen retentions were achieved by the addition of dried milk sufficient to yield one-fourth of the total protein of a mixture that included whole ground nuts, whole maize flour, sucrose and cottonseed oil; there was some evidence that the retentions were less if the proportions of the milk protein were smaller or larger. In the freely-chosen diets of the children of British families investigated between 1935 and 1939, most of whom were in comfortable economic circumstances, over half of the total protein was derived from milk and other animal sources at all ages (Widdowson 1947). In developing countries only a far more modest proportion is practicable at the present time, and it is to be hoped that even our one-fourth will prove to be more than enough.

The day of the inferior substitute, if it ever really dawned, is already passing. If milk cannot be made available in the required amounts, some other source of protein must be found that will be as effective, as acceptable, and of similar prestige. The examples of people who rear fine children on diets that do not include the milk of animals are rare and little known: most of them take the children direct from breast milk to meat or fish.

To some extent, knowledge of technology that could make cheap high-protein foods available has outrun knowledge of how to apply new foods, or how to persuade parents to alter the proportions of the foods they already know, to the best advantage of the children. A recent conference on malnutrition and food habits (Burgess and Dean 1962) succeeded in little more than a statement of the difficulties and of the need for a great deal of research. It met in the shadow of the realisation that extensive efforts to find new foods and to introduce them, sponsored by the International Organisations, had achieved very little. Is it possible that the approach has been fundamentally wrong? Is it good enough to assume that anything less than what is believed to be best will be gratefully taken, even for a short time? The vegetable-protein mixture Incaparina (Scrimshaw *et al.* 1961), introduced as a cheap supplementary food, has run into a difficulty that might seem extraordinary: the economically ill-favoured families for whom it is intended, and whose children are appallingly badly fed, will not buy it because they think it is intended for the poor. This may be an extreme example, but a recognition of the principle involved may be fundamental for the success of other schemes. The deliberate satisfaction of snob values in nutrition, although at first sight ridiculous, and sure to be costly, may eventually prove to be more effective, and even cheaper, than attempts to ensure the acceptance of the second-rate.

REFERENCES

ALBANESE, A. A., ORTO, L. A., ZAVATTARO, D. N. (1958) Biochemical significance of plasma amino nitrogen in man with a comparison of other criteria of protein metabolism. *Metabolism*, **7**, 256

ALLEN, D. M. (1964) The anemia of kwashiorkor in Uganda. *Trans. roy. Soc. trop. Med. Hyg.*, in the press

ALLEN, D. M., WHITEHEAD, R. G. (1964) The excretion of imidazole acrylic acid and formiminoglutamic acid in megaloblastosis accompanying kwashiorkor. *Blood.* In the press

ANNUAL REPORT (1961–62) The Nutrition Research Laboratories Hyderabad (Deccan)

ARROYAVE, G. (1961) Biochemical evaluation of nutritional status in man. *Fed. Proc.*, **20**, 39

ARROYAVE, G. (1963) Biochemical signs of mild-moderate forms of protein-calorie malnutrition. *Symposia Swedish Nutr. Foundation*, **1**, 32

ARROYAVE, G., WILSON, D. (1961) Urinary excretion of creatinine of children under different nutritional conditions. *Amer. J. clin. Nutr.* **9**, 170

ARROYAVE, G., WILSON, D., BEHAR, M., SCRIMSHAW, N. S. (1961) Serum and urinary creatinine in children with severe protein malnutrition. *Amer. J. clin. Nutr.* **9**, 176

ARROYAVE, G., WILSON, D., CONTRERAS, C., BEHAR, M. (1963) Alterations in serum concentration of vitamin A associated with the hypoproteinemia of severe protein malnutrition. *Pediatrics*, **62**, 920

ARROYAVE, G., WILSON, D., DE FUNES, C., BEHAR, M. (1962) The free amino acids in blood plasma of children with kwashiorkor and marasmus. *Amer. J. clin. Nutr.* **11**, 517

AWWAAD, S., ATTIA, M., REDA, M. (1960) Electrocardiographic studies in nutritional œdema in Egyptian children. *J. Egypt. med. Ass.*, **43**, 164

AWWAAD, S., EISA, E. A. (1959) Studies on blood amino acid nitrogen in normal Egyptian infants and children and in cases of nutritional edema. *Arch. Pediat.* **76**, 395

BADR EL-DIN, M. K., ABOUL WAFA, M. H. (1961) Galactose intolerance in kwashiorkor. *J. trop. Med. Hyg.*, **64**, 110

BAILEY, K. V. (1961) Rural nutrition studies in Indonesia 1. Background to nutritional studies in the cassava areas. *Trop. geogr. Med.* **13**, 216

BAKER, R. W. R., MACDONALD, I. (1961) Liver and depot fatty acids in kwashiorkor. *Nature*, **189**, 406

BECKER, W., NAUDÉ, W. DU T., KIPPS, A., MCKENZIE, D. (1963) Virus studies in disseminated herpes simplex infections. Association with malnutrition in children. *S. Afr. med. J.* **37**, 74

BENNETT, M. A. E., WATSON, K. C. (1962) The universal serologic reaction in kwashiorkor. *S. Afr. J. lab. clin. Med.* **8**, 113

BERMAN, M. C., KENCH, J. E. (1963) Excretion of amino acids in the bound form in the urine of patients suffering from kwashiorkor. *S. Afr. med. J.* **37**, 86

BHAGAVAN, R. K., DORAISWAMY, T. R., SUBRAMANIAN, N., NARAYANA RAO, M., SWAMINATHAN, M., BHATIA, D. S., SREENIVASAN, A., SUBRAMANYAN, V. (1962) Use of isolated vegetable proteins in the treatment of protein malnutrition (kwashiorkor). *Amer. J. clin. Nutr.* **11**, 177

BOWIE, M. D., BRINKMAN, G. L., HANSEN, J. D. L. (1963) Diarrhœa in protein-calorie malnutrition. *Lancet*, **2**, 550

BROCK, J. F. (1961) *Recent Advances in Human Nutrition.* Churchill, London

BURGESS, A., DEAN, R. F. A. (1962) *Malnutrition and Food Habits.* London

BURGESS, H. J. L., BURGESS, A. P. (1962) Reinforced milk for the prevention of malnutrition. 1. Preparation and qualitative trials. *E. Afr. med. J.* **39**, 427

CADDELL, J. (1963) *Personal communication.* Address: Dept. of Pædiatrics, Makerere University College Medical School, Kampala, Uganda

CHATTERJI, A., SEN GUPTA, P. C. (1960) Adrenals in malnourished and undernourished infants. *Indian J. Pediat.* **27**, 355

CLEGG, K. M., DEAN, R. F. A. (1960) Balance studies on peanut biscuit in the treatment of kwashiorkor. *Amer. J. clin. Nutr.* **8**, 885

COHEN, S., HANSEN, J. D. L. (1962) Metabolism of albumin and γ-globulin in kwashiorkor. *Clin. Sci.* **23**, 351

CRAVIOTO, J., ROBLES, B. (1963) The influence of protein-calorie malnutrition on psychological test behavior. *Symposia Swedish Nutr. Foundation*, **1**, 115

CRAWFORD, M. A. (1963) *Personal communication.* Address: Dept. of Physiology, Makerere University College Medical School, Kampala, Uganda

CRONJE, R. E., PRETORIUS, P. J. (1963) The electrocardiogram in kwashiorkor. *S. Afr. J. lab. clin. Med.* **9**, 11

CRONJE, R. E., SAVAGE, D. J., THERON, J. J. (1961) Iron metabolism in kwashiorkor. *Proc. Nutr. Soc. S. Afr.* **2**, 27

DEAN, R. F. A. (1952) The treatment of kwashiorkor with milk and vegetable proteins. *Brit. med. J.* **2**, 791

DEAN, R. F. A. (1957) Digestion in kwashiorkor. *Mod. Probl. Pœdiat.* **2**, 133

DEAN, R. F. A. (1960) Treatment of kwashiorkor with moderate amounts of protein. *J. Pediat.* **56**, 675

DEAN, R. F. A. (1961a) Kwashiorkor in Malaya: the clinical evidence. *J. trop. Pediat.* **7**, 3

DEAN, R. F. A. (1961b) Nitrogenous constituents of urine in kwashiorkor. *Fed. Proc.* **20**, 202

DEAN, R. F. A. (1961c) The effects of malnutrition on the growth of young children. *Mod. Probl. Pœdiat.* **5**, 111

DEAN, R. F. A. (1961d) Utilization of indigenous foods rich in protein for the prevention and treatment of malnutrition. In *Meeting Protein Needs;* p. 77. Washington, D.C.

DEAN, R. F. A. (1962a) Nutrition and growth. *Mod. Probl. Pœdiat.* **7**, 191

DEAN, R. F. A. (1962b) Reinforced milk for the treatment of malnutrition. II. Trials in the Medical Research Council Unit, Kampala. *E. Afr. med. J.* **39**, 425

DEAN, R. F. A. (1963a) Historique de l'education nutritionelle. In *Séminaire sur l'education en matière de santé et de nutrition en Afrique au sud du Sahara.* (Edited by I. Paul-Pont and M. J. Bonnal); p. 200. Paris

DEAN, R. F. A. (1963b) Production and control of œdema. *Symposia Swedish Nutr. Foundation,* **1**, 60

DEAN, R. F. A., SWANNE, J. (1963) Abbreviated schedule of treatment for severe kwashiorkor. *J. trop. Pediat.* **8**, 97

DEAN, R. F. A., WHITEHEAD, R. G. (1963a) The metabolism of aromatic aminoacids in kwashiorkor. *Lancet,* **1**, 188

DEAN, R. F. A., WHITEHEAD, R. G. (1963b) Free amino acids in the blood of malnourished children: A simplified method of analysis. *Programme, 6th Int. Congr. Nutr., Edinburgh,* p. 79

DE LA TORRE, J., BERBER, S., DURAN, L. (1949) Alteraciones electrocardiograficas en niños desnutridos multicarenciados. *Bol. méd. Hosp. infant. (Méx.)* **6**, 317

DORAISWAMY, T. R., SWAMINATHAN, M., SREENAVASAN, A., SUBRAMANYAN, V. (1961) Use of calcium caseinate in the treatment of protein malnutrition in children. *Indian J. Pediat.* **29**, 226

DUMM, M. E., WEBB, J. K. G., PEREIRA, S., BEGUM, A., ISAAC, T. (1963) Moderate protein, high-calorie diets in the treatment of kwashiorkor. *Programme, 6th Int. Congr. Nutr., Edinburgh,* p. 87

DUTRA DE OLIVEREIRA, J. E., ROLANDO, E. (1963) Fat absorption studies in undernourished children fed cow's milk or soya milk. *Programme, 6th Int. Congr. Nutr., Edinburgh,* p. 125

EDITORIAL (1962) Kwashiorkor—a notifiable disease. *S. Afr. med. J.* **36**, 801

EDOZIEN, J. C., PHILLIPS, E. J. (1961) Partition of urine nitrogen in kwashiorkor. *Nature,* **191**, 47

EDOZIEN, J. C., PHILLIPS, E. J., COLLIS, W. R. F. (1960) The free amino acids of plasma and urine in kwashiorkor. *Lancet,* **1**, 615

EDOZIEN, J. C., UDEOZO, I. O. K. (1960) Serum copper, iron and iron-binding capacity in kwashiorkor. *J. trop. Pediat.* **6**, 60

EL GHOLMY, A., ABOUL-DAHAB, Y. W., EL ESSAWI, M., ABDEL RAHMAN, Y., MALEK, A. (1962) Biochemical studies in anæmia in malnourished infants: a comparison of marasmic and kwashiorkor cases. *J. trop. Med. Hyg.* **65**, 64

EXPERT COMMITTEE (1963) Expert Committee on Medical Assessment of Nutritional Status. *Wld. Hlth. Org. techn. Rep. Ser.* **258**

FARMER, A. P. (1960) Malnutrition as an ecological problem. *E. Afr. med. J.* **37**, 399

FOLLIS, R. H. (1961) Studies on a kwashiorkor-like syndrome in monkeys. In *Meeting Protein Needs,* Washington, D.C., p. 377

FOY, H., KONDI, A., MACDOUGALL, L. (1961) Pure red-cell aplasia in marasmus and kwashiorkor treated with riboflavine. *Brit. med. J.* **1**, 937

GANDRA, Y. R., SCRIMSHAW, N. S. (1961) Infection and nutritional status. II. Effect of mild virus infection induced by 17-D yellow fever vaccine on nitrogen metabolism in children. *Amer. J. clin. Nutr.* **9**, 159

GARROW, J. S., PICOU, D., WATERLOW, J. C. (1962) The treatment and prognosis of infantile malnutrition in Jamaican children. *W. Indian med. J.,* **11**, 217

GEBER, M., DEAN, R. F. A. (1956) The psychological changes accompanying kwashiorkor. *Courrier,* **6**, 8

HANNA, S., HARRISON, M., MACINTYRE, I., FRASER, R. (1960) The syndrome of magnesium deficiency in man. *Lancet,* **2**, 172

HANSEN, J. D. L., BRINKMAN, L., BOWIE, M. D., FRIIS-HANSEN, B. (1963) Body water compartments and body composition in kwashiorkor. *Programme, 6th Int. Congr. Nutr., Edinburgh,* p. 80

HANSEN, J. D. L., BROCK, J. F. (1954) Potassium deficiency in the pathogenesis of nutritional œdema in infants. *Lancet*, **2**, 477

HASSAN, M. M. (1960) Kwashiorkor in Sudanese children. *J. trop. Pediat.* **6**, 98

HENLEY, K. S., SCHMIDT, F. W., SCHMIDT, E. (1963) Serum enzymes during recovery from malnutrition. *Lancet*, **1**, 390

HOLT, L. E., SNYDERMAN, S. E., NORTON, P. M., ROITMAN, E., FINCH, J. (1963) The plasma aminogram in kwashiorkor. *Lancet*, **2**, 1343

JAYALAKSHMI, V. T., MUKUNDAN, R. (1961) Clinical trials with roasted groundnuts in cases of protein malnutrition (kwashiorkor). *Ind. J. med. Res.* **49**, 6

JELLIFFE, D. B., JELLIFFE, E. F. P. (1960) The prevalence of protein-calorie malnutrition in Haitian pre-school children. *Amer. J. publ. Hlth.* **50**, 1355

JELLIFFE, D. B., JELLIFFE, E. F. P. (1963) The assessment of protein-calorie malnutrition of early childhood as a community problem. *Symposia Swedish Nutr. Foundation*, **1**, 131

JELLIFFE, D. B., JELLIFFE, E. F. P., GARCIA, L., DE BARROS, G. (1961) The children of the San Blas Indians of Panama. *J. Pediat.* **59**, 271

JELLIFFE, D. B., SYMONDS, B. E. R., JELLIFFE, E. F. P. (1960) The pattern of malnutrition in early childhood in southern Trinidad. *J. Pediat.* **57**, 922

JELLIFFE, D. B., WELBOURN, H. F. (1963) Clinical signs of mild-moderate protein-calorie malnutrition of early childhood. *Symposia Swedish Nutr. Foundation*, **1**, 12

JONES, P. R. M., DEAN, R. F. A. (1956) The effects of kwashiorkor on the development of the bones of the hand. *J. trop. Pediat.* **2**, 51

JONES, P. R. M., DEAN, R. F. A. (1959) The effects of kwashiorkor on the development of the bones of the knee. *J. Pediat.* **54**, 176

KAHN, E., STEIN, H., ZOUTENDYK, A. (1957) Isohemagglutinins and immunity in malnutrition. *Amer. J. clin. Nutr.* **5**, 70

KAHN, E., WAYBURNE, S. (1961) Hypoglycæmia in patients suffering from advanced protein malnutrition (kwashiorkor). *Proc. Nutr. Soc. S. Afr.* **1**, 21

KARIKS, J. (1962) Some observations on serum protein levels in kwashiorkor and their changes during treatment. *Med. J. Aust.* **2**, 411

KERPEL-FRONIUS, E. (1960) Volume and composition of the body fluid compartments in severe infantile malnutrition. *J. Pediat.* **56**, 826

KINNEAR, A. A., PRETORIUS, P. J. (1962) Sulphobromphthalein clearance and porphyrin excretion in kwashiorkor. *S. Afr. J. lab. clin. Med.* **8**, 65

KONDI, A., MACDOUGALL, L., FOY, H., MEHTA, S., MBAYA, V. (1963) Anæmias of marasmus and kwashiorkor in Kenya. *Arch. Dis. Childh.*, **38**, 267

KONDI, A., MEHTA, S. H., FOY, H. (1962) Red-cell aplasia in marasmus and kwashiorkor. *Brit. med. J.* **1**, 110

LAHEY, M. E., BEHAR, M., VITERI, F., SCRIMSHAW, N. S. (1958) Values for copper, iron and iron-binding capacity in the serum of kwashiorkor. *Pediatrics*, **22**, 72

LEONARD, P. J., MACWILLIAM, K. M. (1963) Cortisol binding in the serum in kwashiorkor. *Biochem. J.* **89**, 77P

LEWIS, B., HANSEN, J. D. L., WITTMAN, W., STEWART, F. (1963) Lipid metabolism in kwashiorkor. *S. Afr. J. Med.* **37**, 161

LINDER, G. C., HANSEN, J. D. L., KARABUS, C. D. (1963) The metabolism of magnesium and other inorganic cations and of nitrogen in acute kwashiorkor. *Pediatrics*, **31**, 552

LOWENSTEIN, F. W. (1962) Kwashiorkor in the Congo. *Bull. Wld. Hlth. Org.*, **27**, 151

LOWENSTEIN, F. W. (1963) The vicious circle mechanism in the production of protein-calorie malnutrition. *Symposia Swedish Nutr. Foundation*, **1**, 107

LUHBY, A. L., COOPERMAN, J. M., TELLER, D. M. (1959) Histidine metabolic loading test to distinguish folic acid deficiency from Vitamin B_{12} in megaloblastic anemias. *Proc. Soc. exp. Biol. N.Y.*, **101**, 350

LURIE, A. O., JACKSON, W. P. U. (1962a) Aldosteronuria and the edema of kwashiorkor. *Amer. J. clin. Nutr.* **11**, 115

LURIE, A. O., JACKSON, W. P. U. (1962b) Adrenal function in kwashiorkor and marasmus. *Clin. Sci.* **22**, 259

McCULLOCH, H. (1920) Studies on the heart in nutritional disturbance in infancy. *Amer. J. Dis. Childh.* **20**, 486

MACDONALD, I. (1960) Hepatic lipid of malnourished children. *Metabolism*, **9**, 838

MACDONALD, I. (1962) Fat metabolism in malnourished tropical children. *Amer. J. clin. Nutr.* **10**, 111

MACDONALD, I., HANSEN, J. D. L., BRONTE-STEWART, B. (1963) Liver, depot and serum lipids during early recovery from kwashiorkor. *Clin. Sci.*, **24**, 55

McLEAN, A. E. M. (1963) Hepatic failure in malnutrition. *Lancet*, **1**, 772

McLEAN, A. E. M., CHAN, H. V. (1963) Glutamic pyruvic transaminase activity in the liver and serum of malnourished children. *Programme, 6th Int. Congr. Nutr., Edinburgh,* p. 79

MacWILLIAM, K. M. (1964) Hæmoglobin combining power of the serum in kwashiorkor. To be published

MAJAJ, A. S., DINNING, J. S., AZZAM, S. A., DARBY, W. T. (1963) Vitamin E responsive megaloblastic anæmia in infants with protein-calorie malnutrition. *Amer. J. clin. Nutr.* **12,** 374

MAJAJ, A. S., DINNING, J. S., DARBY, W. J. (1963) Vitamin E responsive megaloblastic anæmia in protein-calorie malnutrition. *Programme, 6th Int. Congr. Nutr., Edinburgh,* p. 81

MAMEESH, M. S., ABDOU, K. A., GALAL, O. M., SHOUKRY, A. S., ALI HASSAN (1963) A study of diet and kwashiorkor in Egypt. *Programme, 6th Int. Congr. Nutr., Edinburgh,* p. 80

MATTHEW, C. E., DEAN, R. F. A. (1960) The serum lipids in kwashiorkor. II. The relation of diet to total serum cholesterol. *J. trop. Pediat.* **5,** 135

METZ, J., STEIN, H. (1959) Iron deficiency anæmia in Bantu infants, and its association with kwashiorkor. *S. Afr. med. J.* **33,** 624

MEY, H. S., PRETORIUS, P. J., SMIT, Z. M., DU TOIT, C. V. (1961) The effect of prolonged skim-milk therapy on the levels of certain constituents of the blood in kwashiorkor. *S. Afr. J. lab. clin. Med.* **7,** 137

MEY, H. S., SMIT, Z. M., LABUSCHAGNE, C. J., PRETORIUS, P. J. (1961) Effects of diets containing different types of fat and protein on the levels of certain constituents of the blood serum of convalescent kwashiorkor patients. *S. Afr. J. lab. clin. Med.* **7,** 141

MILNE, M. D., MUEHRCKE, R. C., AIRD, I. (1957) Primary aldosteronism. *Quart. J. Med.* **26,** 317

MODY, N. J., SMITH, C. E. (1964) Glutathione concentration, glutathione stability and glucose-6-phosphate dehydrogenase activity in the erythrocytes of children with kwashiorkor. To be published

MONCKEBERG, F., BEAS, F., PERRETTA, M. (1956) Funcion suprarenal en distróficos. *Rev. chil. Pediat.* **27,** 187

MONCKEBERG, F., DONOSO, G., OXMAN, S., PAK, N., MENEGHELLO, J. (1963) Human growth hormone in infant malnutrition. *Pediatrics,* **31,** 58

MONCKEBERG, F., VILDOSOLA, J., FIGUEROA, M., OXMAN, S., MENEGHELLO, J. (1963) Hematologic disturbances in infantile malnutrition. Values for copper, iron, paraphenylene diamine oxidase and iron-binding capacity in the serum. *Amer. J. clin. Nutr.* **11,** 525

MONTGOMERY, R. D. (1960) Magnesium metabolism in infantile protein malnutrition. *Lancet,* **2,** 74

MONTGOMERY, R. D. (1961) Magnesium balance studies in marasmic kwashiorkor. *J. Pediat.* **59,** 119

MONTGOMERY, R. D. (1962a) Muscle morphology in infantile protein malnutrition. *J. clin. Path.* **15,** 511

MONTGOMERY, R. D. (1962b) Urinary radio-iodine excretion in the malnourished infant. *Arch. Dis. Childh.* **37,** 383

MONTGOMERY, R. D. (1962c) Changes in the basal metabolic rate of the malnourished infant and their relation to body composition. *J. clin. Invest.* **41,** 1653

MOODIE, A. (1961) Kwashiorkor in Cape Town: the background of patients and their progress after discharge. *J. Pediat.* **58,** 392

NAISMITH, D. J. (1963) The role of the essential fatty acids in the ætiology of kwashiorkor. *Programme, 6th Int. Congr. Nutr., Edinburgh,* p. 88

NATIONAL ACADEMY OF SCIENCES (1961) Meeting protein needs. *Publication No. 843 Nat. Acad. Sci.*—Nat. Res. Coun., Washington, D.C.

NELSON, G. K. (1959) The electroencephalogram in kwashiorkor. *Electroenceph. clin. Neurophysiol.* **11,** 73

NELSON, G. K., DEAN, R. F. A. (1959) The electroencephalogram in African children: effects of kwashiorkor and a note on the newborn. *Bull. Wld. Hlth. Org.* **21,** 779

OLARTE, J., CRAVIOTO, J., CAMPOS, B. (1956) Immunidad in el niño desnutrido 1. Producción di antoxina diftérica. *Bol. med. infant. (Méx.),* **13,** 467

PATEL, B. D., PATEL, J. C., GAITONDE, B. B., RAO, G. S. (1960) Blood volume and plasma volume studies in marasmic malnutrition. *Indian J. Child Hlth.* **9,** 407

PEETOOM, F. (1962) Immuno-electrophoretic analysis of the serum in kwashiorkor. *Trop. geogr. Med.* **14,** 193

PHILP, J. R., GRODSKY, G. M., CARBONE, J. V. (1961) Mercaptide conjugation in the uptake and secretion of sulphobromphthalein. *Amer. J. Physiol.* **200,** 545

PIBURN, M. F. (1960) Kwashiorkor: Treatment with cortisone and diamox. *Cent. Afr. J. Med.* **6,** 149

PLATT, B. S. (1961) Experimental protein malnutrition. In *Meeting Protein Needs*, Washington, D.C., p. 383

PRETORIUS, P. J., DE VILLIERS, L. S. (1962) Antibody response in children with protein malnutrition. *Amer. J. clin. Nutr.* **10**, 379

PURVES, L. R., HANSEN, J. D. L. (1962a) The rate of synthesis of albumin before and after treatment in cases with kwashiorkor. *Proc. Nutr. Soc. S. Afr.* **3**, 24

PURVES, L. R., HANSEN, J. D. L. (1962b) Protein-losing enteropathy in kwashiorkor. *Lancet*, **1**, 435

RAMALINGASWAMI, V., DEO, M. G., SOOD, S. K. (1961) Protein deficiency in the rhesus monkey. In *Meeting Protein Needs*, Washington, D.C., p. 365

RAO, G. P. (1960) Treatment of kwashiorkor with vegetable protein diets. *Indian J. Child Hlth.* **9**, 207

RUSSO, G. (1961) Ulteriori osservazioni di kwashiorkor in Sicilia con particulare riguardo alla etiopatogenesi ed alla terapia. *Pediatria, Naples*, **69**, 247

SABRY, Z. I., COWAN, J. W., CAMPBELL, J. A. (1963) The development of protein food mixtures for infant feeding in the Middle East. *Programme, 6th Int. Congr. Nutr., Edinburgh*, p. 128

SATOSKAR, R. S., KULKARNI, B. S., MEHTA, B. M., SANZGIRI, R. R., BAMJI, M. S. (1962) Serum vitamin B_{12} and folic acid (P.G.A.) levels in hypoproteinæmia and marasmus in Indian children. *Arch. Dis. Childh.* **37**, 9

SATYANARAYANA, N. S. (1963) Plasma vitamin B_{12} levels in some nutritional deficiency states. *Indian J. med. Res.* **51**, 103

SCHENDEL, H. E., HANSEN, J. D. L. (1961) Studies of fat metabolism in kwashiorkor II. Serum polyunsaturated fatty acids. *Amer. J. clin. Nutr.* **9**, 735

SCHENDEL, H. E., HANSEN, J. D. L. (1962) Study of factors responsible for the increased aminoaciduria of kwashiorkor. *J. Pediat.* **60**, 280

SCHWARTZ, R. (1958) *Personal communication.* Address: M.R.C. Infantile Malnutrition Research Unit, Kampala, Uganda

SCHWARTZ, R., DEAN, R. F. A. (1957) The serum lipids in kwashiorkor. 1. Neutral fat, phospholipids and cholesterol. *J. trop. Pediat.* **3**, 23

SCHYNS, CH., DEMAEYER, E. M. (1957) Recherches electrocardiographiques dans le kwashiorkor. *Acta cardiol. (Brux.)*, **12**, 413

SCRAGG, J., RUBIDGE, C. (1960) Kwashiorkor in African children in Durban. *Brit. med. J.* **2**, 1759

SCRIMSHAW, N. S. (1961) Panel summary. Proteins and amino acids. *Fed. Proc.* **20**, Supplement No. 7, 111

SCRIMSHAW, N. S., BEHAR, M., WILSON, D., VITERI, F., ARROYAVE, G., BRESSANI, R. (1961) All-vegetable protein mixtures for human feeding V. Clinical trials with INCAP mixtures 8 and 9 and with corn and beans. *Amer. J. clin. Nutr.* **9**, 196

SCRIMSHAW, N. S., TAYLOR, C. E., GORDON, J. E. (1959) Interactions of nutrition and infection. *Amer. J. med. Sci.* **237**, 367

SCRIMSHAW, N. S., WILSON, D., BRESSANI, R. (1960) Infection and kwashiorkor. *J. trop. Pediat.* **6**, 37

SELYE, H. (1958) The chemical prevention of cardiac necrosis. New York

SHAH, P. M. (1961) Blood volume changes in edematous children IV. Malnutrition, severe anemia and infantile cirrhosis of liver. *Indian J. med. Sci.* **15**, 129

SIMSON, J. C., MANN, N. M. (1961) The treatment and prevention of kwashiorkor. *S. Afr. med. J.* **35**, 825

SMITH, C. E. (1962) Serum transaminases in kwashiorkor. *J. Pediat.* **61**, 617

SMITH, R. (1960) Total body water in malnourished infants. *Clin. Sci.* **19**, 275

SMITH, R. (1963) Hyponatræmia in infantile malnutrition. *Lancet*, **1**, 771

SMITH, R., WATERLOW, J. C. (1960) Total exchangeable potassium in infantile malnutrition. *Lancet*, **1**, 147

SMYTHE, P. M., SWANEPOEL, A., CAMPBELL, J. A. H. (1962) The heart in kwashiorkor. *Brit. med. J.* **1**, 67

SNYDERMAN, S. E., HOLT, L. E., NORTON, P. M., ROITMAN, E., FINCH, J. (1963) The plasma aminogram in kwashiorkor. *Amer. J. clin, Nutr.* **12**, 333

SOMESWARA RAO, K. (1962) In *Malnutrition and Food Habits*, edited by A. Burgess and R. F. A. Dean, London, p. 29

STIRLING, G. A. (1962a) The thyroid in malnutrition. *Arch. Dis. Childh.* **37**, 99

STIRLING, G. A. (1962b) Renal pathology in malnourished infants. *Arch. Dis. Child.* **37**, 378

STOCH, M. B., SMYTHE, P. M. (1963) Does undernutrition during infancy inhibit brain growth and subsequent intellectual development? *Arch. Dis. Childh.* **38**, 546

TROWELL, H. C., DAVIES, J. N. P., DEAN, R. F. A. (1954) *Kwashiorkor.* London

TROWELL, H. C., DAVIES, J. N. P., DEAN, R. F. A. (1955) Kwashiorkor and malnutrition. *Acta Pœdiat.* **44**, 487

TROWELL, H. C., SIMPKISS, M. J. (1957) Intramuscular iron in the treatment of anæmia associated with kwashiorkor. *Lancet*, **2**, 264

VASANTGADKAR, P. S., VENKATACHALAM, P. S., TULPOLE, P. G. (1963) Partition of urinary nitrogen in children with kwashiorkor treated with animal and vegetable proteins. *Amer. J. clin. Nutr.* **12**, 150

VELEZ, H., GHITIS, J., PRADILLA, A., VITALE, J. J. (1963) Cali Harvard nutrition project. 1. Megaloblastic anæmia in kwashiorkor. *Amer. J. clin. Nutr.* **12**, 54

VENKATACHALAM, P. S., SRIKANTIA, S. G. (1961) Clinical trials with vegetable protein foods. *Proc. Symposium on Proteins, Aug. 1960*, C.F.T.R.I., Mysore

VENKATACHALAM, P. S., SRIKANTIA, S. G., MEHTA, G., GOPALAN, C. (1956) Treatment of nutritional œdema syndrome (kwashiorkor) with vegetable protein diets. *Indian J. med. Res.* **44**, 539

VIS, H. L. (1963) Aspects et mécanismes des hyperaminoaciduries de l'enfance. Bruxelles

VIS, H., DUBOIS, R., LOEB, H., VINCENT, M., BIGWOOD, E. J. (1958) Le profil des chromatogrammes d'aminoacidurie en pathologie de l'enfance. *Ann. Soc. belge Méd. trop.* **38**, 991

VITALE, J. J., GHITIS, J., CANOSA, C. (1963) Folic acid requirements for the prevention of megaloblastic dysplasia seen in kwashiorkor. *Programme 6th Int. Congr. Nutr., Edinburgh*, p. 86

WACKER, W. E. C., VALLEE, B. L. (1958) Magnesium metabolism. *New Engl. J. Med.*, **259**, 431, 475

WALT, F., HATHORN, M. (1960) High protein feeding in kwashiorkor. *Arch. Dis. Childh.* **35**, 455

WALT, F., TAYLOR, J. E. D., MAGILL, F. B., NESTADT, A. (1962) Erythroid hypoplasia in kwashiorkor. *Brit. med. J.* **1**, 73

WATERLOW, J. C. (1961a) Oxidative phosphorylation in the livers of normal and malnourished human infants. *Proc. roy. Soc., B*, **155**, 66

WATERLOW, J. C. (1961b) The rate of recovery of malnourished infants in relation to the protein and calorie levels of the diet. *J. trop. Pediat.* **7**, 16

WATERLOW, J. C. (1962a) Protein malnutrition and replenishment with protein in man and animals. In *Protein Metabolism*. Edited by F. Gross, Berlin

WATERLOW, J. C. (1962b) Protein metabolism in human protein malnutrition. *Proc. roy. Soc. B*, **156**, 345

WATERLOW, J. C. (1963a) The partition of nitrogen in the urine of malnourished Jamaican infants. *Amer. J. clin. Nutr.* **12**, 235

WATERLOW, J. C. (1963b) Metabolic disturbances in protein-calorie malnutrition. *Symposia Swedish Nutr. Foundation*, **1**, 47

WATERLOW, J. C. (1963c) The assessment of marginal protein malnutrition. *Proc. Nutr. Soc.*, **22**, 66

WATERLOW, J. C., CRAVIOTO, J., STEPHEN, J. M. L. (1960) Protein malnutrition in man. *Advanc. Protein Chem.* **15**, 131

WATERLOW, J. C., WILLS, V. G. (1960) Balance studies in malnourished Jamaican infants 1. Absorption and retention of nitrogen and phosphorus. *Brit. J. Nutr.* **14**, 183

WAYBURNE, S. (1963) Hepatic failure in malnutrition. *Lancet*, **1**, 447

WESTALL, R. G., ROITMAN, E., DE LA PENA, C., RASMUSSEN, H., CRAVIOTO, J., GOMEZ, F., HOLT, L. E. (1958) The plasma amino acids in malnutrition. *Arch. Dis. Childh.* **33**, 499

WETTERFORS, J., GULLBERG, R., LILJEDAHL, S.-O., PLANTIN, L.-O., BIRKE, G., OLHAGEN, B. (1960) Role of the stomach and small intestine in albumin breakdown. *Acta med. scand.* **168**, 347

WHITEHEAD, R. G. (1962) Histidine metabolism in kwashiorkor. *Lancet*, **2**, 203

WHITEHEAD, R. G. (1964a) Amino acid metabolism in kwashiorkor I. Metabolism of histidine and imidazole derivatives. *Clin. Sci.*, **26**, 271

WHITEHEAD, R. G. (1964a) Rapid determination of some plasma amino acids in subclinical kwashiorkor. *Lancet*, **1**, 250

WHITEHEAD, R. G. (in the press) Amino acid metabolism in kwashiorkor I. Metabolism of histidine and imidazole derivatives. *Clin. Sci.*

WHITEHEAD, R. G., ARNSTEIN, H. R. V. (1961) Imidazole acrylic acid excretion in kwashiorkor. *Nature*, **190**, 1105

WHITEHEAD, R. G., DEAN, R. F. A. (1964a) Serum amino acids in kwashiorkor I. Relationship to clinical condition. To be published

WHITEHEAD, R. G., DEAN, R. F. A. (1964b) Serum amino acids in kwashiorkor II. An abbreviated method of estimation and its application. To be published

WHITEHEAD, R. G., MATTHEW, C. E. (1960) The analysis of urine of children suffering from kwashiorkor. *E. Afr. med. J.* **37**, 384

WHITEHEAD, R. G., MILBURN, T. R. (1962) Metabolites of phenylalanine in the urine of children with kwashiorkor. *Nature*, **196**, 580

WHITEHEAD, R. B., MILBURN, T. R. (1964) Amino acid metabolism in kwashiorkor II. Metabolism of phenylalanine and tyrosine. *Clin. Sci.*, **26**, 279

WIDDOWSON, E. M. (1947) A study of individual children's diets. *Spec. Rep. Ser. med. Res. Coun. (Lond.)*, No. 257

WILSON, D., BRESSANI, R., SCRIMSHAW, N. S. (1961) Infection and nutritional status. I. The effect of chicken-pox on nitrogen metabolism in children. *Amer. J. clin. Nutr.* **9**, 154

WOODHAM-SMITH, C. (1962) *The Great Hunger. Ireland 1845–9*, London, p. 193

WRAY, J. D. (1961) Kwashiorkor and marasmus in Turkey. In *Meeting Protein Needs*, Washington, D.C., p. 189.

CHAPTER 11

ASPECTS OF CANCER IN CHILDHOOD

MARTIN BODIAN*

with the assistance of

B. G. OCKENDEN

THIS chapter on malignancies in childhood will be divided into two principal portions: the one dealing with general remarks concerning this group of diseases and how they differ in childhood from adult life, and the other concerning four selected diseases which have in more recent years attracted increasing attention both from pædiatricians and pathologists—*histiocytic reticulo-endotheliosis; embryonic sarcoma; neuroblastoma; nephroblastoma*.

The material used in this chapter is based on personal observations dating from 1925 to 1962 at The Hospital for Sick Children, Great Ormond Street, London; the earlier part of this period was retrospectively, the remainder prospectively collected. During that time we have seen a total of 1168 histologically confirmed cases of malignant disease excluding leukæmia. The latter condition amounting to 36% of all malignant disease in childhood, the overall total would be about 1820 children. Neoplasms of various kinds arising from the central nervous system accounted for 25%, sympathetic nervous tumours for 10%, and nephroblastoma for 7·5% of all tumours.

Embryonic Tumours

I like to divide the neoplasms in childhood into two groups—those arising from embryonic cells, i.e. non-teratomatous and teratomatous *embryonic tumours*, and those arising from "adult" type cells, "*adult tumours*". The embryonic neoplasms have, in common with normal embryonic cell groups, the propensity to differentiate gradually and widely into various types of mature cells. Those which are teratomatous have a completely unselected and "uninhibited" range of differentiation; whilst non-teratomatous embryonic neoplasms have already been submitted to the influence of the

* Dr Martin Bodian died in September 1963. He had worked as a pathologist at The Hospital for Sick Children, Great Ormond Street since 1943, and for the last ten years of his life had devoted a great part of his energies to studying the cancers of childhood. Seven months before his death he was operated on for cancer of the bowel; immediately after this he set to work with feverish energy to place on record his massive and meticulously studied collection of material, of which this chapter is one of the fruits. The draft was completed by him only a few days before his death, enabling his colleague Dr Barbara Ockenden to prepare it for publication. Much of its contents has not previously been published. It is surely fitting that this, his last contribution to medical literature, should be a distillate of that part of his work which he regarded as of most importance.

D.G.

so-called organising substances, hence their range of maturation is restricted to the organ of origin.

The following tumours are embryogenic and non-teratomatous:

1. In the central nervous system—*the medulloblastoma*
2. In the sympathetic nervous system—*the neuroblastoma*
3. In the kidney—*the nephroblastoma*
4. In the liver—*the hepatoblastoma*
5. In the urogenital sinus and outside it—*the embryonic sarcoma*
6. In the retina—*the retinoblastoma*

The teratoma is most frequently found in the sacrococcygeal region; second in frequency are the ovarian and testicular teratoma, and more rarely the intracranial, basicranial, cervical, mediastinal and retroperitoneal teratoma.

The following 1168 neoplasms were verified at Great Ormond Street Hospital between 1925 and 1962 (excluding leukæmia).

1. *C.N.S. Tumours* (excluding intracranial teratoma), 478 cases

	Cases
Nodular astrocytoma .	137
Diffuse astrocytoma .	47
Subependymal glioma	50
Differentiating medulloblastoma .	170
Meningioma	33
Other intracranial tumours .	28
Retinoblastoma .	3
Spinal cord neoplasms.	10

2. *Sympathetic Nervous Tumours*, 184 cases

Neuroblastoma .	165
Ganglioneuroma .	18
Phæochromocytoma	1
3. *Hepatoblastoma*	20
4. *Embryonic sarcoma*	43
5. *Nephroblastoma*	125

6. *Teratoma*, 96 cases

Sacrococcygeal .	50
Testicular .	14
Ovarian .	13
Intracranial	5
Basicranial	2
Cervical .	4
Mediastinal	3
Retroperitoneal .	5

7. *Tumours of Connective Tissues*, 53 cases

Soft tissue sarcoma incl. synovioma	42
Osteosarcoma	11

8. *Tumours of Lympho-Reticular System*, 125 cases

Lymphosarcoma.	36
Giant follicular lymphoblastoma	1
Reticulosarcoma.	22
Hodgkin's disease	25
Histiocytic reticulo-endotheliosis	41

9. *Miscellaneous Tumours*, 44 cases

Adrenal cortical tumours	16
Basal cell carcinoma of skin.	2
Malignant melanoma	4
Carcinoma ? branchial	1
„ of colon	1
„ of small intestine	1
„ of kidney	2
„ of liver	3
„ of parotid	1
„ of thyroid	2
„ of vagina/cervix	3
„ of larynx	1
Maxillary "retinal anlage" tumour	1
Interstitial cell tumour of testis	1
Granulosa cell tumour of ovary	1
Chordoma	1
Pancreatic islet tumour	1
Parathyroid tumour	1
Paraganglioma	1

Of the total of 1168 cases, 641 (55%) were teratomatous or non-teratomatous embryonic; 527 (45%) were "adult" type tumours. It follows that in childhood about 3 out of 5 cases are of embryonic origin if leukæmia is excluded, or 2 out of 5 cases including leukæmia. Embryogenic tumours are exceedingly rare in adult life where carcinoma prevails (a type of tumour only rarely seen in childhood), and here lies one of the most important differences between neoplasms in the child and in the adult.

A further important difference is the incidence of the sites of origin. In childhood 4 out of 5 tumours arise from the nervous systems, urinary system or lymphohæmopoietic system. In adults, on the other hand, 4 out of 5 tumours take origin from the alimentary, genital or respiratory systems—a totally different distribution (Table 1).

Malignant disease in childhood is proportionately a considerable cause of childhood mortality in this country, in France, in the U.S.A., and in other countries of similar economic status. The percentages of deaths from malignant neoplasms in relation to all deaths from natural causes between the ages of 1 and 14 years in England and Wales are as follows: in 1949, 10%; in 1952, 16%; in 1953, 17%; in 1954, 19%; in 1956, 20%; in 1957, 16%; in 1958, 22·6%; in 1959, 20·2%; in 1960, 21·2%; and in 1961, 20·3%. The absolute figures are relatively constant.

TABLE 1. THE APPROXIMATE SITE INCIDENCE OF PRIMARY
MALIGNANT NEOPLASMS

Systems	Relative Distribution	
	in Adults	in Children
Nervous.	1·4%	31%
Urinary	3·6%	11%
Lympho-hæmopoietic . .	2·3%	40%
Alimentary	38%	2·5%
Genital	30%	3·3%
Respiratory	10%	0·4%

Histiocytic Reticulo-endotheliosis

Hand-Schüller-Christian disease was originally established as a syndrome comprising skull defects, exophthalmos and diabetes insipidus. It has subsequently been realised that the characteristic lesions may be present not only in the skull but elsewhere in the skeleton, as well as in the viscera and the skin. The disorder has usually an insidious onset and runs a protracted course. Fom a histological standpoint, many authors have considered that the lesions consist predominantly of xanthoma cells, and there has been a considerable body of opinion that the disease process is essentially an anomaly of lipid metabolism, or "xanthomatosis," akin to Gaucher's and Niemann-Pick's disease.

The condition characterised by *Letterer* (1924) *and Siwe* (1933), sometimes known as "non-lipid-reticulosis," has as its main features a widespread involvement of the reticulo-endothelial system, with conspicuous splenomegaly, usually enlargement of liver and lymph nodes, cutaneous hæmorrhages and sometimes bony lesions. The disorder typically affects very young children and runs an acute course with fever and progressive anæmia, usually with a fatal termination. The microscopic picture in affected organs is described as a diffuse proliferation of reticulo-endothelial cells containing little or no lipid, together with a scanty and inconstant leucocytic infiltration.

The remaining member of this group, only widely recognised as a specific entity within recent years, is the condition described by Lichtenstein and Jaffe (1940) as *eosinophilic granuloma of bone*. The lesions are focal, either solitary or multiple, and may develop in most regions of the skeleton. The disease has been observed to run a relatively short course without causing constitutional disturbances, and to heal either spontaneously or after local therapy. The accepted histological criteria are reticulo-endothelial proliferation with eosinophilic infiltration, necrosis and fibrosis. The lesions containing a variable amount of fat.

Several authors in more recent years have suggested that these conditions which are classified under three designations are in fact closely related. The present survey, based upon a pathological study of 41 cases occurring at The Hospital for Sick Children during the past 38 years, has afforded further evidence that these disorders represent clinico-pathological variants of a condition whose basic feature is a histiocytic proliferation which appears to be neoplastic rather than reactive in nature.

Some difficulty has been encountered in deciding the most satisfactory mode of presenting the material studied, because it was found that the clinical pictures were by no means rigidly distinctive, and because features usually considered typical of one disease were sometimes associated with features suggestive of another. For these reasons the cases have been subdivided according to the distribution of lesions, in preference to the conventional grouping.

Classification of cases according to distributions of lesions

1. *Cases with a solitary bone lesion* (Table II). Seven children came under medical attention with a solitary bony lesion affecting the femur (2), skull (4) and cervical vertebra (1), respectively. In no instance was there any clinical evidence of involvement elsewhere in the skeleton, or in the viscera, nor were there any complications. All recovered, 6 within one year and another $2\frac{1}{2}$ years after onset.

2. *Cases with multiple bone lesions (with or without skin lesions)* (Table III). Multiple lesions apparently limited to the skeleton (with or without skin lesions) were present in 9 cases and these were distributed as shown in Table III. In this group there were, in addition to multiple bony involvement, skin changes in 3 cases. Subsequently 2 of the children in this group developed exophthalmos and diabetes insipidus as complications: 5 of the others recovered fully within 7 months to 8 years and one remained stationary; the average recovery period being about 4 years. There was no death but the course of the illness tended to be more prolonged than in Group I.

3. *Cases with multiple visceral involvement with or without bone lesions* (Table IV). The remaining 25 patients exhibited during the course of their illness visceral lesions, in addition to involvement of the skeleton and/or marrow in 11 instances. The clinical course in this group varied considerably. The conventional diagnosis of Letterer-Siwe disease could have been made in 18 children. All but 2 had a clinical onset during the first year of life (several from birth) and the remaining 2 in the second year; 1 of the 18 children went into a leukæmic phase terminally; 11 of the 18 children succumbed to the disease; 3 have recovered (one spontaneously); 4 are stationary or fair. Three cases (Nos. 14, 18, 30) were transitional forms, from eosinophilic granuloma to Hand-Schüller-Christian syndrome in one instance, and from Letterer-Siwe disease to Hand-Schüller-Christian syndrome in the other 2 cases. There was in this series also a case of acute histio-reticulosis with marked erythrophagocytosis, leaving one case which remained unclassifiable according to the conventional criteria, which proved therefore quite unsatisfactory.

Skin lesions were seen in virtually all children, lung lesions in 15 instances (five of these were of honeycomb lungs). Lymphadenopathy and hepatosplenomegaly were found in a large number of these children. Otorrhœa, seborrhœa and a curious nodular thymic enlargement noticeable on chest radiographs were not uncommon. Therapy with various steroids seemed sometimes to produce regression or arrest of progress of the condition, but

TABLE II

Histiocytic Reticulo-endotheliosis

Cases with a Solitary Bone Lesion

Chronological serial no.	Name	Sex	Age at onset (yrs.)	Histological diagnosis	Skeletal lesions	Skin lesions	Lung lesions	Lymph node lesions	Liver lesions	Spleen lesions	Other lesions	Mode of therapy	Duration of active disease (yrs.)	Outcome	Conventional clinical type	Follow-up (yrs.)
3	A.M.	M.	3.6/12	Bone	F.	—	—	—	—	—	—	Immobilization	6/12	Recovered	E.G.	16½
4	R.W.	M.	2.3/12	Bone	F.	—	—	—	—	—	—	Radio-therapy	10/12	Recovered	E.G.	16½
8	J.D.	M.	12	Bone	Sk.	—	—	—	—	—	—	Curettage	12/12	Recovered	E.G.	13½
13	V.T.	F.	1.11/12	Bone	C2	—	—	—	—	—	—	Immobilization	10/12	Recovered	E.G.	13
25	C.I.	F.	7	Bone	Sk.	—	—	—	—	—	—	Curettage + Radio-therapy	10/12	Recovered	E.G.	7
27	S.H.	F.	1.10/12	Bone	Sk.	—	—	—	—	—	—	Curettage	4/12	Recovered	E.G.	7
32	B.R.	M.	7.4/12	Bone	Sk.	—	—	—	—	—	—	Curettage	2.6/12	Recovered	E.G.	1

ABBREVIATIONS: F. (Femur), Sk. (Skull), C2 (2nd Cervical vertebra), E.G. (Eosinophilic Granuloma of Bone).

spontaneous remission was also seen in one instance of typical Letterer-Siwe disease. This group carried undoubtedly the most serious prognosis as no less than 16 of the 25 children died.

Pathology. In the course of the investigation, tissues were available for pathological examination from surgical specimens and from autopsies.

A review of the lesions exhibited a common basic feature which showed no consistent distinctions in association with the clinical grouping. The fundamental pathological process is a proliferation, local or widespread, of the cells of the reticulo-endothelial or macrophage system.

The observed cells may occur singly, in syncytial arrangement, or as multinucleate giant cells. The mononuclear and giant multinuclear forms have a well-developed eosinophilic cytoplasm, but in syncytial areas the cytoplasm is less conspicuous. The most characteristic feature of these cells is the morphology of their nuclei, which vary considerably in shape from round or ovoid to lunate, horseshoe or convoluted forms with a distinct crinkling and creasing of the nuclear membrane. The nuclei are moderately large in size and more or less vesicular. More primitive forms may also be observed, including reticulum cells and "pro-histiocytes." The frequency of mitotic figures varies, and in general is greater in cases with an acute clinical course and widely disseminated lesions.

Histiocytic proliferation being the fundamental process, the actual histological structure may be influenced by secondary phenomena. In somewhat larger lesions, it is usual to encounter extensive degeneration or frank necrosis. The latter leads to the liberation of lipid as cells break down, and this is phagocytosed by histiocytes in the vicinity which consequently acquire a foam cell appearance; some of these may lead to the development of typical foamy giant cells. The histiocytes also exhibit erythrophagocytosis, seen in the one case of acute histiocytic reticulosis, and not uncommonly hæmosiderosis as iron, another cellular breakdown product, is phagocytosed.

Probably in part as a reaction to cell breakdown and necrosis, there is also a variable degree of inflammatory cellular infiltration. The presence of eosinophil leucocytes has been emphasised, and is indeed usually most conspicuous, but neutrophil polymorphs, lymphocytes and plasma cells are also frequently encountered.

A further feature is the development of fibrosis, probably as a reaction to cell breakdown. A varying amount of reticulin is formed, in some instances enclosing individual cells, but more often a coarser mesh. Sometimes collagen fibres are prominent, and even scar-like areas are seen.

It must be stressed that multiple lesions at autopsy do not necessarily exhibit a uniform histological structure. There may even be variation from one lesion to another. In one child, for instance, tissue from the skull and subdural region consisted mainly of foam cells filled with sudanophilic fat with slight inflammatory cell infiltration. The pulmonary lesions were largely fibrosed, with very few foam cells persisting. The skin, however, showed histiocytic aggregates, almost entirely devoid of fat, while in the spleen, the site of recent necrosis, plump multinucleate cells containing hæmosiderin prevailed.

The more rapid the clinical evolution, the more widespread the lesions, the

TABLE III

Histiocytic Reticulo-endotheliosis

Cases with Multiple Bone Lesions (with or without Skin Lesions)

Chronological no.	Name	Sex	Age at onset (yrs.)	Histological diagnosis	Skeletal lesions	Skin lesions	Lung lesions	Lymph node lesions	Liver lesions	Spleen lesions	Other lesions	Mode of therapy	Duration of active disease (yrs.)	Outcome	Conventional clinical type	Follow-up (yrs.)
5	E.S.	F.	4.2/12	Bone + Skin	Sk. (m)	+	—	—	—	—	—	None	5/12	Residua	H.S.C.	16
7	T.H.	F.	2.5/12	Bone	Sk., L.F., D.9., R.F., D.7., L.5.	A few spots	—	—	—	—	Otorrhœa	Immobilization	1.8/12	Recovered	E.G.	15
9	H.B.	M.	2.5/12	Bone	Sk. (m)	—	—	—	—	—	—	Radiotherapy + Cortisone	6 +	Symptomatic relief	E.G. then— H.S.C.	12.9/12
12	K.C.	F.	7/12	Marrow	R.Il., R.T., R.F., L.F., 6th and 8th Ribs	+	—	—	—	—	—	None	2.2/12	Recovered	E.G.	10½
15	S.R.	F.	1.6/12	Bone	Sk., R.H., L.H., Spine, Pelvis, Ribs	—	—	—	—	—	—	Immobilization	8	Recovered	E.G.	10½
16	J.B.	F.	1.5/12	Bone	Sk., Ribs	—	—	—	—	—	—	None	7/12	Recovered	E.G.	9½
22	N.A.	F.	11	Bone	Sk., R.Il., L.Il., Spine, L.F.	—	—	—	—	—	—	Radiotherapy + Cortisone + Aminopterin	2 +	Stationary	E.G.	7½
24	P.C.	M.	2.10/12	Bone	Rt. and Lt. Ribs, Talus, Sternum.	—	—	—	—	—	—	Prednisone	5	Recovered	E.G.	7
31	R.C.	M.	1	Bone	L.Il., Sk.	—	—	—	—	—	—	Prednisone	3½	Recovered	E.G.	4½

ABBREVIATIONS: M.—Male. F.—Female. E.G.—Eosinophilic Granuloma of Bone. H.S.C.—Hand-Schüller-Christian syndrome. Sk.—Skull. F.—Femur. H.—Humerus. Il.—Ileum. T.—Tibia. D.—Dorsal vertebra. L.—Lumbar vertebra. (m)—multiple. R.—Right. L.—Left.

TABLE IV

Histiocytic Reticulo-endotheliosis

Cases with Multiple Visceral Involvement with or Without Bone Lesions

Chronological no.	Name	Sex	Age at onset (yrs.)	Histological diagnosis	Skeletal lesions	Skin lesions	Lung lesions	Lymph node lesions	Liver lesions	Spleen lesions	Other lesions	Modes of therapy	Duration of active disease (yrs.)	Outcome	Conventional clinical grouping	Follow-up (yrs.)
1	G.R.	M.	3/12	Lymph node P.M.	× (m)	+	+	+	—	—	—	None	3.7/12	Fatal	?	
2	P.K.	F.	3	P.M.	Sk. Femora Sternum 6th rib.	+	+	—	—	+	—	Radiotherapy	6/12	Fatal	H.S.C.	
6	P.S.	M.	5/12	Lymph node Bone. Skin	Sk. Ribs. R.H., L.F., R.T.	+	—	+	+	+	—	None	2/12	Spontaneous recovery.	L.S.	15
10	I.N.	F.	2/12	Skin. Spleen	—	+	+	—	+	+	—	Cortisone	7	Recovered	L.S.	12
11	C.O.	F.	2/12	Skin P.M.	Marrow	+	+	+	+	+	Thymus	None	5/12	Fatal	L.S.	
14	D.O.B.	M.	2.2/12	Bone. Skin P.M.	+ (m)	+	+ Honeycomb	+	+	+	+	Curettage Cortisone Radiotherapy	4.5/12	Fatal	E.G., then H.S.C.	
17	L.H.	F.	8/12	P.M.	—	+	+ Honeycomb	+	Biliary Cirrhosis.	—	Thymus	None	1/12	Fatal	L.S.	
18	C.L.	F.	1.9/12	Bone. Skin	Sk. Pelvis. Rib. scapula Spine.	+	+	—	—	—	—	Cortisone	3+	Stationary	L.S. then H.S.C.	8½
19	B.W.	F.	Birth	Skin	—	+	+	—	—	+	Otorrhoea	Steroids	7.6/12	Stationary	L.S.	
20	S.H.	M.	1/12	Bone. Skin	Sk. (m)	+	+ Honeycomb	+	+	+	Otorrhoea	Cortisone	11/12	Fatal	L.S.	7½
21	J.P.	M.	5/12	Skin. Lymph node. P.M.	Marrow	+	—	+	+	+	—	Antibiotics	4/12	Fatal	L.S. → Leukaemia	

No.	Initials	Sex	Age	Biopsy site	Marrow								Treatment	Duration	Result	Diagnosis	
23	D.L.	M.	3.6/12	Lymph node P.M.	+ (Marrow)	+	—	+	+	+	—	+	None	5/12	Fatal	Acute Histio-reticulosis.	
26	P.W.	M.	2.4/12	Bone. Lymph node P.M.	R. & L. Mastoid Sphenoid R.T.	+	—	+	+	+	+	+	Radiotherapy	1.6/12	Fatal	H.S.C.	
28	C.C.	F.	6/12	P.M.	—	+	Honeycomb	+	+	+	+	Thymus	None	2/12	Fatal	L.S.	
29	C.G.	F.	1	P.M.	—	+	Honeycomb	+	+	+	+	+	None	1/12	Fatal	L.S.	
30	J.H.	M.	1.2/12	Skin		+	+	—	—	—	—	—	Prednisone	2	Still active	L.S. ? H.S.C.	5½
33	R.B.	M.	2/12	Skin	—	+	—	+	+	+	—	Otorrhoea Seborrhoea Gums.	Cortisone	3½/12	Fatal	L.S.	
34	S.L.	M.	2	Lymph node Skin	—	+	—	+	+	+	+	—	Steroids	3½+	Stationary	L.S.	1
35	M.B.	M.	Birth	P.M.	—	+	—	+	+	+	+	Seborrhoea	Steroids	4/12	Fatal	L.S.	
36	C.W.	F.	Birth	P.M.	—		+	—	+	+	+	Otorrhoea Thymus	Prednisone	3/12	Fatal	L.S.	
37	S.M.	F.	9/12	Spleen. Lymph node	—	+	—	—	+	+	+	—	Steroids	10/12	Fatal	L.S.	
38	G.P.	F.	1½	Lung. Spleen	—	—	+	—	+	+	+	—	—	3.5/12	Stationary	L.S.	1
39	H.S.	F.	1/12	Skin	—	+	—	—	+	—	—	—	Prednisone	8/12	Well	L.S.	1
40	N.B.	M.	6/52	P.M.	+	+	+	+	+	+	+	Otitis	Prednisone	7½/12	Fatal	L.S.	
41	D.R.	M.	1	Palate	—	+	—	+	—	—	—	Palate	Excision	7/12	Fair. Alive	L.S.	1

ABBREVIATIONS.—M.—Male. F.—Female. P.M.—Post Mortem. (m)—Multiple. Sk.—Skull. H.—Humerus. F.—Femur. T.—Tibia. E.G.—Eosinophilic Granuloma. L.S.—Letter-Siwe Disease. H.S.C.—Hand-Schüller-Christian syndrome.

more uniformly is found the proliferating histiocyte, other features being relatively inconspicuous.

Special features of lesions according to site. In the *skin* the lesions observed take the form of a maculo-papular eruption predominantly over the trunk, sometimes with some vesiculation and hæmorrhage; sometimes the lesions are very scanty slightly yellowish papules which regress and leave inconspicuous whitish small scars. Microscopically, the "granulomatous" tissue lies in the superficial dermis, usually without lipid or necrosis but sometimes with some eosinophil leucocytes. The overlying epidermis tends to show non-specific changes of pressure atrophy, parakeratosis or even ulceration. The skin lesions, when discovered, are a useful means of histological confirmation of the diagnosis.

Affected *lymph nodes* are moderately enlarged and discrete. Microscopically, the involvement takes the form of a sino-medullary proliferation with gradual obliteration of the original architecture.

The *thymus* was found to be affected in four of the autopsy cases. The organ was considerably enlarged and of distinctive appearance. The surface was irregularly nodular and variegated in colour, individual nodules being greyish-white, yellowish or purplish. In one section the tissue was seen to be intersected by fibrous strands. Microscopically, the proliferating tissue showed appreciable hæmorrhage and necrosis to account for the variety in colour.

The *spleen* was sometimes moderately to markedly enlarged, and microscopically the specific cellular infiltration appeared to be multicentric rather than diffuse.

In the *skeleton* the reticulo-endothelial proliferation is of course in the marrow, and secondary changes in the bony architecture are not invariably present. Grossly, the lesions are characteristically focal and circumscribed, either uni- or multi-centric, but sometimes with more acute and widely disseminated forms the process may be more diffuse. The proliferating tissue may be soft and pale or firmer and distinctly yellowish. The expansion of the lesion leads to circumferential bone resorption, with the production of rounded or ovoid cavities seen on a radiograph. It is not uncommon to see occasional trabeculæ of new bone formation in cases where the skeletal lesions undergo resolution with reconstitution of bony architecture.

The *liver* was sometimes observed to be affected at autopsy. The lesions were multifocal and widespread, leading to generalised enlargement of the organ and accentuation of the portal areas. Microscopically, the proliferating histiocytic tissue was especially prominent around the portal tracts, and in two cases there was irregular involvement throughout the liver lobules themselves. In one child the gross appearances resembled those of an early biliary cirrhosis, with dilatation and mural thickening of the biliary tree, and some retention of bile. This histiocytic proliferation involved the duct walls themselves, with considerable proliferation of bile ducts and cholangitis, evidently the result of the biliary obstruction.

The *lungs* were affected in 15 children in the third group with multiple visceral lesions. In 10 instances miliary nodules were widely distributed throughout all lobes; 5 of these cases were fatal, four are stationary, and one was still active; 5 further children, all fatal, showed the gross cystic change designated by Oswald and Parkinson (1949) as honeycomb lungs.

Microscopically the primary lesions in all cases submitted to histological examination consisted of a cellular proliferation situated in the interstitium, chiefly in relation to the components of the primary pulmonary lobule and as a rule not affecting the larger bronchi to any significant degree. Although involving the lungs widely, this proliferation showed a distinct tendency to focal aggregation. In most of the cases the lesion consisted predominantly of histiocytes, whilst in two the aggregates were composed largely of fibro-blastic cells with fibre formation and clusters of foam cells.

Changes in the pulmonary architecture secondary to the interstitial cellular infiltration was a particularly striking feature in the honeycomb lungs. The giant air spaces appeared to be largely the result of over-expansion of structures in the primary lung lobules, i.e. alveolar ducts, terminal and respiratory bronchioles and sometimes the alveoli themselves. Mostly, they were devoid of any distinct epithelial covering and were lined by proliferating reticulo-endothelial cells with occasional giant multinucleate cells. The development of these secondary cystic changes seems to be the result of structural weakening by the interstitial infiltrate and probably also of obstruction.

Discussion. From the clinical standpoint it seems useful to segregate cases in the manner already suggested, because the distribution of lesions is to some extent related to the age of onset, acuteness of the disease process, and the ultimate prognosis.

Those children with extensive visceral lesions usually present symptoms at an early age and the ensuing illness commonly but not invariably runs an acute course and ends fatally. Patients with solitary bone lesions, together with some having multiple and predominantly or exclusively skeletal manifestations, usually come under attention at a rather later age and the disorder runs a subacute course with ultimate resolution, even in the absence sometimes of any active therapeutic intervention. In other cases of this group the course is more chronic and intractable, and complications of diabetes insipidus may appear as a result of lesions involving the para-pituitary region.

A comparison of clinical and histological features, however, renders untenable the idea that there is any absolute correlation between symptomatic manifestations and the cellular structure of the lesions. From the pathological standpoint the common denominator underlying these apparently distinct clinical entities is *a proliferation of histiocytes*. In considering the nature and pathogenesis of such a process, consideration must be given to the possibility that it represents a reactive condition in response to infection or metabolic disturbances. No infective agent has been detected in the diseases under consideration. The fact that some children with extensive visceral involvement suffer from mucosal infections is almost certainly due to the gross disturbances in the reticulo-endothelial system and interference with normal protective mechanisms.

An error of metabolism akin to Gaucher's and Niemann-Pick's disease has been suggested, particularly in cases of Hand-Schüller-Christian's disease with "xanthomatosis." However, the occurrence in such cases of histiocytic foci devoid of fat renders such an explanation untenable.

Having regard to these considerations, it is suggested that the disorders under discussion represent a process of histiocytic neoplasia involving one or multiple foci, or in its severest form the greater part of the reticulo-endothelial system. The fact that many of the lesions run a benign course may be due to the cell involved, a phagocytic cell which may undergo necrosis in the course of its phagocytic activity. On the other hand, widespread proliferation of the histiocytes, following multifocal origin rather than metastasis, represents frank malignancy and is not without a parallel in other neoplasms of the reticulo-endothelial system such as Hodgkin's disease.

Embryonic Sarcoma

The material on which the following discussion is based is derived from The Hospital for Sick Children, Great Ormond Street, between 1925 and 1962 and consists of 43 cases, 34 of which have arisen from the *urogenital sinus*, and 9 from *outside* this area. The urogenital sinus tumours comprise neoplasms of the bladder (19), the prostate (8), the vagina (3), the broad ligaments (2) and the epididymis or tunica (2). The 9 tumours arising from outside the urogenital sinus were derived from the palate (2), the nasopharynx or ethmoid (3), the parotid region (2), the eyelid (1) and the retro-peritoneal region (1).

The two principal sub-groups will be discussed separately.

Embryonic sarcoma of the urogenital sinus. This is a well-defined group of tumours arising in the genital and lower urinary tract in children, consisting largely of embryonic mesenchyme of densely or loosely cellular consistency and showing evidence of differentiation to rhabdomyoblasts. Where the tumours grow into a cavity they present as loosely cellular grape-like structures with relatively narrow pedicles. Where they infiltrate the prostate for instance, they are much more cellular and present with enlargement of the organ of origin. Willis (1948) suggested that, "perhaps the embryonic mesenchyme around the upper part of the urogenital sinus is, in both sexes, prone to the development of embryonic tumours." The conception of diffuse field origin is supported by this study.

The pathology and pathogenesis of the tumours. The tumours arising in the bladder and vagina present as smooth polypoid masses of slightly translucent tissue, with long slender pedicles, the so-called "grape-like" sarcoma (botryoides). The polypoid tumours are largely localised without any definite invasion.

In the prostate, the growth of the tumour tissue is mainly into the periurethral tissues and into the substance of the prostate, so that there is either displacement of the prostate by the tumour mass or else the prostate is diffusely enlarged owing to neoplastic permeation of the glandular stroma.

Histologically, the tumours consist of embryonic mesenchyme with some degree of differentiation to collagen and to striated muscle fibres. The embryonic mesenchymal cells are fusiform or stellate with scanty cytoplasm in a mucoid ground substance, thus often producing a pseudomyxomatous appearance. Rhabdomyoblasts in varying number may be seen either as straplike cells or as large multinucleate cells sometimes with more or less

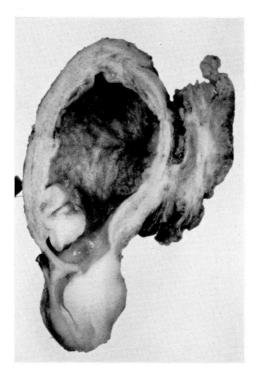

Fig. 1. Embryonic sarcoma of urogenital sinus, to show multicentric
origin in bladder trigone and prostate.
(Sagittal section)

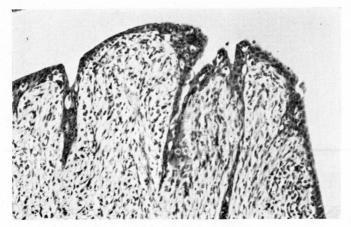

Fig. 2. Bladder tumour shown in Fig. 1. Embryonic mesenchyme covered
by attenuated transitional epithelium.
(H & E × 160)

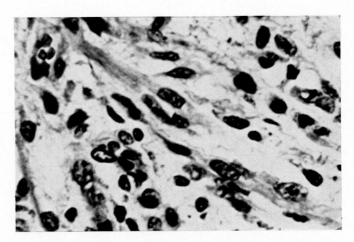

Fig. 3. Prostatic tumour shown in Fig. 1. Embryonic mesenchyme
showing differentiation to rhabdomyoblasts.
(PTAH × 470)

distinct fibrillation and/or cross striation. In the anaplastic growth phase, the mesenchymal cells are pleomorphic, with bizarre and multinucleate forms and increased numbers of mitotic figures.

On purely histological grounds there is a close resemblance between the tumours irrespective of their site of origin. They form essentially one group of embryonic tumours, within which there is a variable degree of differentiation. In support of this conception is the observation in some cases, in which both bladder and prostate (Fig. 1) were involved, of predominantly embryonic mesenchymal areas in the vesical neoplasms (Fig. 2), whereas there was a considerable differentiation of rhabdomyoblasts in the prostatic region (Fig. 3). These tumours never undergo complete differentiation. They are of diffuse field origin and potentially malignant from their inception, though they may have a fairly long phase during which they are only locally "invasive." At a later stage usually, though sometimes quite early in their evolution, they show anaplastic changes and it is then that they metastasise, frequently to the skeleton, lungs and lymph nodes. The prolonged locally "invasive" phase in many tumours is the result of an extension of the field of origin not necessarily clearly defined on gross inspection of the growth. It follows therefore that excision must be wide and based on the conception of radical excision of the total potential tumour bearing field.

From the embryological standpoint it has been suggested by White (1955) that the origin of these tumours may be closely related to an abnormality of the Wolffian duct epithelium in regions which are associated with that structure during their development. Equally, the development of tumours of the metanephros—nephroblastomata—may be similarly explained.

Embryonic sarcoma of the bladder. Of 19 cases, 13 children were male, 6 female. The ages at clinical onset were at birth in 2 cases, within the first 2 years in 10 cases, from 3 to over 10 years in 7 cases. Onset was usually with symptoms due to urinary obstruction, often with hæmaturia.

At the time of presentation the bladder was as a rule considerably distended. Radiological examination usually showed a filling defect and on cystoscopy the typical polypoid appearance was seen. The site of origin of the polypi was not always clear, but there was a marked predilection for the trigone, base and vicinity of the internal meatus.

The tumours may penetrate the bladder wall and invade neighbouring structures such as vagina, prostate and pelvic tissues, while remote metastases are rare.

The treatment of choice appears to be radical surgery as already indicated. Radiotherapy has shown no effect in slowing the progress of the disease.

Both bladder and prostate were involved in three fatal cases, the bladder and vagina in one fatal case. All the other children showed bladder involvement only. Nine children in this group are known to be alive 23, 15, 15, 14, 5, $3\frac{1}{2}$, $2\frac{1}{2}$, $1\frac{1}{2}$ and 1 year respectively after operation. All but three deaths occurred within 1 year of operation, two within less than 3 years, and one after more than 5 years. The two who survived for 23 and 15 years had local operations only.

Since that time radical excision of the total potential tumour bearing field has been carried out, i.e. cystectomy with excision of the posterior urethra and hysterectomy where indicated. Thirteen such operations were performed, with survival as stated above from 1 to 15 years in seven instances, and six fatalities. One of the survivors was shown to have involvement of both seminal vesicles and bladder.

Embryonic sarcoma of prostate. Eight children were seen and all succumbed to the disease within less than 1 year.

The first clinical manifestation was commonly acute urinary retention, sometimes associated with constipation, never with hæmaturia, and a large tumour was found to arise from the pelvis and to be palpable per rectum. The growth may be smooth or nodular and is usually firm. The bladder may be displaced. Five children were inoperable at the time of clinical presentation, one tumour could only be partially excised; in the remaining two cases excision of bladder, prostate and seminal vesicles was followed by recurrence a few months later.

Embryonic sarcoma of vagina. There were three cases in this group. All presented with protruding polypoidal masses at the labia at 13, 2 and 6 months respectively. The tumours were found to arise from the vaginal wall and in the last case hard inguinal glands were also present. The first two cases were only treated locally with radium needles or diathermy. This was followed by death within a few months. The third case was radically treated by complete excision of inguinal lymph nodes, vulva, vagina, tubes and bladder. There was no recurrence 15 months later, when last seen.

Embryonic sarcoma of epididymis and/or tunica. Two cases were in this group. Both were over 8 years old when first admitted. The first presented with enlargement of the left testis which was removed together with the spermatic cord. This was followed by two courses of Actinomycin D. The child was very well 2 years later, when last seen. Pathological examination showed the testis to be normal, but embryonic sarcoma involved both tunica and epididymis. The other case with involvement of the tunica in neoplastic growth, was also treated by radical surgery and found to be alive and well $1\frac{1}{2}$ years later. Testis and epididymis (both normal) were excised with the tumour. Actinomycin D was also given.

Embryonic sarcoma of the broad ligaments. Two children were seen and both succumbed to the disease within 6 months of clinical onset. They were 6 and 4 years old at onset of symptoms. Both proved to have inoperable masses in the pelvis which were thought on pathological examination, to have risen from the broad ligaments. Radiotherapy was given to the second child without success.

Embryonic sarcoma arising from outside the urogenital sinus. Two children had embryonic sarcoma of the *soft palate*. Both were girls, and admitted at the age of 9 years, one with a history of 21 months duration and the other with a growth first observed at the age of 18 months. Local removal and radiotherapy were carried out in both instances several times, each time followed by recurrence and increased growth rate, as well as metastasis to a lung and cervical lymph nodes in the second case. Though the final issue is not known in either case, death must be presumed.

Four girls and one boy were afflicted with embryonic sarcoma apparently arising from the *nasopharynx* with considerable extension to the base of the skull, various antra (maxillary, ethmoid, etc.), and metastases. The four girls presented with symptoms at 4, $2\frac{1}{2}$, $5\frac{1}{2}$ and 8 years of age and although treated with radiotherapy, surgery being impossible, they died after 2, 3, 7 and 7 months, respectively.

The boy presented at $1\frac{1}{2}$ years symptomatically and died 8 months later in spite of intra-arterial perfusions with methotraxate. Two of the children initially presented with apparent *parotid* involvement but it soon became clear that they belonged to the same group of nasopharyngeal sarcoma with widespread extension to the base of the skull and to facial structures.

One of these children had a peculiar pedigree in that a younger sister had been treated for anæmia and two more distant members of the family had died from leukæmia and nephroblastoma respectively at Great Ormond Street.

One girl was admitted at $4\frac{1}{2}$ years with marked frequency of micturition and nocturnal enuresis. At laparatomy a large growth was found, of about 15 cm. diameter, adherent to the anterior abdominal wall and to the fundus of the bladder. Many peritoneal metastases were present. As much of the growth as possible was removed and radiotherapy given. The child died 3 months later, and at autopsy the embryonic sarcoma was confirmed to have arisen from the lower *retroperitoneal region* unrelated to the urogenital sinus.

Finally, there was one girl in this group who is now alive and well at the age of 10 years. The history had dated from the age of $6\frac{1}{2}$ years when a lump presented in the outer angle of the right eye which was excised. It recurred and was again excised at the age of $8\frac{1}{4}$ years. A second recurrence was excised at 9 years and 2 months. The child was then treated with radiotherapy. The diagnosis was embryonic sarcoma of the *eyelid*.

In conclusion, of the 9 cases in this group 7 arose in the region of the nasopharynx variably extending to the base of skull, facial structures (e.g. parotid) and facial bones. They all succumbed. One solitary case arose from the lower retroperitoneal tissue unassociated with urogenital sinus. This girl succumbed. There is only one survivor with a localised sarcoma of the eyelid which had recurred twice but was treated, successfully so far, by local surgery and radiotherapy.

Neuroblastoma

Tumours arising from the sympathetic nervous system, i.e. neuroblastoma, ganglioneuroma and phæochromocytoma, accounted for about 10% of the neoplasms seen at The Hospital for Sick Children during the period from 1925 to 1962 inclusive. During that time, the number of verified cases of neuroblastoma was 165, that of ganglioneuroma 18 and phæochromocytoma 1.

The great majority of neuroblastoma cases (133) presented with symptoms during the first four years of life, and the first year (infancy) accounted for 63 or nearly 40% of the total. The sex distribution was about equal (79 male and 86 female).

Neuroblastoma may arise either in the medulla of the suprarenal glands or anywhere along the sympathetic nervous chains which are of similar embryogenic origin. In 68% of the cases, the tumour arose either in the adrenal medulla or from the upper abdominal sympathetic chain. Cervical tumours were found in 7, thoracic neoplasms in 20 and pelvic tumours in 13 cases. In one instance four apparently independent primary growths were found arising in the chest, adrenal, upper abdomen and pelvis. In 12 cases the site of the primary neoplasm could not be definitely ascertained.

Pathology. Neuroblastoma has certain distinctive features.

1. The tumours are highly invasive and infiltrate the surrounding tissues. They may involve and surround vital structures such as major vessels and nerves and thus render complete surgical removal difficult or impossible.

They tend to extend and to metastasise rapidly, mainly by lymphatic and blood-borne dissemination. The mode of spread is principally (a) to lymph nodes, local and/or distant, (b) to the liver, (c) to the skeleton and (d) by epidural extension. Except during the first year of life, spread to the skeleton is very common. This has, as will be shown, an important bearing on the different prognosis in the first year of life and thereafter. Dissemination to the liver is particularly frequently encountered during the first year of life. That the so-called Pepper's syndrome is more commonly encountered from right than from left-sided adrenal primary tumours, has been confirmed in our series; this is entirely due to the fact that lymphatic extension to the liver takes place more readily due to the proximity of the right-sided tumour to the liver. Blood-borne dissemination, however, is equally frequent from tumours in both adrenal glands, and the alleged predominance of the so-called Hutchinson's syndrome from tumours of the left adrenal gland has not been confirmed. The large group of neoplasms of the two suprarenal glands and of the extra-adrenal abdominal sympathetic chain (68% of the total) show the highest tendency to metastasise, whereas cervical, thoracic and pelvic tumours are less likely to disseminate and least of all the pelvic tumours.

2. The neuroblastoma has a considerable tendency to necrose, so much so that only little viable tissue may remain on occasion. Complete extinction of this type of tumour (spontaneous complete regression) is, however, exceedingly rare and accounts for about 1% of the cases in the world literature. We ourselves have observed only one instance in our 165 cases, and only one such occurrence has been noted at the Cancer Memorial Hospital in New York in more than 200 cases of neuroblastoma (Dargeon, personal communication).

3. All embryonic tumours, including neuroblastoma, are characterised by a tendency to differentiate. Thus all stages of differentiation, including fully mature ganglioneuroma, may be encountered in different areas of any neuroblastoma. It is thus clear that serial biopsies from different areas of a tumour cannot be used as evidence of differentiation associated with any form of therapy.

Clinical manifestations. Two-thirds of the children in our series showed clinical evidence of dissemination at their first examination by a doctor, while symptoms due to the primary tumour may not have been obvious.

Constitutional disturbances were frequently a presenting feature, such as fever, anæmia, vomiting, malaise. These are frequently misinterpreted as evidence of infection when they are really due to tumour necrosis.

Paralysis of the sympathetic nervous system may produce a Horner's syndrome in tumours of the neck or upper chest, and cœliac disease may be simulated in neoplasms arising from the upper abdominal sympathetic chain. Spinal cord compression may be caused by the epidural portion of a dumb-bell tumour of chest or abdomen.

Rarely, neuroblastoma is an incidental finding at autopsy; we have encountered four such examples. In one instance hypertensive encephalopathy was explained by the finding of an adrenal neuroblastoma at autopsy. The neoplasm contained excessive quantities of noradrenaline and its breakdown products.

The natural evolution of neuroblastoma as evidenced by a series of untreated children. It has already been shown that neuroblastoma shows a remarkable tendency to disseminate widely at an early stage of its clinical evolution. Thus an attitude of hopelessness was generally displayed by the practising pædiatricians, including those in this hospital. Therefore we have been able to collect a series of 58 children in whom no treatment whatsoever was undertaken. All the cases, however, have been histologically established, by biopsy and/or at autopsy. This distribution of primary tumours and of metastases was representative of the entire series of 165 neuroblastoma cases. Among the 58 children included, no less than 20 showed a symptomatic onset in the first year of life. In all, 57 of the 58 children have succumbed to the disease, and the average survival period of the untreated children was only 4 months from symptomatic onset of the illness. One child survived 14 months, all the other 56 children succumbed within 1 year of onset. The one solitary survivor is the only instance of complete and spontaneous regression in our series. This was a 4-month old boy who presented in 1947 with a mass in the chest, a markedly enlarged liver, and a subcutaneous nodule which was biopsied and proved to be a deposit of neuroblastoma. No treatment was given, and the child is alive and well, aged more than 15 years now. The only clinical abnormality present is residual calcification, seen radiographically, in liver and thorax. The primary tumour was presumably in the thorax.

Accepting that there may be a biological advantage in neuroblastoma during the first year of life, it has not manifested itself clinically in the series of untreated children, excepting the sole instance of spontaneous regression in the 4-month-old infant.

A selected series of cases of neuroblastoma treated with surgery and/or radiotherapy. A highly selected group of 25 children was treated by surgery, radiotherapy, or a combination of both. Preference was given to children with no, or limited evidence of dissemination, to children in the younger age groups and to cases with extra-adrenal primary tumours.

Of the 25 children, 17 succumbed to the disease within 6½ months of symptomatic onset, and there have been 8 long-term survivors for 3 to 25 years: 4 of the 8 survivors had pelvic tumours (the site with least metastases). Secondary spread was found only once among the 8 favourable cases. This patient had been admitted to hospital in 1933, aged 4¾ years, with an axillary tumour, which was excised and treated with radium needles. At the age of 26 years, the young lady was re-traced and found to be very well. Clinically and radiologically there was no abnormality at all and the site of the original primary tumour remains unknown. It must be assumed that the primary neoplasm regressed spontaneously.

Nine children in this group of 25 showed a symptomatic onset of the illness within the first year of life: 5 fell into the group of survivors, whereas 4 have succumbed as did 13 older children. Most of the children showed widespread dissemination of the tumour at the time of their death.

Finally, it should be stressed once more that our experience in this group was confined to a highly selected series and it is not within our competence to judge the limitations or usefulness of such localised forms of treatment as surgery and radiotherapy in a usually widely disseminated disease. It is not our intention to review the extensive literature on this subject, but to confine ourselves to our own experiences with a large group of cases of neuroblastoma. Nevertheless, observations such as those by Koop *et al.* (1955) in Philadelphia, with partial surgery going as far as possible and subsequent regression of some residual tumours, are of considerable interest in the study of a most remarkable neoplasm.

Cases of neuroblastoma treated with massive doses of vitamin B_{12} with or without additional therapy. In November 1950 a new form of treatment of neuroblastoma was introduced into the The Hospital for Sick Children. The reasoning behind this decision of the Tumour Committee of the hospital to use massive concentrations of vitamin B_{12} was the thought that it might induce maturation of neuroblasts to ganglioneuromatous cells, as indeed it was already known to be an essential factor in the maturation of hæmopoietic cells. From then on, an unselected series of 74 patients was given this treatment, either solely or in addition to surgery and/or radiotherapy. The dosage was 1 mg. (1000 μg.) intramuscularly on alternate days for at least two years, survival permitting. This was varied in 1957 to 1 mg. per 7 kilos (1 stone) of body weight at similar intervals for 3 years. The dose was experimental, the duration of treatment was based on the observation that recurrence of the tumour after more than 3 years is quite exceptional.

The results were as follows: 32 children responded with "permanent" clinical remission. Of these 29 were alive and well for from more than 2 years to 12 years. 1 child survived and was well for $1\frac{1}{2}$ years. 2 children have succumbed to intercurrent disease, namely poliomyelitis after 2 years and acute intussusception after $3\frac{1}{2}$ years. At autopsy no residual tumour was found in either.

Another 8 cases have responded to the treatment temporarily for periods of from 6 months to $2\frac{1}{2}$ years, yet all of these have ultimately succumbed to the disease. One child, at present alive and well, has been followed for less than 1 year, and is therefore not evaluated. Finally, 33 children, all treated with vitamin B_{12} for more than 4 weeks, with or without conventional forms of therapy, have been complete failures. (Another 8 children, have not been included in the series at all, for most of them have died after less than 3 weeks therapy of one kind or another.)

Conclusions. 1. No case with bone metastases has shown "permanent" clinical remission. 2. The group with "permanent" clinical remission included 23 infants and 9 older children at symptomatic onset of the disease; the temporary remission group 6 infants and 2 older children; the clinical failures 2 infants only and 31 older children. There is no doubt that, given therapy, infants have a far better chance to respond than the older children in whom bone metastases are common.

Details of 9 children with neuroblastoma treated successfully with vitamin B_{12} solely (see also Bodian 1959, 1963). Five of these children were derived from the above series of our hospital, another four from outside sources. I am greatly indebted to the clinicians who have given me permission to record their cases.

Case 1

A male infant, aged 7 months, presenting with retention of urine of recent onset. After decompression of the distended bladder by suprapubic cystotomy, a large fixed pre-sacral mass was palpable which extended around the rectum and almost filled the pelvis projecting upwards into the left iliac fossa. Biopsy of the mass through the rectal wall showed on two occasions neuroblastoma.

There was persistent urinary infection and the child's condition was poor. The massive tumour was considered inoperable and the radiotherapist's opinion was that radiotherapy was unlikely to be successful. Metastases were not found. It was then decided to give this child (the first in our series) 1 mg. vitamin B_{12} on alternate days intramuscularly. After 4 months' treatment the tumour was no longer palpable through the abdominal wall, but on rectal examination there was some infiltration in the prostatic region. The suprapubic tube was removed and urine was voided normally.

After 15 months treatment a laparotomy was performed in the hope of finding a residual ganglioneuroma. Only two minute nodules were palpable, but not visible, to the left of the sacrum and biopsy was not possible. Treatment with vitamin B_{12} was maintained for 2 years. The child is well and free from recurrence or metastases, more than 12 years from clinical onset of the illness.

Case 2

This female infant presented at 4 months with weakness of both lower limbs, left more than right, with suspected double sphincter weakness. At 9 months the child was admitted to the Beilinson Hospital in Israel where a left sided retro-peritoneal tumour was found in the region of the lumbar spine infiltrating muscle and extending through intervertebral foramina into the spinal canal. The tumour was considered inoperable and a biopsy was obtained which proved it to be neuroblastoma (confirmed by the author). A month later, the child was admitted to The Hospital for Sick Children at Great Ormond Street, with gross paralysis of both lower limbs. Laminectomy was carried out but the tumour was found to be too extensive and only a biopsy of neuroblastoma in the epidural space was obtained. Vitamin B_{12} in 1 mg. doses on alternate days intramuscularly was then given for 2 years. One year later the child was brought again to London from Israel. Her general condition was excellent. The abdomen was not distended. There was moderate power in the lower limbs, but the tone was diminished and the reflexes absent. There were no further metastases.

After 2 years' treatment with vitamin B_{12} she developed the bulbar form of poliomyelitis. She succumbed to the inter-current infection within 30 hours of admission to hospital. At autopsy only a fibrous scar was found at the site of the former tumour, and complete regression of the tumour was established by an exacting histological examination, confirmed by the author.

Case 3

A three-day-old female infant had a huge nodular abdominal mass on the right side, extending from the costal margin to the inguinal ligament, across to the left flank and indistinguishable from the liver. The mass was palpable per rectum. At laparotomy, the mass was identified in the liver as being massive neoplastic nodules. A biopsy showed massive replacement of liver parenchyma by neuroblastoma and infiltration of portal lymphatics by tumour. There was no evidence of metastasis to skeleton or lungs. Vitamin B_{12} therapy in 1 mg. doses on alternate days was given for a total of $2\frac{1}{2}$ years as the sole form of therapy. After transient increase in the size of the abdomen the mass was definitely decreasing after 2 months. Four months later the liver edge was barely palpable and an intravenous pyelogram was normal. The child has made uninterrupted progress, and is well, without any evidence of recurrence or metastases at the age of 8 years. Vanillylmandelic acid (VMA) output in the urine is now normal.

Case 4

A male infant who was noted at birth to have extreme flaccidity of lower limbs and a tumour was felt in the right loin. At 3 weeks of age he was in a good general condition and admitted to hospital. X-ray of abdomen and spine and palpation revealed a large firm mass in the right costo-lumbar angle with widening of the spinal canal and thinning of the pedicles. A biopsy of the tumour was performed by posterior retroperitoneal approach with the result that the diagnosis of neuroblastoma was made, with extension into the epidural space. Vitamin B_{12} in 1 mg. intramuscular doses was given every second day for a total of 3 years. The mass became impalpable. The erosion of the pedicles of vertebrae had disappeared and X-rays of long bones and skull were normal. There was still flaccid paraplegia in both legs. The child is now aged 7 years. There is no return of motor power to the lower limbs. A uretero-ileostomy has been performed for recurrent urinary infection. The VMA output in the urine is normal.

Case 5

A female infant was noticed at 5 months to have an enlarged abdomen. She was referred to Great Ormond Street under Sir Wilfrid Sheldon where a gross liver enlargement was found with a slightly nodular firm surface. The right lobe extended down to the right iliac fossa. The baby was somewhat wasted, Hb 69%, platelets 33,000 per cmm. IVP showed downward and medial displacement of the left kidney. Laparotomy at the age of 8 months revealed that the mass was an enlarged liver with numerous secondary deposits. A biopsy showed diffuse replacement of liver parenchyma by neuroblastoma with intervening fibrosis. Vitamin B_{12} therapy in 1 mg. intramuscular doses was given for a total of 3 years as the sole form of therapy. After 4 months some regression of the liver was noticed and improvement continued progressively. One year after commencement of vitamin B_{12} therapy only slight liver enlargement was noticed and the consistency appeared normal. After $2\frac{1}{2}$ years the liver was of normal size. At the end of the three years course, the IVP was found to be normal on the left and there was slight calcification in the left adrenal area. A second laparotomy was performed: the liver was of normal size and appearance except for several small whitish firm areas of scar formation. In the left adrenal region a lump about the size of a walnut was felt. Two biopsies were taken: one from normal appearing liver tissue (microscopy was normal) and one from a white scar. Microscopically the latter was fibrous tissue, with Schwann cells and a few mature ganglion cells, but no neuroblasts. Urinary VMA was normal at the end of treatment. The child is now perfectly well with no signs of recurrence of tumour, about $4\frac{1}{2}$ years after symptomatic onset.

Case 6

A male infant, born on June 14th, 1962, was admitted under Drs Lightwood and Oppé at St Mary's Hospital on the second day of life and found to be pale with a distended abdomen and enlarged firm liver. There was slight œdema of lower abdomen and legs. In the next few days the liver progressively enlarged until it reached the right lower quandrant. IVP showed normal calyces and a possible slight downward displacement of the right kidney. At 2 weeks, laparatomy was carried out and multiple small nodules were found all over the enlarged liver. Biopsy showed a primitive neuroblastoma. The radiotherapist considered irradiation inadvisable and the infant was treated with 1 mg. vitamin B_{12} intramuscular injections on alternate days from June 29th, 1962. His hæmoglobin tended to fall and he required small blood transfusions. VMA output in urine was 21 mg. and 17·4 mg./24 hours respectively at Great Ormond Street and at Queen Charlotte's Hospital (Dr Sandler). Homovanillic acid (HVA) was 9·4 mg./24 hours. On August 13th he had improved and was discharged home, the vitamin B_{12} to be continued.

Subsequently he did well. Abdominal distension and œdema slowly disappeared, the liver slowly decreased in size, the hæmoglobin levels were between 11 and 12 g. Further urine collections have shown a progressive fall in VMA and HVA excretion. On August 16th and 17th VMA was 6·5 mg./24 hours and HVA 7·5 mg. (Dr Sandler). On September 25th and 26th VMA was 1·9 mg. and HVA approximately 0·045 mg./24 hrs.

On October 6th a bilateral inguinal herniotomy was performed and a smooth much smaller liver (except for a few small nodules) was palpated through the herniotomy.

On April 26th, 1963 the liver was reported palpable one finger breadth below the right costal margin. He was well. Hb 11·5 g., HVA 1 mg./24 hours (Dr Sandler) i.e. normal. The child continues to progress very well.

Case 7

A male infant, born on December 27th, 1961 in France. Increase in the size of the abdomen from the age of 1 month. At 2 months, the abdomen was very large and a liver biopsy was found to be positive for neuroblastoma. At 3 months, the infant was admitted in Paris under the care of Professor Marcel Lelong and Dr O. Schweisguth with an enormous abdomen with numerous subumbilical venous anastomoses. The liver reached down to the symphysis pubis. Cyanosis and respiratory difficulties were present. RBC 2·75 m. An IVP showed a downward displacement of the left kidney. The VMA output on April 17th, 1962 was 9·6 mg./24 hours (VMA 169·3 µg./mg. creatinine, and HVA 289·2 µg./mg. creatinine, Dr Käser, Bern). From March 31st, 1962, the child was put on 1 mg. vitamin B_{12} intramuscularly on alternate days. In addition he received three blood transfusions. Slowly the general condition improved and at the end of the first month's treatment there was already some regression in the size of the liver. VMA and HVA levels decreased progressively to 77·5 µg./mg. creatinine for VMA and 95·4 µg./mg. creatinine for HVA on May 27th, 1962. At the age of 10 months he looked a well baby. The liver edge was 1·5 cm. below the costal margin. The IVP was normal. VMA was 17·3 µg./mg. creatinine and HVA 25·6 µg./mg. creatinine (normal range). When last seen, at one year of age, he was very well.

Case 8

A male infant under the care of Dr Mary Wilmers at The Belgrave Hospital for Children. Born December 8th, 1956. Admitted aged 18 months with loss of weight for 5 weeks and reluctant to walk. There was a lower dorsal kyphosis. Knee-jerks were slightly impaired. An indefinite swelling over the lower dorsal spine and neck stiffness were noted. IVP showed a downward displacement of the left kidney. Myelogram showed a complete block on the lower border of T12. A biopsy revealed neuroblastoma. Treatment with vitamin B_{12} was commenced 1 mg. on alternate days intramuscularly for a total of 3 years, till June 1961. At the age of 2 years and 2 months he was running around without any abnormal physical signs or any neurological deficit. At the end of therapy, June 1961, the IVP was quite normal. Some calcification was visible at the level of T12. The child is now perfectly well.

Case 9

A male infant, born in August 1958, first seen at 4 months when several small subcutaneous nodules were removed which, histologically, were typical of neuroblastoma metastases. He was admitted under the care of Professor J. K.

Martin of Edmonton, Alberta, Canada. Physical examination apart from one or two skin nodules was negative. IVP was attempted but failed. The bone marrow of the tibia showed metastatic tumour cells consistent with neuroblastoma. The child was started on 1 mg. vitamin B_{12} intramuscularly on alternate days early in October 1958.

Subsequently, the two nodules on the back disappeared but a new skin nodule was discovered. Repeated bone marrow examination again showed abnormal cells, thought to be neuroblastoma. By October 1960, he had completed a two years course of vitamin B_{12}, he remained very well and was clinically normal. The skin nodules had all disappeared and none recurred. He was last seen in June 1962 when he was physically quite normal. The bone marrow was also normal. VMA output was normal in September 1961.

Nephroblastoma (Wilm's Tumour)

A total of 125 cases in which histological proof of the diagnosis has been obtained represents the series seen at Great Ormond Street during the period 1925 to 1962. The composition of the series is shown below.

Sex distribution. 70 male, 55 female.

Site distribution. Right-sided tumours, 58; left-sided tumours, 65; bilateral tumours, 2.

Age incidence

Age on admission 0—1—2—3—4—5—6—7—8 years
Number of cases   17 35 26 16 15 7 4 5 **125**

It will be seen that nearly two-thirds of the cases occurred below the age of 3 years. There was no proven case of a congenital tumour, although this was suspected in at least two of those admitted in the first year of life.

Symptomatology. The incidence of various symptoms and their frequency as presenting complaints are shown in the following table.

	Total No.	Presenting Complaint
Abdominal swelling .	67	58
Hæmaturia .	35	29
Pain . .	27	26
Vomiting . .	16	16
Other symptoms .	18	13

It will be seen that in about a half of the cases the presence of a local or generalised abdominal swelling was the first and only sign of illness; it is also of interest that gross hæmaturia occurred in another quarter of this series; the possibility of Wilm's tumour should therefore be seriously considered in young children with unexplained hæmaturia. One case presented with heart failure due to the extension of the growth along the inferior vena cava to the right auricle; a further two children showed a similar direct extension of the neoplasm. Hypertension was noted in a significant number of cases.

Methods of treatment. The efficiency of different methods of treatment in this condition is the subject of much controversy. During the period 1925–1948, 57 cases came under our care. The methods of treatment then were not standardised. Some cases were inoperable and possibly given no treatment or only radiotherapy; others were given pre-operative irradiation, followed by surgery; and others surgery as well as pre- and post-operative irradiation. The surgical approach was also variable; in some cases lumbar and in others transperitoneal. In common with other authors we have adopted the term "two-year cure," for it is very seldom that recurrences or metastases occur later than 2 years after surgical removal of the tumour.

During the period 1925–1948 we had 7 long-term survivors out of a group of 57 children (12%).

From 1949 a uniform attitude was adopted in regard to management. A child with suspected Wilm's tumour is admitted to hospital and the mass is palpated only once. Thereafter an intravenous pyelogram is performed as soon as possible and if the suspected diagnosis is thus confirmed, immediate surgery is carried out without pre-operative irradiation. We have only rarely encountered the situation that the tumour has seemed inoperable, in which event irradiation is given to shrink the growth before a second attempt is made to remove it. Nephrectomy is carried out by the transperitoneal route, using a generous abdominal incision and with minimal handling of the tumour. This operative approach is suitable for even the largest tumours, it enables the vessels of the renal hilum to be ligated at an early stage and exposes the regional lymph nodes for examination and, if necessary, excision. By thus reducing palpation and manipulation of the tumour to a minimum, it is hoped to avoid as far as possible the dissemination of tumour emboli, which seems to constitute a definite danger.

The second group in this series, treated as outlined above, now comprises a total of 58 cases to the end of 1960, with a two years or longer survival of 26 children, i.e. 45%.

Our present results are consistent with the view that the age of the patient is an important factor in the prognosis.

The following tables show the survival in relation to age in the two groups, 1925–1948 and 1949–1960 and for the whole period.

GROUP I 1925–1948

Age (yrs) on admission	. 0–1	−2	−3	−4	−5	−6	−7	−8	Total
No. of cases .	7	12	17	5	9	2	3	3	57
Survivors .	1	3	1	2	0	0	0	0	7

GROUP II 1949–1960

Age (yrs) on admission	. 0–1	−2	−3	−4	−5	−6	−7	−8	Total
No. of cases .	10	20	8	8	5	4	0	3	58
Survivors .	8	9	5	2	0	2	—	0	26
% survivors .	80	45	63	25	0	50	—	0	

GROUPS I AND II 1925–1960 (115 CASES)

Age (yrs) on admission	0–1	−2	−3	−4	−5	−6	−7	−8	Total
Both groups	9/17	12/32	6/25	4/13	0/14	2/6	0/3	0/5	33/115
% survivors	53	38	24	31	0	33	0	0	

The results in Group II (1949–1960) can also be stated as follows:

> In the first year of life   8/10 or 80% survive.
> Between 1 and 4 years of life 16/41 or 39% survive.
> 5 years and over   2/7   or 29% survive.

Pathology. In about half the cases the relationship of the tumours to the residual kidney was ascertainable, and there was no appreciable difference in the incidence of tumours arising in the vicinity of the upper or lower renal pole. The combined weight of the tumour and residual renal parenchyma was recorded; with the exception of one enormous tumour of approximately 11,000 grams present at autopsy, the weight ranged from 250 to about 2000 grams, with an average value of 900 grams. There was no correlation between the size of the tumour and the age of the patient at the time of removal.

Nephroblastomata arise within the renal parenchyma, and usually remain enclosed within a stretched and atrophic rim of kidney (Fig. 4). This results in the characteristic pseudocapsule formation, which discloses on microscopic examination the presence of a few atrophic nephrons, notably glomeruli. In a few instances, where the tumour had apparently arisen in a superficial portion of the kidney, the latter remains largely intact and the bulk of the tumour projects outside the contour of the kidney. To this type the somewhat misleading description "extra-renal" has been applied. Uncommonly, the tumour appeared to have ruptured through its pseudocapsule.

In some instances there was evidence of recent or old hæmorrhage within residual renal tissue, with distension of the neoplasm by extravasated blood, and sometimes it was possible to prove that this was the result of thrombosis of the renal vein, presumably due to pressure by the enlarging tumour, and it appears likely that this was the factor leading to hæmaturia in most, if not all, cases which presented with this symptom. In no case was there any apparent developmental abnormality of the renal parenchyma (except in one case with horseshoe kidney), and it was apparent that prior to the formation of the tumour, renal development had proceeded normally.

In three instances, there was massive extension of new growth into the renal vein, thence into the inferior vena cava and into the right auricle.

As a result of expansion of the tumour the renal pelvis suffers considerable and progressive distention. In some instances the renal pelvis was filled with blood as a result of hæmorrhage from the kidney, and sometimes there is extension of tumour into the pelvis and ureter.

Commonly the tumour is largely composed of moderately firm creamy-white tissue which microscopically is seen to be nephric blastema (Fig. 10).

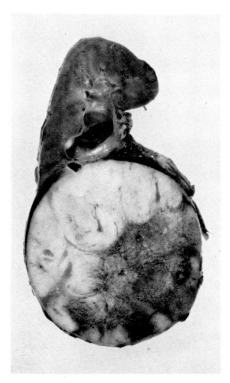

Fig. 4. Nephroblastoma arising in lower pole of right kidney with characteristic pseudocapsule of compressed renal tissue indicating that the
tumour has a renal origin.
(Coronal section × 1/4)

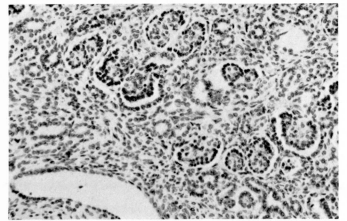

FIG. 5. Nephroblastoma.
Type A. Reniform.
(H & E × 40)

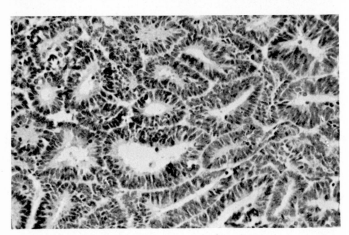

FIG. 6. Nephroblastoma.
Type B. Tubular.
(H & E × 40)

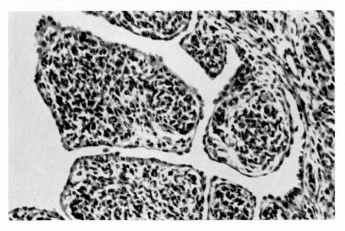

FIG. 7. Nephroblastoma.
Type C. Papillary.
(H & E × 40)

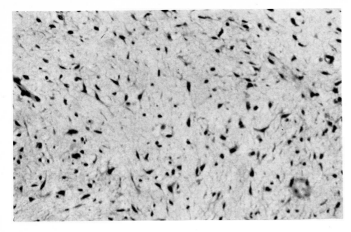

Fig. 8. Nephroblastoma.
Type D. Mesenchymal.
(H & E × 40)

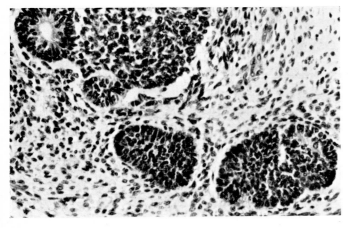

Fig. 9. Nephroblastoma.
Type E. Focal-blastemal.
(H & E × 40)

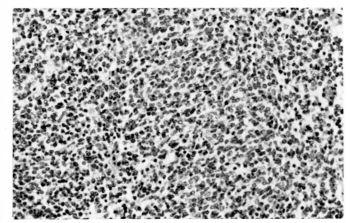

Fig. 10. Nephroblastoma.
Type G. Massive blastemal.
(H & E × 40)

In a proportion of tumours, however, firmer tissue of greyish colour is present showing an obvious fibrous texture and whorling, representing mesenchymal elements within the tumour. Necrosis is of common occurrence, sometimes focal, sometimes massive. Hæmorrhage is also a common feature, and thrombosis of vessels within the tumour was sometimes observed. An appreciable number of tumours, less than a quarter, were cystic; usually this appeared to be the result of necrosis and liquefaction of the tumour, occasionally the cysts were minute and microscopically they appeared to be dilated tubules. Rarely, the cystic spaces presented a papilliferous appearance, and microscopic examination showed the cyst wall and papilliferous extensions to be covered by pelvic epithelium, suggesting that the condition was of developmental origin.

Embryonic tissue of more or less undifferentiated microscopic appearance was observed in virtually all tumours. It usually consisted both of loose embryonic mesenchyme and of renal blastema. It is of doubtful validity to base any quantitative relationship between these two elements on chance sections.

The commonest finding was that of minimal differentiation, but moderate and considerable differentiation were also observed. Mesenchymal differentiation would give rise to collagenous connective tissue; smooth muscle, adipose tissue and metaplastic change would produce striated muscle, cartilage and osteoid material. Smooth muscle included in Wilm's tumours is usually a derivative of the renal pelvis rather than a true constituent of the differentiating embryonic tumour tissue. Differentiation of nephric blastema gives rise to renal tubules (Fig. 6) and these may further produce glomerular-structures (Fig. 5). Tubules within a nephroblastoma of lower nephron or collecting tubular type are outgrowths from the embryonic pelvis and not derivatives of the blastema (Nicholson 1931). Such tubules are commonly surrounded by masses of renal blastema and it has been suggested that their function is to evoke differentiation of the blastema.

Occasionally pelvic (transitional) epithelium is included within the nephroblastoma, sometimes showing squamous transformation and keratinisation. The association of pelvic epithelium with the cystic papilliferous type of nephroblastoma has already been mentioned.

L. L. R. White while working at Great Ormond Street made an attempt to find a natural histological classification of nephroblastoma, in order to find any factor of tissue pattern which might be of prognostic significance.

The following seven decreasingly differentiated tissue types can be distinguished:

A. *Reniform:* The tumour has differentiated into a tissue showing a marked resemblance to normal kidney (Fig. 5).

B. *Tubular:* Tumour in which little or no undifferentiated tissue is present, and the vast bulk consists of tubules of varying maturity (Fig. 6).

C. *Papillary:* The tumour masses are papilliferous, covered by pelvic epithelium, and project into the pelvis or into single large or numerous small cysts (Fig. 7).

D. *Mesenchymal:* The tumour consists predominantly of mesenchymal elements with differentiation into connective tissue, muscle, etc. (Fig. 8).

E. *Focal blastemal:* Spherical blastemal masses embedded in young mesenchymal tissue and closely associated with budding collecting tubules (Fig. 9).

F. *Mixed mesenchymal—blastemal:* There is a close intermixture of both embryonic elements, but no isolation of blastemal clumps by mesenchyma as in Type E.

G. *Massive blastemal:* The tumour is composed almost entirely of blastema with minimal differentiation to tubules (Fig. 10).

The above classification was applied to our series of 125 cases (1925–1962). Of these 36 cases had to be excluded for various reasons such as radiation effects, insufficient material, extensive necrosis or, as in 3 cases only, an unclassifiable mixture of tissue types were present. The distribution of types and their relationship to age and survival are shown in the following tables. In the case of the second table, 7 cases occurring after 1960 have been excluded in accordance with a survival time of 2 years or more.

RELATION OF TISSUE TYPE TO AGE OF PATIENT 1925–1962

Type	Age (yrs) of patient at time of removal of tumour								Total
	0–1	—2	−3	−4	−5	−6	−7	−8	
A	1	0	0	0	0	0	0	0	1
B	6	2	2	0	0	1	1	1	13
C	2	2	0	0	0	0	0	0	4
D	1	1	3	1	0	0	0	0	6
E	2	2	2	1	1	1	1	0	10
F	2	10	4	5	2	2	0	2	27
G	1	5	9	5	5	0	1	2	28
Total	15	22	20	12	8	4	3	5	89

RELATION OF TISSUE TYPE TO SURVIVAL OF PATIENT 1925–1960

Type .	A	B	C	D	E	F	G
Alive .	0	9	4	2	3	6	2
Dead .	1*	3	0	4	6	18	24
% Survival .	0	75	100	33	33	25	8

* Cause of death unrelated to the tumour.

These tables show that there is a tendency for the more differentiated tumours (types A, B and C) to occur in the first three years of life and, as has already been shown earlier in this chapter, the prognosis is better in the early age groups. The majority of nephroblastoma, however, fall into the poorly differentiated groups (types F and G) and here the prognosis appears unfavourable.

REFERENCES

BODIAN, M. (1959). Neuroblastoma. *Ped. Clin. N. Amer.* **6**, 449

BODIAN, M. (1963) Neuroblastoma—An evaluation of its natural history and the effects of therapy, with particular reference to treatment by massive doses of vitamin B_{12}. *Arch. Dis. Childh.* **38**, 606

DARGEON, H. W. (Personal communication)

KOOP, C. E., KIESWETTER, W. B., and HORN, R. C. (1955) Neuroblastoma in childhood. Survival after major surgical insult to the tumour. *Surgery,* **38**, 272

LETTERER, E. (1924) Aleukämische Retikulose. (Ein Beitrag zu den proliferativen Erkrankungen des Retikuloendothelial Apparates.) *Frankfurt. Z. Path.* **30**, 377

LICHTENSTEIN, L., JAFFE, H. L. (1940) Eosinophilic granuloma of bone. *Amer. J. Path.* **16**, 595

NICHOLSON, G. W., (1931) An embryonic tumour of the kidney in a fœtus. *J. Path. Bact.* **34**, 711

OSWALD, N., PARKINSON, T. (1949) Honeycomb lungs. *Quart. J. Med.*, **18**, 1

SIWE, S. A. (1933) Die Reticuloendotheliose—ein neues Krankheitsbild unter den Hepatosplenomegalien. *Z. Kinderheilk.* **55**, 212

WHITE, L. L. R. (1955) *Embryonic Sarcoma of the Urogenital Sinus.* M.D. Thesis, University of Wales

WILLIS, R. A. (1948) *Pathology of Tumours*, 1st Ed., Butterworth, London, p. 751

CHAPTER 12

STEROID TREATMENT IN ASTHMA

A. P. NORMAN

IT became apparent soon after their introduction into medical use that the corticosteroid group of drugs had a remarkable inhibiting effect on the manifestations of allergy. To possess a drug that suppressed all the symptoms of bronchial asthma, leaving the child alert and lively, would seem too good to be true. From the very first it was realised that the side effects of cortisone itself greatly diminished its value in the treatment of asthma. The evolution of more refined products with less obvious side effects has enabled use to be made of the corticosteroids in the treatment of asthma on a fairly wide scale, but in the absence of any clear indications as to how and when they can best be used, in a somewhat haphazard manner.

A number of carefully documented papers on the long term treatment of chronic asthmatics, adult and child, have however been published, and some general guidance can be obtained from them. A problem which besets any attempt to evaluate treatment in asthma is in the difficulty of any uniform assessment of severity; this is even more difficult in the case of milder or intermittent attacks of asthma, as subjective aspects make it almost impossible to assess whether or not treatment is justifiable, when, as with steroids, this carries an element of risk.

Mode of action. The general activities of the corticosteroids in enhancing the feeling of well-being and increasing the appetite are well known. The glucocorticoids have been described (Lanman 1962) as appearing to "enhance the capacity of the organism to adjust to environmental changes and to maintain homeostasis in the face of adverse conditions . . . favour the deposition of depot fat particularly over the trunk, and depress the circulating eosinophil and lymphocyte count . . . glucocorticoids inhibit inflammation due to infection, hypersensitivity, or other cause." This would seem a good description of their effects in asthma, but it is likely that a major factor in the relief of allergic symptoms by corticosteroids lies in their effect on histamine production.

Experiments with rats (Telford and West 1963), to find out the mechanism of the protective action of corticosteroids in animals, showed that deoxycortone, a mineralocorticoid, was inactive in the tests. A range of other corticosteroids, including prednisolone, dexamethasone and fludrocortisone, all possessing both glucocorticoid and mineralocorticoid activity gave the following results. These consisted of marked reduction of either 5-hydroxytryptamine or histamine activity in the skin and various organs, or of both. There was also a marked reduction of histidine decarboxylase in the liver, following the administration of glucocorticoids. Histidine decarboxylase is required in the formation of histamine. It was also shown that amine levels in the tissues were raised after adrenalectomy and that treatment with glucocorticoids reduced these levels to normal. The ability of adrenalectomised animals to form histamine was not altered and as histaminase activity was almost unaltered, Telford and West suggest that the binding of the amines with their tissue components may be modified. They sum up by suggesting that "the therapeutic effects of the glucocorticoids in allergy and inflammation may be partly the result of an action on histamine metabolism or the binding mechanisms for histamine in the tissues."

Prognosis in asthma. The choice of a drug which will suppress symptoms but will not cure, and which can produce harmful complications, must be related to the prognosis of the disease itself. Common experience and some recent studies (Ryssing and Flensborg 1963, Kraepelien 1963) suggest that whilst a considerable percentage of children with *mild* asthma will become symptom-free or virtually symptom-free by the age of 15, this is not so with *severe* asthma. Ryssing and Flensborg found 49% of those with mild asthma to be symptom-free by the age of 15 years, but only 27% of those with more severe asthma. They felt that the prognosis was worse not only for those with already severe asthma, but for those with "a familial predisposition to atopic illness, or with associated allergies." Kraepelien found 29% of his group of 528 children to be symptom-free by the age of about 15 years, and 47% to be considerably improved. He concluded that the beneficial effect of puberty tends to be over-estimated, and that it was necessary to be cautious in any conclusions about prognosis, especially if derived from apparently good clinical results based on the patient's own subjective opinion.

The mortality in childhood seems to be about 1%, but it is almost impossible for such a figure to mean anything in such a common disease with such a wide range from the very mild to very severe. Severe asthma does, however, carry a mortality, which, depending on the criterion of severity, is probably in the nature of 1% or rather more.

It can be accepted that apart from any mortality, severe persistent asthma is not very likely to improve spontaneously, that it may lead to general physical disability, permanent pulmonary damage and educational retardation as a result of loss of schooling. Furthermore, the child with severe chronic asthma is not able fully to take part in all the normal activities of childhood, and as a result of broken sleep and the extra physical effort required in breathing is probably always more tired and more under stress than other children.

Mild or intermittent asthma. It may be stated dogmatically that there is no place for the treatment of mild asthma with the corticosteroids at present available. The administration of these steroids carries a risk, which slight though it may be, is greater than that of the asthma itself. Furthermore, it should be possible to prevent mild attacks of asthma to a considerable extent by conscientiously carried out measures to remove allergens from the local environment and sometimes in addition by means of hyposensitisation. The attacks themselves can be relieved to some extent by use of the appropriate drugs, whilst the associated emotional stress and anxiety of the child and parents can be helped by psychotherapy in some form and in its widest sense.

Nevertheless, treatment of even mild asthma is neither satisfactory nor easy and the temptation to use occasional short courses of steroids is great. The trouble is that occasional courses tend to get more frequent and short courses longer unless a very definite and clear plan of action is adopted and adhered to most strictly, and this is by no means easy.

It is probable that there is equally no place for the use of steroids in the treatment of the occasional severe attack, which can usually be relieved by the use of subcutaneous adrenaline or intravenous aminophylline, if oral drugs fail, and by sedation. However, short courses of steroids are sometimes given in such instances and it is less easy to deny that they have a place. It is usual then to give a drug such as prednisone in doses such as 20 mg. on the first day, 15 mg. on the 2nd day, 10 mg. on the 3rd and 4th day, and 5 mg. on the 5th and 6th day, to a child over the age of about 3 years. It may be pointed out here that if the child can swallow and retain the drug, prednisone and most steroids are more rapidly absorbed and effective by the oral route than by intramuscular injection. If the child is unable to swallow, or vomits, then initially intravenous hydrocortisone should in any case be given.

The risk attached to the occasional use of such courses of steroids is probably very slight. There is no evidence that adrenal function will be depressed, at least quantitatively; whether any qualitative disturbance of adrenal function occurs is merely speculative. It has been held, particularly by anæsthetists, that sudden adrenal shock may occur up to a year or more after such a course, during surgery or under any other form of trauma or stress. Objective evidence of adrenal inadequacy (Robinson, Mattingly and Cope 1962), in such emergencies is difficult to obtain, but numerous such cases have been reported.

Status asthmaticus. Hydrocortisone sodium succinate, or prednisolone disodium phosphate, administered intravenously in a dose of 20–50 mg., repeated if necessary, or by drip transfusion, 50–100 mg. over the course of a few hours, may be extremely effective in status asthmaticus. Indeed, it may be life saving if the child has been on a course of steroids or if steroid treatment has been terminated during the previous year. Oral treatment, prednisone 10 mg. 8-hourly, should be initiated after 4–6 hours and continued until recovery is obviously recurring, when the dose should be reduced by 5 mg. every 48 hours. The exact manner and rate of tailing off the drug is not of importance.

In any severe instance of status asthmaticus intravenous therapy will probably be required, and the rôle played by acidosis requires emphasis (Bukantz 1963). Buffering solutions should be given (sodium lactate, Tris, etc.) as well as aminophylline and hydrocortisone. It has been suggested (Blumenthal 1961) that it is falling arterial pH which is responsible for the diminished response to adrenaline in severe acute asthma.

A point that must be made is the necessity for a clear and acceptable definition of *status asthmaticus*, for it is a term most loosely used. It should not include the severe acute attack of asthma which clears up with treatment by oral antispasmodics and a sedative, nor the attack which is relieved by admission to hospital without any specific drug treatment. It is probably best to accept as definition (Bukantz 1963), a *persistent, severe, refractory asthma which is adrenaline resistant.* This at least both describes the condition and gives fairly objective criteria. It might be better to define the latter part more closely, as *asthma resistant to an adequate dose of adrenaline given slowly, subcutaneously, over a period of several minutes.* If some such definition is not accepted steroids are likely to be given in many severe attacks of acute asthma which might well have been relieved without undue difficulty by adrenaline or aminophylline alone.

Chronic asthma. The most striking response to steroids is made by the group of children with chronic persistent asthma, or with frequent severe attacks with only short periods of remission. The group is comparatively small in numbers, but the distress caused to the parents and the child is considerable. The appearance of such a child is well known, small, thin with high shoulders, an anxious expression and a fixed, distended chest. They are unable to take part in games and their educational performance is liable gradually to deteriorate as a result of absences from school and inability to concentrate from loss of sleep. Their appetite is poor and they are finicky about their food. There is evidence that all these children and their parents develop some symptoms of anxiety, as might be expected.

In the author's series of 33 children (Norman *et al.* 1964) general anxiety was universal; neurotic fears, phobia and nervous habits were present in a minority; in 3, psychogenic factors in causation seemed pre-eminent; 9 others showed signs of severe emotional disturbance sufficient in itself to account for persistence of asthmatic symptoms, and to have a deleterious effect on any form of treatment. Certain character reactions were typical, presumably representing ways in which the children, not always adaptively, have tried to limit their stress response, and to avoid the asthmatic attack.

Pulmonary function studies show impairment of vital capacity and decrease in forced expiratory volume (Blatman *et al.* 1961, Norman *et al.* 1964). These findings are not always correlated with the severity of the symptoms, although usually of greater degree in the more severe asthmatics.

Effect of Steroid Therapy on Chronic Asthma

Symptoms of asthma disappear within about three days of starting treatment with an adequate dose of steroids. A dose of 5 mg. prednisone given twice daily will completely suppress symptoms in almost all cases. Within a few weeks the parents report a complete change in the child's temperament; he sleeps well and eats well, and becomes boisterous and lively. In most cases the life of the family is revolutionised, and they may realise for the first time what it is to have a normal child in the house.

On physical examination the child looks more confident, holds himself better, and the chest is free of wheeze and rhonchi, with the air entry improved. The weight usually increases, sometimes rapidly, and obesity may prove a complication. There is only occasionally a comparable spurt in height however (see p. 299 and Chapter 8, p. 213).

Associated allergic conditions such as eczema and rhinitis improve very considerably and the child may become completely symptom free.

Pulmonary function. Following steroid therapy there is at first marked improvement in *vital capacity* and in *forced expiratory volume*, but later both fluctuate and deteriorate (Blatman *et al.* 1961). In the author's series of 33 cases in whom pulmonary function studies were carried out at yearly intervals for up to four years, in spite of an increase in vital capacity, there was never any real improvement in forced expiratory volume.

This may be interpreted as suggesting that an obstructive element may persist in spite of an apparently adequate dose of steroids and the absence of symptoms, the improvement in vital capacity being due to the increased self-confidence of the child and loss of the feeling of being unable to achieve any respiratory effort. In several instances it was noted that a child would be boasting of running for the first time successfully in a cross country race or of swimming some long distance, and yet on auscultation the breath sounds remained wheezy and the air entry poor; this would seem to support the pulmonary function findings.

Radiology. There is very little recorded concerning changes in the radiographic appearance of the chest following clinical control of symptoms by steroids in chronic asthma. Interpretation of the radiograph is of course not easy and allowance must be made for the subjective nature of the interpretation of the usual findings. In the author's series before treatment, over distension of the lungs was present in almost every instance; a yearly radiograph during the period of treatment showed very little change in general, although less cases were reported as showing over distension in the latter years of treatment than in the first years. Bronchial wall thickening was noted often before treatment, but less frequently after symptoms had been controlled for a year or two; even this improvement was by no means dramatic. Other changes such as segmental collapse were remarkably infrequent before treatment and not recorded at all during steroid therapy; such changes would only have been picked up by chance as radiological examination was carried out only at the time of annual re-assessment.

Emotional state. An attempt was made in the author's series of severe chronic asthmatic children, to evaluate in 32 of them the effects on their emotional state of steroid therapy over a period of several years. The seriously maladjusted children, particularly if one at least of the parents was neurotic or rejecting in attitude, failed to respond as well as the others to steroid treatment, both in respect to recurrences of asthma and their psychological state. Children who had resorted beyond infancy to "comfort habits" and had become dependent on inhalers and pills, responded well to steroids but developed anxiety and relapse when withdrawal of the drug was attempted.

Generalised anxiety was rapidly reduced; neurotic fears and habits were better tolerated. Asthma with largely psychogenic determination responded well, and the improvement was sustained. All, with the exception of the 9 severely emotionally disturbed children, showed increased tolerance of exercise, excitement, and anger. They became less dependent on their mothers and able to join in group activities, camping, swimming and games. The period of better physical health during steroid therapy seemed to improve the mental health of the children in all except the seriously and neurotically disturbed.

From the educational point of view the effect of steroids in the author's series was most striking. The 32 children tested were of a high range of intelligence, with a mean intelligence quotient of 124 (S.D. 14·9). All, before steroid treatment, were missing more than one-third of school attendances in the school year, and some scarcely attended at all. Nine showed at least two years retardation in basic subjects and 13 were described as generally retarded.

During the period of treatment with steroids only 5 missed as much as two weeks in any one term, and the rest missed only an occasional day. All but one were progressively overcoming their educational retardation at the time of survey; that one child remained depressed as well as asthmatic. Seven are still in junior schools and 9 are suitably placed in secondary modern schools; 10 succeeded in passing into grammar schools. It is likely that steroids not only enable the children to attend school but by reducing their emotional tension, allow them to reach more nearly their intellectual potential.

Complications. The risks of cortisone and ACTH therapy in pædiatric practice were underlined some ten years ago by Good and colleagues (Good *et al.* 1957). They listed among minor hazards, acneiform skin eruptions, striæ, hirsutism, increase in blood pressure, obesity. Among the more severe were major intercurrent infections, thrombosis of central retinal artery, status epilepticus, hypertensive encephalopathy, psychosis, peptic ulceration and intestinal perforation, pathological fractures, compression fractures of spine, sudden death.

The safety of steroid therapy has been increased very considerably with the introduction of the newer corticosteroids which produce far fewer side effects, and the amount of the drug required daily to control asthma is usually much less than the amount given to the cases that suffered the complications listed above. Obesity, linear growth inhibition, hypertension, adrenal shock are still among the complications which may occur in children on prolonged steroid therapy; the risk of cataract cannot be entirely excluded.

Obesity. Excessive increase in weight is mentioned in many papers on the prolonged administration of steroids to asthmatic children, together with development of a cushingoid appearance. The author has seen only 2 instances of asthmatic children who might perhaps have been described as cushingoid, but many instances of rapid increase in weight, which in a few cases became excessive.

Inhibition of growth. The height as well as the weight of children with severe chronic asthma tends to be lower than average. Out of the author's group of 33 children aged 6–12 years only 2 had reached the 90th percentile for height before treatment; 18 were below the 50th percentile, 9 were below the 10th percentile, and of these 5 were below the 5th percentile for both weight and height. Linear growth was consistently diminished following the introduction of steroid therapy; in some cases very little growth occurred in the course of a year or more. The lack of growth was parallelled by stasis of epiphyseal development during the period of treatment, so that bone age lagged further and further behind chronological age. It may be noted that in some cases there was already a discrepancy between bone and chronological age before starting treatment. The treatment in this group consisted of prednisone 10 mg. daily for the first year, and the same or a gradually smaller dose in the succeeding years.

Similar findings have previously been recorded at the Children's Asthma Research Hospital, Denver (Falliers *et al.* 1963a), where 83% of 302 asthmatic children were found below the 50th percentile for height; bone age corresponded with the height rather than with chronological age. However, 84% of these children had already been receiving steroids for some time, and 31% for at least a year, before the measurements were made. These authors comment that the growth inhibition is likely in many cases to be due to the asthma itself. This is especially true of the more severe cases, who are also the most likely to be treated with steroids. The Denver group also, over rather short periods, tried to assess the relative degree of growth inhibition produced by the various steroids in current use, and came to the conclusion that betamethasone (dexamethasone) was possibly the drug that, in a sufficient dose to control symptoms, had least inhibitory effect.

The average daily dose required to produce equivalent control of asthma, was as follows:

Cortisone . . . . . 54·7 mg. per sq. metre of body surface
Prednisone . . . . 8·55 mg. per sq. metre of body surface
Betamethasone (dexamethasone). 0·49 mg. per sq. metre of body surface

The average daily dose which permitted satisfactory linear growth was:

Cortisone . . . . . 50·5 mg. per sq. metre of body surface
Prednisone . . . . 5·12 mg. per sq. metre of body surface
Betamethasone (dexamethasone) . 0·37 mg. per sq. metre of body surface

Growth is resumed at a normal rate when steroid treatment is discontinued, or when the dose is reduced to a lower than effective level. There is some evidence that growth inhibition may then be followed by a growth spurt (Blodgett 1956, Van Metre *et al.* 1960), and this is given some support by the evidence that stunting due to an adrenal tumour in a 4 year old child disappeared following removal of the tumour (Prader, Tanner and von Harnack 1963).

Experimental work on rats some twenty years ago (Evans, Simpson and Li 1943, Becks *et al.* 1944), showed the inhibiting effect of ACTH on the growth of rats, especially in respect to bone growth, effecting both chondrogenesis and osteogenesis. Beck and his colleagues also showed that this growth inhibition did not occur in adrenalectomised animals. They further demonstrated cessation of growth with inactive epiphyses in hypophysectomised rats. Normal activity reappeared in the epiphyseal cartilage following the administration of growth hormone; they do not specify the type of growth hormone used; but if ACTH was administered at the same time as growth hormone, endochondral bone formation was retarded, and irregularity occurred in the arrangement of cartilage columns and bony trabeculæ.

These findings, if substantiated, could have a bearing on the administration of anabolic steroids or growth hormone to children receiving corticosteroid therapy. A further warning that care is necessary before administering androgenic hormones or anabolic steroids for a possibly temporary growth arrest is shown by the finding that sterility can be produced experimentally in female rats to whom these have been given (Jacobsohn 1963).

Anabolic steroids may, nevertheless, be administered to children with growth retardation due to steroids, without apparent harm. Stanozolol (17 β-hydroxy-17 α-methyl-androstano [3.2-c]-pyrazole) in doses of 6 mg. daily over a period of six months (Falliers et al. 1963b, Bukantz 1963) produced "significant acceleration of height and weight" with no evidence "of disproportionate advances in skeletal maturation" (see also pp. 211, 213).

It is evident that whilst growth inhibition is an unwelcome complication of steroid therapy in asthma, it may later be compensated by a growth spurt. Futher knowledge of the way in which steroids inhibit growth and of the way in which severe asthma will itself inhibit growth, is required before the administration of anabolic steroids can be safely advocated.

The eyes. No changes in the optic fundi were noted on regular ophthalmoscopic examination of the author's cases, nor do reports of any abnormality occur in other published series. There have, however, been reports of posterior subcapsular cataract occurring in adult patients treated with long-term steroids. Most of these reports concern patients treated for various rheumatic disorders (Black et al. 1960, Pfahl et al. 1961). In one series (Leibold et al. 1962) of asthmatics of various ages, treated with prednisone 1–16 mg. daily for a period of from one to eight years, no instance of posterior subcapsular cataract was found, although out of a small group of adult chronic asthmatics (Giles et al. 1962) treated with intermittent bursts of steroid therapy, 2 out of 6 under treatment for over four years developed cataract. The risk of cataract in young asthmatics treated with long-term steroids must be small, but obviously the possibility of this and possibly other late or delayed ill effects of the steroids cannot be entirely excluded if treatment is maintained for many years.

Hypertension. A rise in blood pressure is a well known hazard of treatment with large doses of corticosteroids, even over relatively short periods. A significant rise has not been noted in reported series of children on the dosage required to suppress the symptoms of asthma; some mild hypertension may occur, however, and in the author's series a diastolic pressure of 80 mm. or over was recorded at intervals over a period of two years or more in 8 out of 33 cases, who were receiving 10 mg. or less of prednisone daily.

Infections. It seems generally agreed that on the minimum dose usually required to suppress symptoms in asthma, infections are overcome without incident, provided the dose of steroid is maintained (Morrison Smith 1963). This is true of measles, chicken pox and mumps, as well as the common respiratory illnesses. It may still be advisable to increase the dose of the drug used during the height of the illness.

Adrenal shock and adrenal suppression. Adrenal shock as a result of trauma or infection in patients on prolonged courses of steroids, is a very real bogey, and numerous cases have been described (Silove 1962). Two possible instances are known to the author, both in children receiving prednisone 10 mg. daily. In one, a drowsy state associated with tonsillitis alarmed the parents; on admission to hospital the child was not thought to be seriously ill and recovered on a temporarily increased dose of prednisone. In the other instance tonsillitis was complicated by vomiting; the child became drowsy and dehydrated but responded immediately to intravenous hydro-cortisone.

Any child treated with long-term steroids must always carry a card showing that steroids are being administered and suggesting what should be done in an emergency. The necessary precautions should be detailed to the parents and it should be an essential part of the treatment to see that they understand that the child must never interrupt the course, especially in illness; that the dose of steroid should be doubled in any emergency if medical advice is not available; that an injection should be given if vomiting prevents retention of the tablets. If these measures are understood, the risk of untoward events from adrenal shock is very slight indeed.

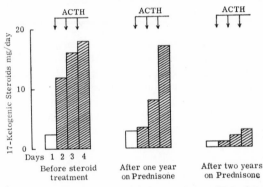

Adrenal response to ACTH stimulation, as shown by urinary output of 17-ketogenic steroids, in an asthmatic child on prednisone therapy. Response graded as *normal* initially, as *reduced* after 1 year, and as *bad* after 2 years.

Adrenal function, as measured by the 17-hydroxycorticoid output in response to three days stimulation with ACTH (Clayton *et al.* 1963), shows a moderate to severe degree of suppression in a large proportion of children treated with prolonged courses of corticosteroids (Fig.). In the author's series 33 children were given prednisone 70 mg. weekly (10 mg. daily) as a maximal dose, gradually reduced to 50 mg. and less during the second or succeeding years of treatment, and the response to ACTH was graded as *normal, reduced, poor* or *bad*. Only 7 showed a *normal* response at each annual re-assessment; 26 showed a *reduced* response, and of these 8 gave a *bad* response at one or other retesting, perhaps indicating a real degree of risk from adrenal suppression (Fig.). The prednisone dosage was always re-duced following the report of a *bad* response, which was only once recorded on two occasions in the same case, although a *reduced* or *poor* response was found several times in the same case. These findings are similar to those recorded in other series of asthmatic children treated with long-term steroids (Siegel *et al.* 1959).

There is therefore no question but that prednisone and other corticosteroids, given in a dose sufficient to suppress the symptoms of asthma, can cause adrenal suppression of a degree sufficient to expose the child to the risk of adrenal shock in time of stress. It must be largely a matter of luck that no cases of adrenal shock have occurred in reported series of steroid treated asthma, and the possibility of its occurrence must be in the mind of anyone treating an asthmatic child with long-term steroids.

A detailed study of a number of adult asthmatics (Harter *et al.* 1963), showed that complete suppression of symptoms was possible with steroids given in a single dose on alternate days, but not at longer intervals. It further suggested that adrenal suppression as indicated by 17-hydroxycorticoid urinary excretion in response to ACTH, was much less in those patients who were given their steroid in a single dose every other day, than in those receiving the same total in daily divided doses. The observation that a 48-hour period was the longest these adult asthmatics remained symptom free when no steroid was given, accords with the author's finding in children. In those cases in whom relapse is going to occur on weaning from steroids, wheezing always begins to reappear if prednisone is omitted for 48 hours, and in some cases after 24 hours. However, in view of the known and often severe degree of adrenal inhibition caused by daily steroids, a single dose on alternate days might prove in many cases to be adequate to suppress symptoms with less effect on the adrenals.

The 17-hydroxycorticoid response to ACTH improves when the dose of steroids is reduced, and returns to normal when they are finally omitted or given in small amount, without the need for administration of ACTH therapeutically. This is, of course, not necessarily true if excessive doses of steroids are given nor if they have been maintained for many years in a dose sufficient to produce adrenal suppression throughout.

The ACTH test gives no information about the state of the pituitary, or its ability to release ACTH (Robinson, Mattingley and Cope 1962). For this the metapiron test is required, but as yet no results of the use of this test in steroid treated asthmatic children have been reported.

Inhalation therapy. It has been suggested that a more effective method of using steroids than the oral would be to deliver the drug directly to the bronchi by inhalation. Some of the effects of this may be due to the topical application of the steroid, but systemic absorption occurs, as shown by a fall in the 11-hydroxysteroid excretion in the urine (Crepea 1963). There is a possible risk of local damage as a result of prolonged inhalation of a dust, but there is no evidence that this has in fact occurred in asthma. Crepea administered dexamethasone phosphate dust in metered doses given in two inhalations four times a day, to 29 children with severe chronic asthma. The total dose in the day was 0·67 mg. (equivalent to about 6·7 mg. prednisone). The results were good and symptoms in most of the group were controlled at first, but tended after a while to recur following respiratory infections.

In a group of 71 adults with chronic asthma (Bickerman 1963), half obtained marked relief from the use of 1 mg. dexamethasone phosphate sodium, with a particle size of less than 5 micrograms, suspended in a mixture of fluorchlorocarbons as propellant, and delivered in a metered spray. Ventilatory function studies in 49 of these patients showed, in 32, significant increases in vital capacity, forced expiratory volume, and maximal expiratory flow rate, as compared with the values before treatment. A careful study of a group of children whose adrenal function was tested following treatment (Siegel *et al.* 1964) has shown that successful suppression of symptoms by inhalation of dexamethasone is definitely associated with adrenal suppression.

It appears that although the results of treatment with steroid aerosols are quite good, they do not avoid the problem of absorption and some degree of adrenal suppression.

Choice of steroid. The choice of steroid currently obtainable seems to lie between prednisone, prednisolone, dexamethasone and triamcinolone.

The equivalent dosage of these drugs and their chemical names are as follows:

Prednisone   = Δ1-dehydrocortisone, 5 mg.
Prednisolone   = Δ1-dehydrohydrocortisone, 5 mg.
Dexamethasone = 9 α-fluoro-16-α-methyl-prednisolone, 0·5 mg.
Triamcinolone = 9 α-fluoro-16-α-hydroxy-prednisolone, 4 mg.

There is some suggestion that prednisone and prednisolone may have a greater growth inhibitory effect than dexamethasone (Falliers *et al.* 1963), and it is generally held that triamcinolone has less growth inhibitory effect than any of the others, although the evidence is not very impressive. Triamcinolone has the defect of producing muscle weakness when given in fairly large doses, but this does not appear to be a real risk in the usual doses given.

Weaning off steroids. It has been said (Knowles 1961), that one of the main problems in the use of steroids in asthma is not whether to give long term treatment to any particular patient, but how to wean a patient off treatment once symptoms have been brought under control. Knowles quoted many papers to illustrate the point that relapse is the usual answer to the withdrawal of steroids, even after many years of treatment. In a large retrospective survey he found that the only (adult) patients weaned off with any ease were those with seasonal asthma, and those who did not benefit. The risk of death in adults from status asthmaticus for at least twelve months after discontinuence of prolonged steroid therapy has been emphasised (Rees and Williams 1962), and must be equally true of children (Morrison Smith 1963).

Symptoms are liable to recur in a large proportion of children treated with long-term steroids, during the process of reducing the dose. A few remain perfectly well, and a few develop symptoms equal to or worse than those they suffered before the course of steroids was started. There is no clear indication as to which child is likely to suffer severe relapses, but some evidence from the author's study suggests that seriously maladjusted children are likely both to fail to respond well during treatment, and to relapse when steroids are finally withdrawn. Another group likely to relapse, but who do well during treatment, are those who show marked signs of anxiety and dependence on comforters in infancy and on inhalers and pills as asthma develops. From the constitutional angle, children with a gross predisposition to allergy are equally liable to relapse.

There is no doubt that reduction of the steroid used should be carried out very slowly, over a period of many months, and contemporaneous efforts should be made to remove the factors likely to cause recurrence of symptoms, either by psychotherapy, removal of potential allergens from the environment or hyposensitisation.

Final termination of a long course of steroids may be made possible by admission to a suitable boarding school.

The present place of steroids. Corticosteroids are of certain value in the treatment of status asthmaticus, and of children who, following previous steroid therapy, are suffering from a severe relapse.

They have at present no place in the treatment of mild asthma, for the complications and risks associated with their use outweigh the advantages.

There is no definite contra-indication to their occasional use during a severe attack or for a short period during a severe exacerbation of asthma, but there is a strong tendency for the courses to become progressively more frequent and more prolonged.

Children with severe chronic asthma are greatly relieved by long-term treatment with corticosteroids, but the complications are such that steroids should be reserved for only the most severely affected. Furthermore, steroids merely suppress symptoms for the period of administration, so that recurrence is probable when treatment is ended. Hence the period of relief should be regarded as a breathing space during which other steps should be taken to afford more permanent relief. These other measures should be of a comprehensive nature, physical and psychological and directed at the child, his family and environment.

The age of the child to be treated is of some importance. There can rarely be sufficient reason for long term treatment with steroids before the age of 5 years, and it is generally possible to refrain from their use for another 2 or 3 years even in severe cases. One of the benefits of steroid therapy is that it gives the child the possibility of obtaining the most benefit from school and of maintaining the educational level he is intellectually capable of reaching; it also allows him to join fully in the life of his fellows. For this reason coverage with steroids over the 8 to 12 year age has particular advantages. Termination of treatment at about the age of 12 years also gives the child a good possibility of further growth before adolescence.

REFERENCES

BECKS, H., SIMPSON, M. E., LI, G. H. EVANS, H. M. (1944) Effects of adrenocorticotropic hormone (ACTH) on osseous system in normal rats. *Endocrinology*, **34**, 305

BECKS, H., SIMPSON, M. E., LI, G. H., EVANS, H. M. (1944) Antagonism of ACTH to action of growth hormone on osseous system of hypophysectomised rats. *Endocrinology*, **34**, 311

BICKERMAN, H. A., ITKIN, S. E. (1963) Aerosol steroid therapy and chronic bronchial asthma. *J. Amer. med. Ass.* **184**, 533

BLACK, R. L., OGLESBY, R. B., VON SALLMAN, L., BUNIM, J. J. (1960) Posterior subcapsular cataracts induced by corticosteroids in patients with rheumatic arthritis. *J. Amer. med. Ass.* **174**, 166

BLATMAN, S., BRAVO, L., PERMUTT, S. (1961) Pulmonary function studies in asthmatic children. *Amer. J. Dis. Child.* **102**, 529

BLODGETT, F. M., BURGIN, L., IEZZONI, D., GRIBETZ, D., TALBOT, N. B. (1956) Effect of prolonged cortisone therapy on the statural growth. *New Engl. J. Med.* **254**, 636

BLUMENTHAL, J. S., BLUMENTHAL, M. N., BRAIN, E. B., CAMPBELL, G. S., PRESAD, A. (1961) Effect of changes in arterial pH on the action of adrenalin in acute adrenalin-fast asthmatics. *Dis. Chest.* **39**, 516

BUKANTZ, S. C. (1963) Residential study and treatment centre for children with intractable asthma. *J. Amer. med. Ass.* **185**, 75

CLAYTON, B. E., EDWARDS, R. W. H., RENWICK, A. G. C. (1963) Adrenal function in children. *Arch. Dis. Childh.* **38**, 49

COHEN, M. B., WELLES, R. R., COHEN, S. (1940) Anthropometry in children. *Amer. J. Dis. Child.* **60**, 1058

CREPEA, S. B. (1963) Inhalant corticosteroid management of chronic asthmatic children. *J. Allergy*, **34**, 119

DREIZEN, S., STONE, R. E., SPIES, T. D. (1961) Influence of chronic undernutrition on bone growth in children. *Postgrad. Med.* **29**, 182

FALLIERS, C. J., SZENTIVANYI, J., McBRIDE, M., BUKANTZ, S. C. (1961) Growth rate of children with intractable asthma. *J. Allergy*, **32**, 421

FALLIERS, C. J., TAN, L. S., SZANTIVANYI, J., JORGENSEN, J. R., BUKANTZ, S. C. (1963a) Childhood asthma and steroid therapy as influences on growth. *Amer. J. Dis. Child.* **105**, 127

FALLIERS, C. J., JORGENSEN, J. R., TAN, L. S., BUKANTZ, S. C. (1963b) Anabolic effects of stanozolol: reversal of growth arrest and possible changes in adult height prognosis among children with intractable asthma treated with corticosteroids. *Amer. J. Dis. Child.*, **106**, 388

GILES, C. L., MASON, G. L., DUFF, I. F., McLEAN, J. A. (1962) Association of cataract formation and systemic corticosteroid therapy. *J. Amer. med. Ass.* **182**, 719

GOOD, R. A., VENNIER, R. L., SMITH, R. T. (1957) Serious untoward reactions to therapy with cortisone. *Pediatrics*, **19**, 95

HARTER, J. G., REDDY, W. J., THORN, G. W. (1963) Studies on intermittent corticosteroid dosage regimen. *New Engl. J. Med.* **269**, 591

HELM, W. H., HEYWORTH, F. (1958) Bronchial asthma and chronic bronchitis treated with hydrocortisone acetate inhalers. *Brit. med. J.* **2**, 765

HERXHEIMER, H., McALLEN, M. K., WILLIAMS, D. A. (1958) Local treatment of bronchial asthma with hydrocortisone powder. *Brit. med. J.* **2**, 762

HUGHES, E. R., SEELY, J. R., KELLY, V. C., ELY, R. S. (1962) Corticosteroid levels before and after cortico-tropin. *Amer. J. Dis. Child.* **104**, 605

JACOBSOHN, D. (1963) The effect of anabolic steroids on rats. *Brit. med. J.* **2**, 1128

KNOWLES, J. P. (1961) Difficulties in weaning in steroid treatment of asthma. *Brit. med. J.* **2**, 1396

KRAEPELIEN, S. (1963) Prognosis of asthma in children. *Acta pœdiat., Suppl.* **140**, 92

LANMAN, J. T. (1962) In *Pediatrics*, ed. Holt, L. E., MacIntosh, R., Barnett, H. L. 13th Ed. Appleton, New York, p. 686

LEIBOLD, J. E., ITKIN, I. H. (1963) Cataracts in asthmatics treated with corticosteroids. *J. Amer. med. Ass.* **185**, 448

MORRISON SMITH, J. (1963) Prolonged treatment with prednisolone in children with asthma. *Tubercle*, **44**, 281

NORMAN, A. P., STEPHEN, J. M., EDWARDS, R. W. H., GANDERTON, M. A. (1964) Severe asthma in childhood; the effect of long-term steroids. To be published

PFAHL, S. B., MAKLEY, T. A., ROTHERMICH, N. O., McCOY, F. W. (1961) Relationship of steroid therapy and cataracts in patients with rheumatoid arthritis. *Amer. J. Ophthal.* **52**, 831

PRADER, A., TANNER, J. M., VON HARNECH, G. A. (1963) Catch-up growth following illness or starvation. *J. Pediat.* **62**, 646

REES, H. A., WILLIAMS, D. A. (1962) Long term steroid therapy in chronic intractable asthma. *Brit. med. J.* **1**, 1575

ROBINSON, B. H. B., MATTINGLY, D., COPE, C. L. (1962) Adrenal function after prolonged corticosteroid therapy. *Brit. med. J.* **1**, 1579

RYSSING, E., FLENSBORG, E. W. (1963) Prognosis after puberty for asthmatic children. *Acta pœdiat.* **52**, 97

RYSSING, E., FLENSBORG, E. W. (1963) Prognosis for asthmatic children. *Acta pœdiat., Suppl.* **140**, 92

SIEGEL, S. C., HEIMLICH, E. M., RICHARDS, W., KELLY, V. C. (1964) Adrenal function in allergy. IV. Effect of dexamethasone aerosols in asthmatic children. *Pediatrics*, **33**, 245

SILOVE, E. D. (1962) Coma as presenting sign of adrenal failure after steroid withdrawal. *Brit. med. J.* **1**, 515

TANNER, J. M. (1958) In *Modern Trends in Paediatrics*, ed. Holzel, A. and Tizard, J. P. M. Butterworth, London

TELFORD, J. M., WEST, G. B. (1963) Allergy and adrenal corticosteroids. *Int. Arch. Allergy*, **22**, 106

VAN METRE, T. E., NIERMANN, W. A., ROSEN, L. J. (1960) Comparison of the growth suppressive effect of cortisone, prednisone and other adrenal cortical hormones. *J. Allergy*, **31**, 531

CHAPTER 13

RENAL BIOPSY

J. A. BLACK and R. H. R. WHITE

THE contribution which renal biopsy could make to the study of diseases of the kidney was originally shown by Castleman and Smithwick (1943) who removed specimens of kidney tissue from hypertensive patients during the operation of lumbar sympathectomy. The first attempts at percutaneous needle biopsy of the kidney are attributed to Alwall who, in 1944, experienced a fatality which discouraged him from further development of the technique. He did not publish his findings until eight years later (Alwall 1952): by this time Pérez Ara (1950) and Iversen and Brun (1951) had reported their own experiences.

Percutaneous renal biopsy failed to gain widespread acceptance until Kark and Muehrcke (1954) described their improved technique, with the patient in the prone position. The technique was soon adapted for the investigation of renal disease in children; Galán and Masó (1957) and Vernier and his colleagues (Farquhar et al. 1957) first reported its use. Vernier's group (Vernier et al. 1958) obtained adequate material in 70% of their cases and (Vernier 1960) have had no deaths in their series. Dodge et al. (1962) have also recently analysed a series of 205 biopsies in children. We started doing percutaneous biopsies in 1959, and record here our experiences of the procedure as used at The Hospital for Sick Children, London and at the Children's Departments of Guy's Hospital, London, and the Mulago Hospital, Kampala, Uganda.

Percutaneous Biopsy

Choice of method. Either general or local anæsthesia may be used; it is best for each operator to accustom himself at first to one method. The use of general anæsthesia has the advantage that complete control over respiration can be obtained by muscle relaxants such as succinyl choline, thus minimising the chance of tearing the capsule or renal tissue by unexpected respiratory movements. The disadvantages are that a general anæsthetic with relaxants requires the resources of an operating theatre and that the respiratory movements produced by pressure on the bag are often smaller than those in a conscious patient; this may sometimes increase the difficulty in identifying the kidney by the movements of the needle. A further drawback to a general anæsthetic is that special precautions are required in children who are under treatment with corticosteroids, or who have recently been treated with these drugs. One of the advantages, therefore, of the use of local anæsthesia is that it simplifies the whole procedure. Nevertheless, for the relatively inexperienced operator general anæsthesia is perhaps preferable, as it allows a greater margin of safety when there is difficulty in finding the kidney or in obtaining an adequate specimen.

Contraindications. The following are absolute contraindications: a single functioning kidney, ectopic kidney, suspected tumour of the kidney, hydronephrosis or pyonephrosis, the form of polycystic disease with large cysts, bleeding diseases and disorders of the clotting mechanism. A biopsy should not be done, unless the indications are extremely urgent, in the early stages of acute pyelonephritis or in severe hypertension with retinal hæmorrhages and exudates. When a biopsy is required for diagnostic purposes in acute renal failure, dialysis should be performed before the biopsy, in order to reduce the risk of bleeding.

Preparation. A plain radiograph of the abdomen is first obtained, to show the renal outlines. This may show or exclude an ectopic kidney and if it is a good film the actual size of both kidneys can be measured, and difference in size is noted. A simple method of marking the approximate place for introducing the needle is to place an opaque marker over the proposed site before exposing the film, and to observe its position in relation to the lower pole of the kidney. This is useful in fat or œdematous patients or in those in whom the last rib is difficult to palpate. We have noticed, however, that the position of the kidneys, as seen radiologically in the supine child, may be much lower than when the anæsthetised or heavily sedated child is placed prone with a sandbag under the abdomen. If it is not possible to see at least part of both kidneys by plain radiography, a single film taken 10 minutes after an intravenous injection of 45% "Hypaque" will show their position. Particular care should be paid to a history of any abnormal tendency to bruise or bleed excessively after cuts or operations, and the bleeding time and prothrombin index should be estimated in each patient. As a further precaution the Hb is estimated and one pint of blood is cross-matched, to be available on the day of operation. If local anæsthesia is used, a simple explanation to the child on the day before the operation is important in order to establish confidence and to obtain cooperation; in the very young, to whom a verbal explanation is not possible, a few minutes spent playing with the child on the days before the biopsy may be rewarding. Special precautions must be taken in cases involving past or present treatment with corticosteroids and a definite plan for steroid cover must be worked out beforehand.

Biopsy technique. The actual technique of locating the kidney has been previously described (Kark and Muehrcke 1954, White 1963). When local anæsthesia is used pre-medication is necessary. At first we used a combination of pethidine, chlorpromazine and promezathine, or occasionally paraldehyde (White 1963), but further experience has shown that better results are obtained with a combination of pethidine hydrochloride (2 mg./kg.) and promazine hydrochloride ("Sparine") (2 mg./kg.) with a maximum dose of 100 mg. of either drug, given by intramuscular injection 1 hour before the biopsy. With this pre-medication most young children sleep through the operation, and older ones remain awake but calm. After selecting the site for biopsy, the skin, underlying tissues and muscles are infiltrated with 1% lignocaine; 4–5 ml. is usually sufficient and more than 10 ml. is rarely needed. At this stage resistance may be encountered in the young child, despite sedation, but once analgesia is complete he will usually go to sleep again, and it has only very rarely been necessary to abandon the procedure on account of inadequate sedation. The infiltrating needle can be felt to penetrate the layers of fascia overlying the kidney. We do not infiltrate the renal capsule itself because of the risk of tearing it or of damaging the cortical tissue at the site of biopsy. If it is intended to take two biopsy specimens, as is our usual practice, it is best to infiltrate both perpendicularly to the skin and somewhat obliquely towards the head. With adequate sedation, the respiration remains shallow and regular. Older children will usually cooperate, during the insertion and withdrawal of the inner cutting needle, by holding their breath after shallow inspiration, but in young children who are asleep or are unable to co-operate, the risk of a capsular tear is reduced if the needle is inserted or withdrawn only during the passive expiratory phase of respiration. When the prongs of the inner needle have been closed by advancing the outer needle, the whole instrument should be rapidly withdrawn, for this movement sometimes stimulates a deep inspiration.

When using general anæsthesia the main requirement is a good understanding between operator and anæsthetist. The relaxant is injected as soon as the operator is ready to insert the exploring needle and the anæsthetist ceases pressing on the bag whenever the position of the exploring needle, or later the biopsy needle, is altered. Normally there is little difficulty in obtaining an adequate respiratory excursion of the kidney, but in some older children the amount of movement of the kidney under controlled respiration has been very small.

Post-operative care. After the return of the child to his bed the blood pressure and pulse rate are recorded over the next 12 and 24 hours respectively. The abdomen is examined as soon as the child is conscious or cooperative. Normally there is no abdominal tenderness after a biopsy: the development of marked pain or tenderness in the region of the appropriate kidney, together with any increase in size of the kidney is most suggestive of bleeding into the renal tissue or beneath the renal capsule. The appearance of the urine is noted; massive hæmaturia with clots is likely to be accompanied by ureteric colic and occasionally by vesical distension from obstruction by a large clot. Pethidine may be required, or relief of the obstruction by passing a catheter.

Processing of specimens. Whenever possible two pieces of tissue are removed; it is not to be expected that a length of less than 0·5 cm. would prove of much use diagnostically, and the aim is to obtain two pieces measuring 1–2 cm. in length. The tissue is removed gently from the needle and carefully straightened out on a glass slide, which is then placed in the fixative. If desired fragments may first be cut off and frozen immediately for fluorescence studies for antibodies, or processed for electron microscopy. It is necessary to have the fixatives available in or just outside the operating theatre, as any delay causes shrinkage and distortion of the specimen from drying: 10% neutral buffered formalin or Heidenhain's Susa are both suitable fixatives for light microscopy, but the use of the latter alone precludes the use of silver stains and frozen sections. After embedding the tissue in histological wax, sections should be cut at a thickness of 2 μ and stained for routine purposes with hæmatoxylin and eosin, the periodic acid-Schiff method, Masson's trichrome, and periodic acid silver methenamine stains.

When the number of glomeruli is small, more may be revealed by cutting serial sections.

Results. All the percutaneous biopsies reported here were performed by one of three operators, using with few exceptions the Vim-Silverman needle as modified by White (1962) for use in children. In the few cases in which a Menghini needle was used it proved less satisfactory. The ages of the patients ranged from 1 month to 16 years (see Table). Contrary to expectations it was easier to identify the kidney in the younger children, partly because the kidney is often as little as 1 cm. below the surface of the skin (in older children the kidney was encountered at depths varying from 2 to 6 cm.), and also because the respiratory excursion was well-marked.

TABLE

AGE INCIDENCE AND FAILURES

Age	No. of patients	No. of attempts	Failures	
			No.	%
Less than 12 months . .	5	5	1	20
12–23 months . . .	18	19	2	11
2–5 years	80	92	4	4
6–9 years	62	74	7	10
10–16 years	56	63	7	11
Total	221	253	21	8

Causes of failure. Of the total of 221 cases, there was failure to obtain an adequate specimen in 8%. In many cases when the first attempt was unsuccessful, the biopsy was repeated satisfactorily at a later date. The causes of failure were three.

(i) Inability to identify the kidney. This was due in most instances to inexperience; in a small number of cases a respiratory excursion was not obtained and arterial pulsation was not seen, while in a few cases, particularly those with considerable œdema, it was not possible to identify the kidney by means of movement of the needle or by the sensation of entering the kidney substance. The commonest error, particularly under general anæsthesia, was to insert the needle just below the lower pole which resulted in an apparently satisfactory respiratory excursion but no sensation of resistance on inserting the inner cutting needle. When this occurred the needle was withdrawn slightly and reinserted pointing in a slightly more cranial direction.

(ii) Adequate identification of the kidney, but failure to obtain a specimen at all, or the production of a piece of tissue too small or unsuitable for histological interpretation. Occasionally too deep penetration of the kidney resulted in a specimen consisting solely of medulla, which was useless for diagnostic purposes: this may be expected to occur more frequently if the cortex is particularly thin, as in chronic renal disease. The chief cause of failure to obtain an adequate specimen was the use of a blunt or faulty needle, and for this reason we usually have two needles available at every biopsy. The proper care of the instrument, in order to reduce such failures, has been described elsewhere (White 1962).

(iii) Obtaining a piece of tissue from the wrong organ. This only occurred twice in this series; in one case the needle was directed obliquely upwards towards the head to avoid entering the pelvis of a slightly hydronephrotic kidney and a piece of liver tissue was obtained. The biopsy was successfully repeated at a later date. In the other case splenic tissue was obtained in a child with chronic malarial splenomegaly and nephrotic syndrome, when attempting a biopsy of the left kidney.

Complications. The commonest complication is hæmorrhage, but the risk of this can be reduced by proper selection of patients, and the elimination of any cases with severe anæmia, bleeding disorders, or an abnormal clotting mechanism. Microscopic hæmaturia is invariably found immediately after the biopsy. In this series the following complications were found: hæmaturia visible to the naked eye, 25 cases (11%); massive hæmaturia with clots, 3 cases; perirenal or possibly intrarenal hæmatoma, 2 cases; post-anæsthetic shock requiring transfusion, 1 case; cardiac arrest attributable to general anæsthetic, 1 case (White 1963).

Two complications which have been recorded elsewhere but have not been seen in this series are, massive bleeding into or round the kidney necessitating nephrectomy, and arterio-venous aneurysm of the renal vessels. A review of the literature suggests that most of the fatalities from renal biopsy have resulted from disregard of the recognised contraindications or have occurred in the hands of casual operators.

Open Biopsy

Open renal biopsy may be performed when percutaneous biopsy is contra-indicated, for example, when there is a history of bleeding tendency or when pyelography has shown the kidneys to be very small. A surgical specimen may also be taken during an operation on the kidney. It is sometimes preferable to take a biopsy from a particular area of the kidney under direct vision, as in chronic pyelonephritis with localised abnormalities on pyelography.

In performing the actual biopsy two methods have been used. Originally a wedge of tissue was removed, but it was subsequently found that the use of a burr of internal diameter 1·5 mm. was quicker and easier, and produced a more satisfactory specimen.

During the period under review open biopsies were done in 25 cases, with the following indications: failure to thrive in infancy, 5 cases; chronic pyelonephritis, 4 cases; hypertension, 3 cases; chronic renal failure, 3 cases; renal calculi, 3 cases; nephrocalcinosis (oxalosis), 1 case; hypercalcæmia, 1 case; recurrent hæmaturia with history of easy bruising, 1 case; anaphy-lactoid purpura with episodes of anuria, 1 case; renal vein thrombosis, 1 case; portal hypertension, 1 case; horse-shoe kidney and hydronephrosis, 1 case.

Nephrotic Syndrome

The term *nephrotic syndrome* as used here indicates a clinical state with œdema, usually generalised, gross proteinuria and hypoproteinæmia. The terms *nephrosis, lipoid nephrosis* and *pure nephrosis* are regarded as synony-mous and apply to those children with the nephrotic syndrome which

show, on renal biopsy, normal glomeruli or minimal changes on light microscopy.

Adequate biopsies were obtained in 32 children attending The Hospital for
Sick Children, with the nephrotic syndrome. The age of onset in the majority
was between 2 and 4 years; the youngest was aged 3 months and the oldest
11 years when the disease became obvious. There were 9 females and 23
males. A single biopsy was performed in 29 children and repeat biopsies in 3
children: in 3 other cases an autopsy was later performed which provided a
comparison with the earlier biopsy material. The indications for biopsy
were:

(i) Request for a histological diagnosis in children who had failed to respond satisfactorily to an adequate course or courses of steroids or
ACTH or who had had repeated relapses (15 cases).
(ii) Confirmation of diagnosis to decide whether steroids should be used
(5 cases).
(iii) The further investigation of cases with atypical features, such as
hypertension, hæmaturia, a very early onset, or a family history of
renal disease (12 cases).

The second biopsies were done in 2 of the patients because of continued
or increasing difficulty in controlling the proteinuria with steroids, and also to
discover whether any irreversible changes had developed which were not
present in the first biopsy. Apart from the clinical indications it was hoped
that a study of the biopsy material would provide answers to the following
questions:

(i) Is there any correlation between the histological changes and particular clinical or pathological findings, such as hæmaturia, azotæmia or
hypertension?
(ii) Does the histological appearance indicate whether the disease is
reversible or irreversible?
(iii) Are there any histological changes which are associated with failure
to respond to the corticosteroid group of drugs?
(iv) Is there any evidence that those cases which originally appeared to be
reversible can become irreversible with the passage of time?

It was felt that it would introduce less bias to divide up the cases according
to the histological appearances, and then to see whether there was any
correlation between certain clinical or pathological features and the histology.
The cases were therefore placed in one of two groups, based upon the *glomerular* changes; tubular abnormalities were regarded as secondary and of minor
importance.

Group I: No abnormality or minimal changes, the latter defined as one or
more of the following:

(1) Thickening of the walls of the glomerular tuft capillaries without
endothelial proliferation. Presumably this appearance indicates
thickening of the basement membrane.
(2) Slight degrees of endothelial proliferation of the tuft capillaries.
(3) Not more than an occasional sclerosed or fibrotic glomerulus seen.

Group II: Major changes. That is, one or more of the following:

(1) More than "slight" endothelial or epithelial proliferation of tuft capillaries.
(2) Fibrinoid necrosis of the tuft.
(3) Capsular adhesions.
(4) Epithelial crescents.
(5) More than an occasional sclerosed or fibrotic glomerulus.
(6) Pericapsular or capsular fibrosis.

Assessment of the response to treatment was necessarily somewhat arbitrary. It was decided to grade the response in terms of the reduction in proteinuria resulting from the first course of treatment which was considered to be adequate, both in dosage and duration. The three categories were as follows:

Good: A complete disappearance of proteinuria.
Partial: A reduction in proteinuria by 50% or more, but without complete disappearance of protein from the urine.
None: No change in proteinuria or a reduction of less than 50%.

Such a classification only shows whether the proteinuria was reversible and does not give any indication of the response to treatment of later relapses or of the final outcome of the disease.

Results. In Group I there were 18 cases (16 boys and 2 girls) with an age of onset varying between 1 year 3 months and 9 years 11 months, with a maximum incidence between 2 and 4 years.

In 9 children the onset appeared to be related to various types of upper respiratory infection, while in 7 cases there was no such history nor was there apparently any other precipitating factor. It is however a common observation that an upper respiratory infection will precipitate a relapse or increase in proteinuria in a child in remission and it is therefore difficult to know whether such infections really determined the onset of the disease, or merely caused it to become clinically obvious. The blood pressure at the onset was recorded in all but 3 instances; in 3 children there appeared to be a definite hypertension, but in all of these cases the blood pressure is now normal. This hypertension at the onset was not related to steroid treatment, and it is possible that some of the high readings are artifacts due to the difficulty in obtaining an accurate reading in a child with an arm swollen with œdema. The urine was examined repeatedly in all cases: a definite excess of red cells was not reported in any of this group and in only one child did the urine contain an excess of white cells and hyaline casts. Of the 17 cases in which the blood urea was estimated at the onset of the disease, slightly raised values were found in only 2 children, subsequent readings being normal. In 2 children in this group steroids were never used; one had a spontaneous remission and has remained well, while the other continues to have intermittent proteinuria, but is otherwise well. Of the 16 children treated with steroids, 3 showed a partial response to what appeared to be an adequate course of treatment; in the remaining 13 cases there was a good initial response. Of the treated cases, 4 are now no longer under treatment and have normal urine: 4 are still on steroid treatment and have normal urine and 4 are inadequately controlled by continuous steroids; a further 4 cases have been taken off treatment and have a considerable degree of proteinuria.

In Group II of 14 children there were 6 in whom the onset was apparently related to an infection. 4 cases were hypertensive at the onset; 2 of these died, 1 is normotensive and 1 requires hypotensive drugs; the same considerations of possible artifact in measurement of the blood pressure apply in this group. The results of urine examination showed a marked difference from those in Group I; in all except 2 cases an excess of red cells was found, and an excess of white cells was present in all but 5 cases; hyaline casts were absent in only 4. The initial blood urea levels tended to be higher than in Group I; 5 children had levels above 40 mg./100 ml., and 3 of these later died. Of the 11 cases in which steroids were used there was a good response in only 1 case, a partial response in 4 cases, no response in 5 cases. In one case steroids were used for only a short time and it is uncertain whether the complete clinical remission was related in any way to the treatment. In 3 children steroids were not used; one of these, who later died, was a most unusual case in which a prolonged bacteræmia resulting from an infected Spitz-Holter valve was associated with a nephrotic syndrome with gross hæmaturia; treatment of the bacteræmia, which was due to a coagulase-negative staphylococcus, caused a complete return to normal of the urinary abnormalities and a remission of the nephrotic syndrome (Black and Challacombe, to be published). The family history of one case is of particular interest and may indicate a specific form of renal disorder, probably genetically determined.

Male: born May 21st, 1954. Developed nephrotic syndrome at the age of 5 years: he was started on steroid treatment a year later. There was no response to steroids. A renal biopsy was performed at $6\frac{1}{2}$ years and showed capsular fibrosis with some glomerular fibrosis and sclerosis. There was also cellular proliferation of the tuft, with adhesions and thickening of the stalk. He has now considerable proteinuria and his blood urea is 163 mg./100 ml. His family history is as follows:

Maternal great grandfather died at 82 years from "ruptured heart and uræmia."
Maternal grandfather died of "Bright's disease" at 24 years.
Mother has chronic renal failure and hypertension.
A male cousin of the mother died at 21 years of renal disease.
One sib (female) died at 3 weeks of prematurity and hypothermia.

Discussion. From this series it is not yet possible to answer some of the more important questions concerning the ætiology and prognosis of the nephrotic syndrome in childhood. The evidence from serial biopsies is too scanty to provide any certain indication as to the evolution of the histological changes; in those cases studied in this way there was slight progression in the thickening of the walls of the tuft capillaries; this was remarkable in one case because this child was free from proteinuria and clinically normal without treatment at the time of the second biopsy. There does, however, seem to be a relationship between the histological changes and the likelihood of a response to steroid treatment. In group II, with marked histological changes, the response to corticosteroids was poor. In nearly all cases in this group microscopic hæmaturia and hyaline casts were present at the onset. The poor prognosis in this group is in agreement with the findings of the purely clinical studies of Debré *et al.* (1960) and of Arneil (1961), indicating that the presence of even microscopic hæmaturia at the onset carries a bad prognosis. In view of this association between advanced histological changes in the kidney and hæmaturia, it seems that such cases should be separated from the "pure" nephrosis group, both from the point of view of their poor response to steroid treatment and because of their bad prognosis. Further studies by renal biopsy are needed in order to clarify many of the points raised by these findings; more information is required on the natural history of the histological changes in the various forms of the nephrotic syndrome. More detailed studies of those cases with a family history of renal disease should be made, as the prognosis appears to be poor in such cases (Debré *et al.* 1960, Marie *et al.* 1960); they must be distinguished from the congenital or neonatal form of the nephrotic syndrome which is familial, has an onset at or shortly after birth, and appears to be always fatal (Hallman, Hjelt and Ahvenainen 1956).

Recurrent Hæmaturia

The causes of recurrent hæmaturia are likely to differ in different communities and age groups. All the patients had had two or more attacks of hæmaturia and a renal biopsy was done because it had not been possible to make a diagnosis by other methods. The indications for biopsy were thus primarily diagnostic and, apart from those cases with chronic pyelonephritis, the actual treatment was not greatly influenced by the histological diagnosis. From the point of view of the prognosis however, it was important to be in a position to exclude chronic nephritis. The results reported in this chapter are recorded more fully elsewhere (Bodian *et al.*, in press).

There were 46 cases in this group, 30 boys and 16 girls. They were of British descent with 3 exceptions (Cypriot-Italian, Spanish-Italian, American Indian-British).

The cases were divided into three groups on the basis of the type of onset.

Group I. Onset unrelated to any definite disease. There were 25 males and 11 females in this group. The youngest was aged 14 months at the onset of the hæmaturia and the oldest 11 years. In all cases the first attack of hæmaturia appeared to be identical with subsequent ones and there was no specific illness of onset. The number of attacks varied from 2 to over 400 and the intervals between attacks from 2 days to over a year. The pattern of attacks remained fairly constant in each patient. Two types of history were obtained: in one the hæmaturia was noticed in the evening, after a day of strenuous physical exercise; in the other the hæmaturia was associated with a minor upper respiratory tract infection. Symptoms such as vague abdominal discomfort, frequency of micturition, headache or general malaise occurred in a few cases, but in the majority there was little or no general disturbance during the attacks. Oedema and hypertension were never observed.

In almost half of the patients microscopic hæmaturia persisted between the attacks. In 5 patients pyuria and bacteriuria were found; in three of these the biopsy showed evidence of chronic pyelonephritis. Abnormalities on intravenous pyelography were found in 4 cases, of which 2 were those already mentioned with chronic pyelonephritis. Cystoscopy was done on one occasion in 18 cases and more than once in 7 cases, but no helpful information was obtained. Other investigations provided little clue to the ætiology: β-hæmolytic streptococcal infections were rarely associated with attacks, and an antistreptolysin-O titre greater than 200 units/ml. was found in only 1 case at the onset, and in 8 others during the course of observation. The sedimentation rate was persistently raised in 3 patients, but was normal in the majority. In 2 children the family history gave a possible clue to the ætiology: both were boys who have recently become deaf; in both instances there was a strong family history of "nephritis" or hæmaturia on the maternal side, and it seems probable that these two boys are suffering from the hereditary syndrome of hæmaturia and deafness (Alport's syndrome).

The *histological diagnoses** were as follows:

Focal segmental glomerulonephritis, 21 cases (Fig. 1); focal diffuse glomerulonephritis, 9 cases; focal segmental and focal diffuse glomerulonephritis, 1 case; generalised segmental glomerulonephritis, 1 case (Fig. 2); generalised diffuse glomerulonephritis, 1 case; chronic pyelonephritis, 3 cases.

Group II. Onset with anaphylactoid purpura. All 7 patients had a typical rash and colicky abdominal pain. Hæmolytic streptococci were isolated from the throat swab in only 1 case, and the antistreptolysin-O titres which were estimated in 5 cases were all normal. The initial attack of hæmaturia lasted longer in these cases than in Group I, the duration being weeks or months, while subsequent attacks lasted about a week. There was microscopic hæmaturia between attacks in all cases and proteinuria was often considerable (100–1200 mg./100 ml.). 3 of these children had raised blood urea levels and diminished creatinine clearances and 2 also had hypertension. Pyuria and bacteriuria developed in one case, but this was thought to be due to an intercurrent infection. Intravenous pyelograms were normal in all cases.

Histologically all 7 cases showed evidence of progressive disease, with capsular adhesions, crescent formation and interstitial fibrosis. The distribution of the lesions was as follows: focal segmental glomerulonephritis, 2 cases; focal segmental and diffuse glomerulonephritis, 1 case; generalised segmental glomerulonephritis, 2 cases; generalised diffuse glomerulonephritis, 2 cases.

It is generally agreed that there is great difficulty in giving an exact prognosis in the nephritis associated with anaphylactoid purpura. In this small series there was a high proportion with generalised glomerulonephritis, and with such findings the long-term prognosis is likely to be poor, while in those with focal renal lesions chronic renal insufficiency is less likely to occur or may develop much later.

Group III. Onset with acute nephritis. In these 3 patients the clinical picture at the onset was suggestive of acute nephritis, but the histological appearance in each case was one of focal segmental glomerulonephritis. It is

---

* The terms used require definition. *Focal:* scattered glomeruli abnormal. *Generalised:* all glomeruli abnormal. *Segmental:* part of the glomerular tuft affected. *Diffuse:* the whole of the glomerular tuft affected.

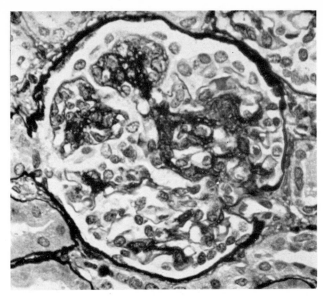

Fig. 1. Glomerulus showing early segmental lesions in a case of focal segmental glomerulonephritis presenting with recurrent hæmaturia.
(Periodic acid-silver methenamine: × 560)

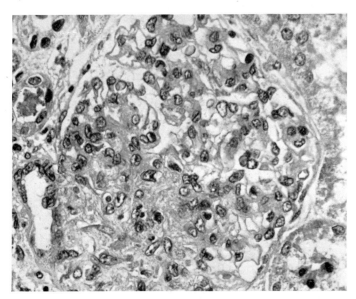

Fig. 2. Glomerulus showing a rather more advanced segmental lesion in a case of generalised segmental glomerulonephritis presenting with recurrent hæmaturia.
(Masson's trichrome: × 400)

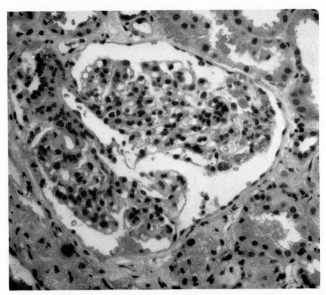

FIG. 3. A representative glomerulus from a 16-year-old boy with hereditary
nephritis and deafness (Alport's syndrome), presenting with recurrent
hæmaturia. The tuft is hypertrophied and lobulated and shows marked
segmental endothelial proliferation. Near the hilum the tuft is hyalinised
and is adherent to the capsule. Red cells in the capsular space and in the
tubule in the top left corner.
(H & E: × 290)

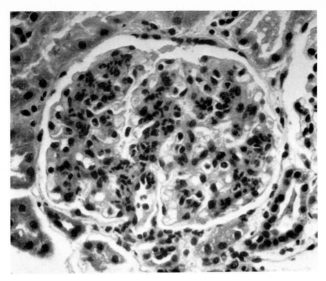

Fig. 4. Glomerulus from a 2-year-old West Indian boy with asymptomatic proteinuria, showing swelling of the tuft due to endothelial proliferation and marked polymorphonuclear leucocytic infiltration. Many of the capillary loops are occluded by the swollen endothelial cytoplasm. Similar changes were present in all 61 glomeruli seen, and are typical of acute diffuse glomerulonephritis.
(H & E: × 360)

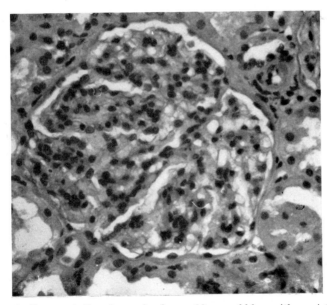

Fig. 5. Representative glomerulus from a 10-year-old boy with persistent proteinuria and transient symptomless hypertension one year before the biopsy. The tuft shows marked thickening of the stalk and localised endothelial proliferation. There are adhesions in several places. Some glomeruli in the same specimen showed diffuse endothelial proliferation and contained up to 10 polymorphonuclear leucocytes. These changes indicate a persistent glomerulonephritis, probably associated with a previous streptococcal infection, in the early chronic phase.
(Periodic acid-Schiff: × 360)

possible, as has been suggested by others (Jennings and Earle 1961), that this may indicate a late subsiding or early chronic stage of acute nephritis.

Conclusions. As might be expected, these cases were not a homogeneous group. In many, the actual history gave no indication of the probable histological appearance, but renal biopsy was able to provide a clear-cut diagnosis. Both from the point of view of treatment and prognosis it seems particularly important to pick out those cases with chronic pyelonephritis.

As a result of Ross' (1960) work with adults it is generally accepted that the prognosis is usually good in cases of recurrent hæmaturia associated with focal glomerulonephritis and our experience supports this. An exception should be made, however, in the two males with Alport's syndrome in whom the histological changes were remarkably slight (focal segmental glomerulonephritis and focal diffuse glomerulonephritis respectively). Two brothers with Alport's syndrome, not included in this series, have been reported elsewhere (White et al. 1964): the younger brother showed focal and segmental endothelial proliferation, while the older brother aged 16 years showed in addition glomerular sclerosis and adhesions (Fig. 3), focal interstitial fibrosis and tubular dilatation. It is evident from the literature (Williamson 1961) that most of the affected males die from renal failure before reaching the age of 30 years.

Glomerulonephritis

Acute nephritis. The principal histological changes in acute diffuse glomerulonephritis are in the glomeruli, and consist of proliferation and swelling of the endothelial cells and infiltration by polymorphonuclear leucocytes (Fig. 4) causing swelling of the glomerular tufts, obstruction of the capillaries and obliteration of the capsular spaces; such changes appear to be completely reversible in most cases. Sometimes polymorphonuclear exudation is very extensive and may be associated with proliferation of the epithelial cells of the tuft and Bowman's capsule, which adhere to each other, and with striking interstitial inflammatory reaction (Jennings and Earle 1961). The appearance of numerous cellular crescents, together with widespread interstitial and tubular lesions and glomerular scars, usually denotes a subacute or rapidly downhill course.

Renal biopsy is not needed for the diagnosis of "classical" acute hæmorrhagic nephritis, but recognition of the features described above has enabled us to identify the disease in children with atypical clinical presentations. Out of 46 East African children presenting with clinical evidence of renal disease or with urinary abnormalities alone, and studied by renal biopsy, 24 were shown to be suffering from acute diffuse glomerulonephritis (Hutt and White, 1964). Evidence of β-hæmolytic streptococcal infection was obtained in 75% of cases. The clinical pattern of these children was frequently modified by disorders such as malnutrition and hookworm infection, so that gross œdema and congestive cardiac failure were prominent features: 4 presented with the nephrotic syndrome, 3 with cardiac failure, and 3 were detected on routine urinalysis. The classical picture was seen in only 14 patients and this observation perhaps partly explains the alleged rarity of acute nephritis in East Africa suggested by previous workers (Luder 1957).

Hendrickse and Gilles (1963) also noted that gross œdema and hypoalbumin-æmia were features of all the cases of acute diffuse glomerulonephritis which they studied in Nigerian children.

Asymptomatic glomerulonephritis. This is probably commoner than is generally believed and may account for some cases of chronic nephritis in which there is no history of a previous acute nephritis. White (1964) has recently published renal biopsy studies of 4 children in whom there was evidence of silent progression towards chronic nephritis. In none of these cases was nephritis suspected until the urine was found to be abnormal on routine testing. In one child the urine was examined because symptomless and transient hypertension was discovered at a minor operation under general anæsthesia. 2 of the patients had persistent proteinuria, 1 had intermittent proteinuria, and 1 had microscopic hæmaturia. The antistrepto-lysin-0 titres were raised in 2 of the children. Renal biopsy was repeated in 2 cases and showed changes ranging from acute diffuse glomerulonephritis (Fig. 4) to early chronic glomerulonephritis (Jennings and Earle 1961) (Fig. 5), and chronic nephritis with interstitial fibrosis.

Chronic glomerulonephritis. In most instances chronic glomerulonephritis can be diagnosed clinically, particularly where there is a previous history of acute hæmorrhagic nephritis, or of the nephrotic syndrome. But renal biopsy may occasionally be of diagnostic value where the previous history is inadequate or atypical, as in the following example.

Female, 13 years. Recurrent hæmaturia which first began following an attack of influenza, together with persistent proteinuria. On examination, a thin, anæmic girl; blood pressure 120/80; Hb 9·9 g.; blood urea 36 mg./100 ml.; urine protein 100 mg./100 ml.; Addis count, 69 million RBC; granular casts present; maximum s.g. 1·031. The history, urinary findings and anæmia suggested chronic nephritis but the absence of hypertension, uræmia and impaired urine concentration were contradictory. Renal biopsy showed fibrosis of Bowman's capsules with hypercellularity of the epithelium and adhesion to the glomerular tufts, some of which showed incipient sclerosis. The findings were consistent with early chronic glomerulonephritis.

Renal biopsy has also helped in the management of chronic nephritis and in assessing prognosis. It will presumably be used increasingly when the problems of renal homografting have been mastered. The following case illustrates the part played by renal biopsy in assessing the usefulness of treatment.

Female, 11½ years. In December 1958, at 7 years of age, headache, fever and sore throat were followed by hæmaturia which decreased but recurred a month later. On admission to hospital in January 1959, she was slightly œdematous but normotensive. The urine contained protein, RBCs and granular casts and the blood urea was 50 mg./100 ml. In spite of prolonged bed rest, hæmaturia continued and treatment with prednisolone was begun in November 1959, the initial dose of 40 mg./day being decreased after four weeks to a dose of 15 mg./day, which was maintained for the next 3½ years. Hæmaturia became microscopic and proteinuria persisted. In October 1961, renal biopsy showed marked lobulation of the glomerular tufts with localised endothelial proliferation, thickening of the lobular stalks and capsular adhesions.

In June 1963 she was stunted, moon-faced and had slight hirsuties. The blood pressure was 115/80. Urine protein 50 mg./100 ml., Addis count 1,350,000

RBCs; no casts; concentration-dilution test, s.g. 1·011–1·006. Hb 17·7 g. Blood urea 34 mg./100 ml. A further renal biopsy showed advanced chronic glomerulonephritis, with partial or complete sclerosis of all the glomeruli present, capsular fibrosis and extensive interstitial fibrosis and tubular atrophy. Comparison with the previous specimen showed that, in spite of the mild clinical course, prednisolone had not prevented progressive destruction of her kidneys. The drug was therefore slowly discontinued, under cover of ACTH, and she has since remained well, showing a considerable spurt in growth.

Miscellaneous Uses

Asymptomatic proteinuria. Renal biopsy is of undoubted value in distinguishing the causes of persistent proteinuria, once a postural effect has been eliminated. We have diagnosed both acute and chronic glomerulonephritis (White 1964) as well as chronic pyelonephritis.

Pyelonephritis. The diagnosis of pyelonephritis is based upon examination of the urine, and few cases should be missed if quantitative cytology (Stansfeld 1962) and bacteriology (Bradley and Little 1963) are employed. In acute cases and the majority of chronic ones the disease is focal and normal tissue may be obtained. However, on one occasion, when normal tissue was obtained from a 6-year-old girl with persistent proteinuria following acute tonsillitis, a clean urine specimen voided four hours after biopsy showed for the first time significant pyuria and gave a positive culture. The post-biopsy urine should be examined microscopically and cultured routinely. If pyelonephritis is suspected the inner biopsy needle can also be dipped in a glucose-broth bottle which is then incubated. We are opposed to culturing renal tissue routinely since it necessarily limits the amount available for histological examination.

We have seen three examples of diffuse bilateral chronic ("primary") pyelonephritis in which the diagnosis was established by means of renal biopsy. The first was a 1-year-old boy who, unlike his twin sister, failed to thrive; the second was a 9-year-old boy with anorexia, excessive thirst and enuresis; and the third was a 9-year-old girl with lassitude and pallor. All three showed similar findings characterised by anæmia, uræmia and failure to concentrate the urine. The urine contained less than 30 mg./100 ml. protein, and pyuria was absent except in one case in which an excess of white cells was found after biopsy. Radiographically the renal outlines were smooth but small and the pelvi-calyceal patterns normal. Renal biopsy showed intense lymphocytic infiltration and interstitial fibrosis; some of the tubules were atrophic while others were dilated and contained "colloid" casts. In some areas there was fibrosis and sclerosis of glomerular tufts, whereas in others the glomeruli were hypertrophied but structurally normal. These changes are believed to be characteristic of chronic pyelonephritis.

Anaphylactoid purpura. In addition to the 7 patients suffering from recurrent hæmaturia already described, we have performed renal biopsies in 3 other cases of anaphylactoid purpura. In a 9-year old girl, the persistent hæmaturia failed to respond to prednisolone therapy and, after 1½ years of treatment, biopsy showed chronic glomerulonephritis. A 2-year-old boy developed a steroid-resistant nephrotic syndrome after a severe bout of purpura; the urine contained RBCs. Renal biopsy showed well-established focal proliferative glomerulonephritis some 6 months after the onset. A 10-year-old girl had a typical attack of acute nephritis, associated with slight purpura, abdominal pain and occult blood in the fæces, and biopsy 1 month after onset showed acute, diffuse glomerulonephritis with marked capsular epithelial proliferation.

Hypertensive encephalopathy. When acute nephritis presents in this way, there are usually sufficient urinary abnormalities to make the diagnosis apparent. In one case, a 10-year-old girl, the only urinary abnormality was slight proteinuria, which vanished within two days of the onset. Addis counts were repeatedly normal, as were the blood urea, urinary catechol amine excretion and intravenous pyelogram. Renal biopsy showed typical acute diffuse glomerulonephritis.

Nephrocalcinosis. Renal biopsy confirmed a suspected diagnosis of nephrocalcinosis in a 6-year-old girl with pyuria and chronic renal failure. Symptoms of vomiting and frequency began 16 months previously and at that time, although urea and creatinine clearances were normal, her maximum urinary s.g. was 1·016. Pyelonephritis was diagnosed and she was treated with sulphafurazole. However, she gained little weight during the next 15 months and developed polyuria and polydipsia. Further inquiry led to the discovery that she had been taking vitamin tablets equivalent to 150,000 units of vitamin D per day during the six months before the onset of symptoms. Her blood urea at the time of biopsy was 61 mg./100 ml. and her serum calcium 13·8 mg./100 ml.

Conclusion

It will have become apparent that there are comparatively few instances in which renal biopsy has led directly to a change of treatment in an individual patient. This reflects our limited knowledge concerning the treatment of many forms of renal disease, and it is to be hoped that the time will come when advances in knowledge will necessitate diagnostic accuracy. However, renal biopsy is at present fulfilling two important rôles. It enables us to answer parents' questions with a precision which was not previously possible. The other major rôle is in research. Comparison of serial biopsy specimens will advance our knowledge of the evolution of the various forms of chronic renal disease, and may help us to understand why some children suffering from the nephrotic syndrome fail to respond to treatment.

There can be no doubt that the incidence of failures and serious complications is reduced with experience. It is also certain that a great deal of time must be devoted to the study of many biopsy specimens before experience in renal pathology can be gained. We not infrequently find, on reviewing a specimen obtained perhaps a year or more previously, that we must modify our interpretation of it in the light of increasing experience. For these reasons we believe that at the present time renal biopsy will be more profitable if its use is confined to a number of larger centres interested in the many aspects of renal disease, in both children and adults, because of the need for long-term studies. In such circumstances its continued use is, we feel, justified even where it cannot be claimed that it will be of immediate benefit to the individual patient.

Acknowledgements

We are greatly indebted to the late Dr Martin Bodian, and to Dr Barbara Ockenden for their help.

REFERENCES

ALWALL, N. (1952) Aspiration biopsy of the kidney. *Acta med. scand.* **143**, 430

ARNEIL, G. C. (1961) 164 children with nephrosis. *Lancet*, **2**, 1103

BLACK, J. A., CHALLACOMBE, D. N. (to be published)

BODIAN, M., BLACK, J. A., KOBAYASHI, N., LAKE, B. D., SHULER, S. E. (in press)

BRADLEY, J. M., LITTLE, P. J. (1963) Quantitative urine cultures. *Brit. med. J.* **2**, 361

CASTLEMAN, B., SMITHWICK, R. H. (1943) The relation of vascular disease to hypertensive state, based upon study of renal biopsies from 100 hypertensive patients. *J. Amer. med. Ass.* **121**, 1256

DEBRÉ, R., MARIE, J., ROYER, P., LÉVÊQUE, B. KAPLAN, L. (1960) Pronostic éloigné du syndrome néphrotique de l'enfant. *Ann. Pediat. (Par.)* **36**, 63

DODGE, W. F., DAESCHNER, C. W., JR., BRENNAN, J. C., ROSENBERG, H. S., TRAVIS, L. B., HOPPS, H. C. (1962) Percutaneous renal biopsy in children; I. general considerations. *Pediatrics*, **30**, 287

FARQUHAR, M. G., VERNIER, R. L., GOOD, R. A. (1957) An electron microscope study of the glomerulus in nephrosis, glomerulonephritis and lupus erythematosus. *J. exp. Med.* **106**, 649

GALÁN, E., MASÓ, C. (1957) Needle biopsy in children with nephrosis. *Pediatrics*, **20**, 610

HALLMAN, N., HJELT, L., AHVENAINEN, E. K. (1956) Nephrotic syndrome in newborn and young infants. *Ann. Pœdiat. Fenn.* **2**, 227

HENDRICKSE, R. G., GILLES, H. M. (1963) The nephrotic syndrome and other renal diseases in children in Western Nigeria. *E. Afr. med. J.* **40**, 186

HUTT, M. S. R., WHITE, R. H. R. (1964) A clinico-pathological study of acute glomerulonephritis in East African children. *Arch. Dis. Childh.* **39**, 313

IVERSEN, P., BRUN, C. (1951) Aspiration biopsy of the kidney. *Amer. J. Med.* **11**, 324

JENNINGS, R. B., EARLE, D. P. (1961) Post-streptococcal glomerulonephritis: histopathologic and clinical studies of the acute, subacute and early chronic latent phases. *J. clin. Invest.* **40**, 1525

KARK, R. M., MUEHRCKE, R. C. (1954) Biopsy of the kidney in prone position. *Lancet*, **1**, 1047

LUDER, J. (1957) Some pædiatric problems in Uganda. *Brit. med. J.* **2**, 1143

MARIE, J., ROYER, P., LÉVÊQUE, B. (1960) Le syndrome néphrotique familial de l'enfant. *Ann. Pediat. (Par.)* **36**, 76

PÉREZ ARA, A. (1950) La biopsia punturel del riñón no megálico. Consideraciones generales y aportación de un nuevo métudo. *Bol. Liga Cancer, Habana*, **25**, 121

ROSS, J. H. (1960) Recurrent focal nephritis. *Quart. J. Med.* **29**, 391

STANSFELD, J. M. (1962) The measurement and meaning of pyuria. *Arch. Dis. Childh.* **37**, 257

VERNIER, R. L., FARQUHAR, M. G., BRUNSON, J. G., GOOD, R. A. (1958) Chronic renal disease in children. *Amer. J. Dis. Child.* **96**, 306

VERNIER, R. L. (1960) Kidney biopsy in the study of renal disease. *Pediat. Clin. N. Amer.* **7**, 353

WHITE, R. H. R. (1962) A modified Silverman biopsy needle for use in children. *Lancet*, **1**, 673

WHITE, R. H. R. (1963) Observations on percutaneous renal biopsy in children. *Arch. Dis. Childh.* **38**, 260

WHITE, R. H. R. (1964) Silent nephritis: a study based on renal biopsies. *Guy's Hosp. Rep.* (in press)

WHITE, R. H. R., PARSONS, V., WALT, F. P. (1964) The renal disorder in Alport's syndrome. *Guy's Hosp. Rep.* (in press)

WILLIAMSON, D. A. J. (1961) Alport's syndrome of hereditary nephritis with deafness. *Lancet*, **2**, 1321

CHAPTER 14

HYDROCEPHALUS OF INFANCY

G. H. MACNAB

Ventricular Drainage Valves

SINCE this chapter in the second edition of *Recent Advances in Pædiatrics* was written, a great amount of knowledge has been gained in the use of valves made from silastic, providing a unidirectional flow of cerebrospinal fluid from the lateral ventricle to the right atrium of the heart. Silastic (silicone rubber) has the property of self-adherence, so that a slit made in a silastic cap will open at a constant pressure and close as soon as the pressure drops, a property which will be maintained throughout the years, as the material does not lose its elasticity. In addition, silastic is water repellent and does not give rise to reaction when placed in the body tissues. However it is highly electro-static and so easily attracts particles to it; it therefore has to be carefully sterilised and the minimum of handling used in setting the valve in the patient, to avoid introducing low-grade infection.

The Holter valve was designed in 1955 by an engineer in co-operation with Dr. Eugene Spitz, neurosurgeon to the Philadelphia Children's Hospital. The valve (Fig. 1) consists of a portion of silastic tubing joined at each end by two stainless steel collars. Two portions of stainless steel tubing pass into the lumen of the silicone tube and are covered by silastic caps forming the inlet and the outlet of the valve. In the silastic cap a slit is made which will open and shut at a defined pressure according to the size of the slit. An angled silastic catheter is placed in the right lateral ventricle of the brain and fitted over the inlet of the valve. The valve itself is placed in a groove made in the right parietal bone and a silicone catheter leads from the outlet down to the right atrium of the heart, passing through the internal jugular vein in the neck. After insertion the valve can be pumped through the scalp. Compression of the tube with failure to refill from above denotes blockage of the ventricular catheter. Non-compressibility of the tube denotes a block in the jugular vein or right atrium due to clot. The fact that there is a constant unidirectional flow of CSF through the valve and the cardiac catheter, prevents reflux of blood or even diffusion of red cells, which would lead to blockage of the valve system.

Rates of flow in vitro and in vivo. The original Holter valve was made to open at a pressure of 42 mm. H_2O, on the assumption that an infant forms CSF at the rate of 25 ml./24 hrs. at a pressure of 60–70 mm. H_2O. However experience has shown that valves with lower opening pressures are needed.

Fig. 2 shows some observations made by Mr Holter with valves opening at three different pressures, 42, 25 and 10 mm. H_2O; the flow of water through these was measured at varying heads of pressure. With a 25 mm. valve, for instance, and a head of pressure of 150 mm. the volume of water

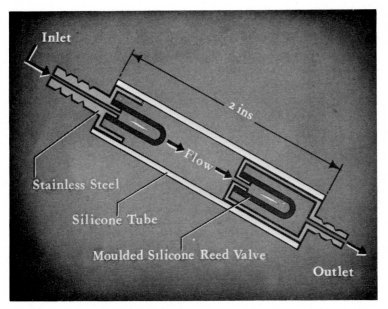

Fig. 1. Spitz-Holter ventriculo-jugular shunt valve.

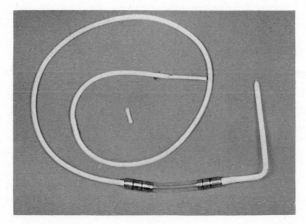

FIG. 3. Holter valve, with modified terminal portion of catheter.

delivered is 240 ml./24 hrs., while if the head of pressure is dropped to 70 mm. only 43 ml./24 hrs. is delivered, equivalent to less than 1 drop/minute from the end of the cardiac catheter.

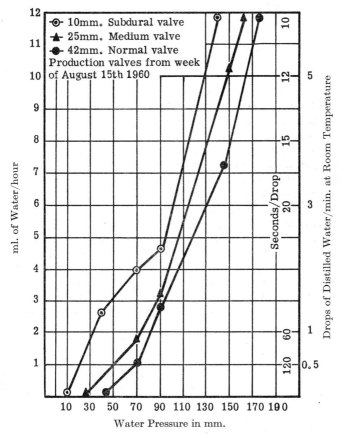

FIG. 2. Rates of flow of water through three Holter valves with different opening pressures (10, 25 and 42 mm. H_2O) at varying heads of pressure.

At operation, tapping the ventricle of a hydrocephalic infant causes a marked fall in pressure, the magnitude of the fall depending upon the amount of CSF removed in comparison with that in the ventricular system. In a typical instance, an original ventricular pressure of 200 mm. would drop to 130 mm. after removal of 10 ml. CSF. On account of this fall in pressure when CSF is drained, in order to give a satisfactory flow of CSF with control of hydrocephalus, in most cases a valve opening pressure of 10 mm. is required.

The valve was next inserted in a two-stage procedure. In the first stage the valve was placed in position and CSF drained from the lateral ventricle through the exteriorised cardiac catheter, allowing 24-hour collections of CSF to be made. The catheter was then clamped off and the pressure allowed to build up again in the ventricle; at the end of 48 hours a new catheter was attached to the outlet valve and passed down the internal jugular vein into the right atrium. This procedure enabled a comparison to be made of the rates of drainage in Holter's *in vitro* tests when the head of pressure was constant, with those obtaining in the hydrocephalic infant when the head of pressure in the ventricles was inconstant. Constant pressure between 200 and 250 mm. produces *in vitro* 300 ml. of water per 24 hours, against 185 ml. CSF from the hydrocephalic infant; while constant pressure between 100 and 150 mm. produces *in vitro* 160 ml. of water, against 55 ml. CSF from the infant. At these pressures the rate of drainage is thus much lower than expected by laboratory tests, due to the fact that secretion of CSF by the choroid plexus must vary according to the CSF pressure. Lowering of this pressure by tapping the ventricle cuts down the rate of formation of CSF until the pressure is built up again. However, with very high and long-standing pressures of over 300 mm., tapping of the ventricle does not lower the rate of formation of CSF, but may allow even more to be secreted.

From these experiments it was concluded that a Holter valve will deal with pressures of up to 300 mm., but that when the pressure exceeds 300 mm. and is of long standing the valve has difficulty in coping with the drainage of adequate quantities of CSF; the small drop in pressure created by insertion of the valve tending to encourage further formation of CSF. In dealing with the problem of the long-standing case of hydrocephalus that appears to be arrested at a very high ventricular pressure, we at one time thought that reduction of the ventricular pressure might somewhat improve the mental status and relieve the degree of spasticity in the limbs. Unfortunately, the insertion of a valve in such a case, because it can lead to an increased formation of CSF, can also lead to coning of the brain stem.

A further practical point is that progressive hydrocephalus is not an orderly procedure, but moves forwards in acute phases interspersed with latent periods. In the acute phase a sudden rise in ventricular pressure may lead to ventricular hæmorrhage and raised CSF protein. If in this phase a valve is inserted, it is liable to become blocked.

Complications that may arise following insertion of the valve. In order to place the end of the cardiac catheter in the right atrium of the heart an incision is made in the neck to expose the internal jugular vein. The proximal portion of the vein is ligated, then a small opening is made in the vein and the catheter passed through it to the heart. Clot formation takes place in the distal portion of the internal jugular vein down to the level of the subclavian vein. If the ligature is not properly applied, the cardiac catheter will work up into the clotted vein and drainage cease. A radiograph of the opaque cardiac catheter should be carried out each 6 months to ensure that body growth has not brought the cardiac catheter out of the right atrium. The cardiac catheter can be easily lengthened by opening the neck wound, sectioning the catheter in the neck and attaching a new elongated distal portion to the proximal portion over a junction tube.

A complication occurring in 10% of cases is the development of a bacteræmia due to a coagulase-negative staphylococcus. For the bacteræmia to occur the valve must be functioning normally. Following insertion of the valve the child develops a temperature which persists over weeks or months, but the child's general condition remains good and the hydrocephalus arrested. After many weeks there is splenic enlargement and a progressive anæmia requiring repeated blood transfusions. Blood culture is positive and the organism can be recovered from the ventricular fluid. Intra-muscular and intra-ventricular methicillin gives temporary control, but the condition will not be cured until the valve is removed. I proved this by exteriorisation of the cardiac catheter after sterilisation of the blood-stream and ventricular fluid with methicillin. Sterile ventricular fluid, which passed through the valve and was collected from the end of the cardiac catheter, still contained the staphylococcus. In the process of removing the valve the tissues around the valve and the outer covering of the valve were not affected, but culture of the material from within the valve assembly was always positive. This means that once bacteræmia is established the infected valve must be removed and a second valve placed in the left side of the head after the ventricular fluid and blood-stream have been rendered sterile. A rarer form of infection occurs when the aseptic clot becomes infected and softens; small portions of septic thrombi break off and are carried to the periphery of the pulmonary circulation setting up septic broncho-pneumonia.

Clot formation leading to cessation of drainage occurs in about 10% of the cases. The clot may form at the opening into the right atrium or in the lower portion of the superior vena cava, and is probably due to trauma set up by the lower end of the cardiac catheter impinging on the endothelial lining. The clot then forms across the level of the opening of the cardiac catheter but does not enter its lumen; the result is that CSF still drains through the catheter and passes upwards in a retrograde fashion in the superior vena cava up to the neck, where it forms a fluid swelling. In order to avoid this complication I have had the lower 3 cm. of the cardiac catheter reduced in diameter down to a lumen of 0·8 mm. (Fig. 3).

Ætiology and Pathology of Hydrocephalus. Laurence (1959) in 100 consecutive post-mortem examinations found that malformation alone accounted for only 14% of cases, but when associated with infection or trauma in the form of hæmorrhage accounted for 46%. Inflammatory reaction due to infection or hæmorrhage without malformation accounted for another 50%, leaving 4% due to tumour formation (Table).

TABLE
AETIOLOGY OF HYDROCEPHALUS
(100 *Post Mortem Examinations*)

Malformations **46**	*Inflamation* . . . **50**
Alone 14	Infection alone . . . 17
With infection . . . 30	Trauma (hæmorrhage alone) . 22
With trauma (hæmorrhage) . 2	Doubtful (infection or trauma) 11
Tumour **4**	

(After Dr. K. M. Laurence)

This means that 46% had a malformation, but in 82% low-grade infection or hæmorrhage was present, capable of setting up a block due to œdema,

debris, or adhesions. *Post mortem* evidence of the site of the block corresponded with the neuro-radiological findings in my series of 200 cases. This site
of the block was as follows: 18% due to aqueduct block, 42% due to basal
cistern block and 40% associated with presence of an Arnold-Chiari malformation leading to basal cistern block. The aqueduct block was temporary in
character in the majority of cases, due to swelling of the ependymal lining
of the aqueduct or to debris passing down from infected lateral ventricles.
The presence of an Arnold-Chiari malformation can set up a block in the
subarachnoid space at the level of the foramen magnum (Fig. 4), where
venous congestion over the malformation sets up an obliterative arachnoiditis,
or at the level of the tentorial opening by the upward extension of the malformation. In addition, it may be associated with a congenital aqueduct
stenosis. When low-grade ascending infection from the sac of the myelomeningocele is present, blockage may occur from the level of the aqueduct of
Sylvius down to the basal cisterns.

Neuro-radiology has to be used to diagnose the level of the block, but as
the pressure in the ventricles is high it is dangerous to perform a lumbar
encephalogram. The presence of an Arnold-Chiari malformation can be
diagnosed by ventriculography. Where the air can pass round the third
ventricle into the elongated fourth ventricle, air will be seen below the level
of the foramen magnum (Fig. 5); while if the air is held up in the third
ventricle there is always evidence of a constant notching of the anterior wall
of the dilated third ventricle.

Natural Arrest

For many years we have been aware that certain cases of progressive
hydrocephlaus undergo spontaneous arrest, and those of us working in the
field in the early days of drainage operations saw many cases in which the
drainage system was blocked but yet the hydrocephalus underwent natural
arrest. Laurence (1962) was granted facilities by Mr. Wylie McKissock to
follow up a group of 182 patients who had been fully investigated as to the
cause of hydrocephalus over a 20-year period, but had not received treatment. The cause of hydrocephalus in 182 cases was: malformation 43,
trauma 59, infection 42, tumour 4 and unknown 34. There was definite
evidence of natural arrest in 81 cases (44·5%), and overall figures showed
that 51% survived and 49% died. A percentage of 51% is a high figure for
survival without treatment, and Laurence (1962) has re-adjusted the figures
of life expectancy on actuarial principles using a life table. He points out
that the chance of a hydrocephalic child seen soon after birth reaching adult
life is 20 or 23% depending upon the method of calculation employed. If a
hydrocephalic infant has reached three months of life he has a 26% chance of
reaching adult life without surgery, and if the infant is between one and two
years he has a 50% chance of reaching adult life. On the other hand, Mc-
Keown and Record (1960) found that only 33% of *all infants born with
hydrocephalus*, and only 10% of those with associated spina bifida cystica,
were alive at the end of the first year of life. It must be remembered that
many infants suffering from hydrocephalus and spina bifida cystica only
survive a few weeks and never reach a clinic for investigation, and so are

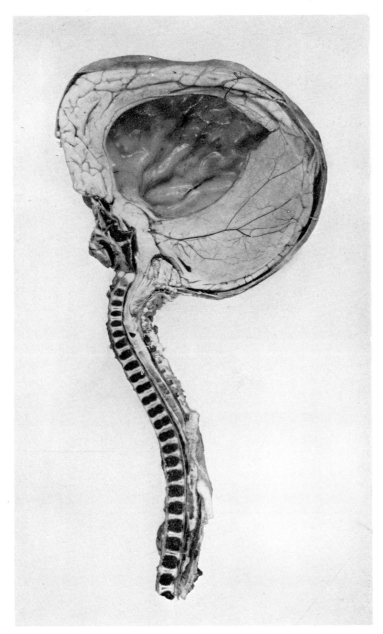

Fig. 4. Hydrocephalus associated with Arnold-Chiari malformation.

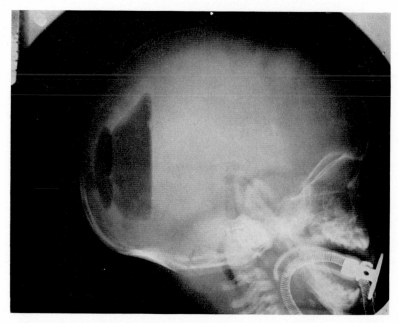

FIG. 5. Ventriculogram showing elongation of fourth ventricle below level of foramen magnum due to Arnold-Chiari malformation.

not included in surveys of a hospital series of cases, such as that of Laurence quoted above. On the other hand, many cases are sent to a clinic with a diagnosis of progressive hydrocephalus, and after investigation and a period of observation undergo natural arrest. In my clinic this group of (unoperated) cases accounted for 16·5% of all those that eventually arrested.

The mode of natural arrest is not truly known, but observations suggest that it is by re-canalisation of the subarachnoid space. We have already shown that the majority of cases of progressive hydrocephalus are due to basal cistern block. The adhesions tend to be fine in character, as they are formed in response to low-grade infection or sub-clinical hæmorrhage. We have noted that where the block is well forward, at the level of the chiasmatic cistern, natural arrest is more likely to occur as the adhesions are few in number and finer in character.

Prognosis for the Arrested Hydrocephalic Child

Intelligence. In the majority of cases the cerebral cortex is thinned out by the dilated ventricular system. As the dilatation proceeds the white matter is stretched out and the gyri containing the grey matter of the cerebral cortex are unfolded, but the nerve cells are left intact although spaced out over a larger area. Cerebral cortex can thus be reduced from 5 cm. to 0·5 cm. without great disturbance of intelligence. On the other hand, where there is clinical evidence of brain damage, such as hemiplegia caused by a severe hæmorrhage disrupting white and grey matter, the level of intelligence will remain low. The level of intelligence will also remain low in cases of severe meningitis which has set up hydrocephalus, because infective thrombophlebitis has spread along the cortical veins and directly damaged the nerve-cells in the grey matter.

Laurence (1962) has shown that the average IQ for patients undergoing natural arrest was 69 and that in the youngest group of ten cases which had reached the chronological age of $3\frac{1}{2}$ years the average tested IQ was 43 with a range from 4 to 82. In my group of ten cases arrested by the insertion of a Holter valve the chronological age was $3\frac{1}{2}$ years and the average IQ was 85 with a range from 71 to 114. Lorber (1961) has analysed a group of 76 infants suffering from hydrocephalus associated with myelomeningocele, where ventriculography in the first few weeks of life showed marked dilatation of the ventricular system: 40 had a valve inserted and 36 acted as controls. As these children grew up the patients with valves showed heads within normal limits of circumference and had good cerebral function in 73% of cases, compared with the control group whose heads were abnormally enlarged and in whom only 50% had good cerebral function. It would appear, therefore, that early insertion of a valve drainage system will preserve intelligence provided the grey matter is intact.

Sight. The fundi of hydrocephalic infants show marked pallor of the optic discs, indicating some degree of primary optic atrophy. This condition does not affect the sight of the child. Loss of vision is usually a terminal affair associated with prolonged high ventricular pressure causing degenerative changes in the region of the basal ganglia and the lateral geniculate body. It is interesting to note that papillœdema is never present in the hydrocephalic infant, but will be present in an infant suffering from a space-occupying lesion, such as a cerebral tumour or papilloma of the choroid plexus. This is due to the fact that in the hydrocephalic infant there is a block in the ventricular system or the subarachnoid pathway, so that CSF cannot pass forward to the subarachnoid space contained in the orbital portion of the optic sheath. There can thus never be a rise of CSF pressure in this portion of the subarachnoid space, where the central vein of the retina leaves the eye to pass across the orbital portion of the subarachnoid space to gain entry to a neighbouring sinus. Dr Hayreh (personal communication) has just completed experimental work on the monkey to prove this point. He inserts balloons into the cerebral substance of the monkey and the attached inflation tubes are brought to the surface. When the wounds are well healed he slowly inflates the balloons and produces papillœdema. He then exposes the orbital portion of the optic sheath on one side and opens the subarachnoid space in the sheath so that CSF can escape. Papillœdema in that eye then disappears. The high ventricular pressure in the hydrocephalic infant does not reach this portion of the optic sheath; only in the long-standing case of hydrocephalus which has undergone natural arrest by opening up of a distorted and narrowed subarachnoid pathway may papillœdema be seen.

Physical disability. Laurence and Coates (1962) re-assessed their 81 survivors by natural arrest and divided them into four groups from the point of view of physical handicap.

Group I included all the cases who were physically normal or had only a slight or intermittent squint, or who had brisk reflexes. 26 such children included a large proportion of cases of reasonable intelligence with basal cistern or aqueduct blocks, but none with spina bifida cystica.

Group II consisted of 16 cases with comparatively slight physical disability which would not always necessitate education in special schools. Disabilities such as slight spasticity, unsteady gait, some impairment of vision or slight incontinence of urine were included.

Group III contained 23 severely handicapped children, all of whom required education in special schools or institutions. Cases with sphincter and limb paralysis and flexion deformities were amongst these, as well as children who were unable to walk because of severe incoordination. These cases usually gave clinical evidence of brain damage or had a myelomeningocele.

There were 16 cases in Group IV in which the child was completely incapacitated with a very low IQ. They were either in institutions or confined to bed at home and had to have home tuition where this was practicable. Many of these had spastic quadriplegia and some were unable to feed themselves.

In my group where drainage operations have been used, the arrest of hydrocephalus occurs at an earlier date so that many cases in Group II move up into Group I. Where the presence of a myelomeningocele places the child in Group III or Group IV, early decapping of the myelomeningocele associated with early arrest of the hydrocephalus has now moved some of these cases from Group III to Group II. The introduction of the operations of ureterostomy and uretero-ileostomy associated with early control of the hydrocephalus has, in many cases, rendered these children continent, and able to attend a normal school. This is well seen in the cases of sacral myelomeningocele, where the nerves to the lower limbs are not affected but the patient has a neurogenic bladder.

Conclusion

Only 14% of cases of hydrocephalus are due to an uncomplicated congenital malformation. In 82% low-grade infection or sub-clinical hæmorrhage leads to a temporary or permanent block; 44·5% are associated with a myelomeningocele which acts as a source of sepsis. Infection and hæmorrhage are usually so mild that the infant presents with an enlarging head and no other clinical signs.

The author's own results, from a series of 200 hydrocephalic children followed for 4 years or longer, are as follows: 16·5% have arrested without treatment, 55% have arrested with valve drainage operation, 10% have died from infection, 10% have died from failure of the drainage operation due to clot formation, and the remaining 8·5% will live on for many years until coning sets up cardio-respiratory failure.

REFERENCES

LAURENCE, K. M. (1959) The pathology of hydrocephalus. *Ann. roy. Coll. Surg. Engl.* **24,** 388

LAURENCE, K. M., COATES, S. (1962) The natural history of hydrocephalus. Detailed analysis of 182 unoperated cases. *Arch. Dis. Childh.* **37,** 345

LORBER, J. (1961) Systematic ventriculographic studies in infants born with meningomyelocele and encephalocele. *Arch. Dis. Childh.* **36,** 381

McKEOWN, T., RECORD, R. M. G. (1960) In *Ciba Symposium on Congenital Malformations,* ed. Wolstenholme, G. E. W. and O'Connor, C. M., Churchill, London

CHAPTER 15

SPINA BIFIDA CYSTICA

G. H. MACNAB

THE term spina bifida cystica is used to describe sacular swellings containing cerebrospinal fluid enclosed by the coverings of the spinal cord and associated with a defect in the spine. A brief review of the development of the spinal cord and spine will help to interpret the clinical findings in this condition.

Developmental Anatomy

Embryological development of the normal spinal cord is well described by Patten (1946), Arey (1954) and Hamilton, Boyd and Mossman (1952). The main stages of development are now summarised (Fig. 1).

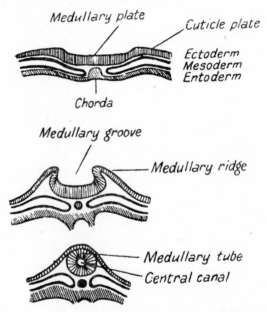

FIG. 1. The development of the spinal cord and spine.

The ectodermal layer of the embryonic (medullary) plate appears as a thickening over the notocord (chorda) in the middle of the third week in the late pre-somite phase, and rapidly becomes a groove and then a tube, which is closed by the end of the fourth week. Formation of the tube proceeds from head to tail, the last part to close being the lumbo-sacral area. The lumen of the tube is large in relation to the thickness of its wall, and this temporary phase of hydromyelia continues until the rhombic roof of the primitive fourth ventricle perforates at about the sixth week. Thereafter, the central canal becomes small in size as the subarachnoid space opens up, although the ventricles of the brain remain relatively hydrocephalic for a longer period because of the large size of the choroid plexuses within. At the end of the fourth week the most ventral part of the neural tube gives rise to the anterior spinal roots, but not until the fifth week will the neural tube close and the neural crests form as columns on either side of the tube. The crest gives rise to the posterior root ganglia and the sensory root. Sections

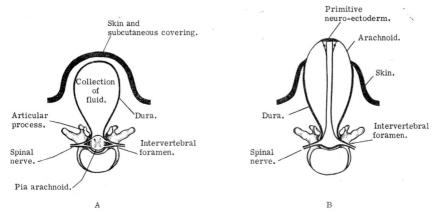

FIG. 2. Diagram of (A) meningocele, (B) myelomeningocele.

have shown normal development of dorsal ganglia and sensory peripheral roots in the presence of gross dysplasia of the spinal cord. Clinical lesions are, therefore, due to dysplasia of the central and not the peripheral nervous system, motor disability being due to dysplasia of the anterior part of the cord, and sensory loss due to failure of the dorsal root ganglia to establish central connections with the cord.

Following closure of the neural tube the mesodermal tissue around the notocord spreads to surround the neural tube and form the bony spinal column. Failure of the neural tube to close gives rise to the spinal cord lying free on the dorsal surface of the newly-born infant, *complete spinal rachischisis*. Where the infant presents with a sacular swelling over the back, it is either in the form of a myelomeningocele or a meningocele. In both conditions there is a defect of the spine due to failure of fusion of the laminæ. In the *meningocele* (Fig. 2A) all the coverings of the spinal cord are intact and the sac contains only CSF; the ectodermal layer forming the skin is always present so the sac is covered by true skin, though it may be stretched and thinned out. In the *myelomeningocele* (Fig. 2B) the dura only lines the sac a portion of the way, being replaced by arachnoid membrane up to the point where the spinal cord, or cauda equina, lies on a free surface forming the fundus of the sac wall, while the ectodermal skin only reaches to the base of the sac. Abnormal blood-vessels ascend with the spinal cord, or cauda equina, to the fundus of the sac and give rise to a serous discharge on its free surface. A scab is formed over this free surface and fibroblastic reaction takes place underneath the scab, leading to healing of the sac by scar formation. The spinal cord, or cauda equina, descends through the sac to pass the spinal nerves out through the intervertebral foramina.

Dysplasia of Spinal Cord Associated with the Presence of a Myelomeningocele

Cameron (1956) has shown that in 50% of cases of myelomeningocele the spinal cord above the level of the lesion shows evidence of hydromyelia, and in 40% of the cases at the level of the myelomeningocele the spinal cord is divided into two portions, a spur of bone projecting from the posterior aspect of the body of the vertebra. This is in contrast to the condition of *diastematomyelia* occurring in spina bifida occulta, where the spur of bone projects from the posterior body of the vertebra and creates a cleft in the spinal cord, the two normal portions of spinal cord uniting below the level of the spur to continue as one cord. As my experience increases I doubt if a pure meningocele can ever be present. Wherever there is a defect in the spine the underlying spinal cord will show some evidence of dysplasia, due to malformation in its formative state. The deficit may be very slight but tends to show itself in later years. Due to the fact that development of the spinal column is dependent upon true formation of the neural tube, 50% of cases of myelomeningocele show bony deformities of the vertebræ. This may show itself as a spur of bone due to the overgrowth of a lamina which has failed to fuse with its opposite number, or hemi-vertebra may be present leading to severe scoliosis or kyphosis.

Incidence

The incidence of spina bifida cystica is of the order of 2 to 3 per 1000 live births. Record and McKeown (1949) found that in Birmingham over a 7 year period it averaged 2·45 per 1000, and Nash (1963) gave a similar figure of 2·3 per 1000 for England and Wales, although Laurence and David (1963) found that in some parts of Wales the incidence was as high as 5 per 1,000.

Doran and Guthkelch (1961) in a survey of 307 cases found a positive family history of spina bifida in 8·14% of cases. The ratio of pure meningoceles to myelomeningoceles was 1 to 3·7 in the series reported by Doran and Guthkelch. A recent survey by Laurence (1964) of 407 cases shows the ratio to be 1 to 10. I am sure that a critical survey of the operative findings and histological examinations and a follow-up for a period of years in relation to neurological function will require revision of this ratio to perhaps 1 to 30.

Clinical Picture in Relation to the Sac

Meningocele. The sac is always covered by skin, even though it is stretched out to the fineness of a transparent membrane. The result is that ulceration is not present, and leakage of CSF does not occur. The neck of the meningocele is narrow but it may be masked by the presence of lipomatous tissue around its base. The narrow neck of the sac will permit, in a small percentage

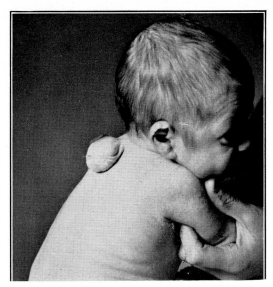

FIG. 3. Meningocele undergoing self-cure by fibrosis at neck of sac.

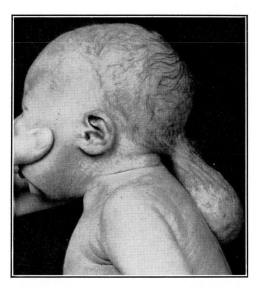

FIG. 4. Occipital encephalocele with narrow pedicle simulating cervical meningocele.

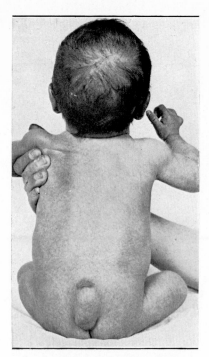

FIG. 5. Sacral myelomeningocele covered by normal skin with hæmangiomatous changes at upper aspect.

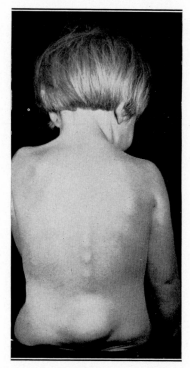

FIG. 6. Lumbo-sacral myelomeningocele covered by true skin overlying
fibro-lipomatous tissue.

of cases, fibrosis to take place across the neck leading to natural cure (Fig. 3). When fibrosis is complete the sac wall collapses and becomes puckered up, but always contains a small amount of residual CSF. On the other hand, the sac may show a rapid increase in size and tension as the newborn infant becomes active. In contrast to a myelomeningocele, it is more common to find a meningocele present in relation to the cervical and upper dorsal spine than to the lumbo-sacral spine, due to the fact that the final closure of the neural tube takes place in that region, leading to a major deformity of the neural as well as the spinal formation. Confusion may arise in differentiating between the pedunculated occipital encephalocele (Fig. 4) and the highly-placed cervical meningocele. A radiograph of the skull in relation to a pedunculated encephalocele will always show a small bony defect in the occipital bone just above the rim of the foramen magnum. This opening permits the passage of the contents of the posterior fossa into the sac, and in many cases the fourth ventricle is drawn out into the sac. Neural content of such a sac usually has to be excised with the sac, as the posterior fossa is not large enough to contain it. This may lead to formation of adhesions at the base of the brain and development of postoperative hydrocephalus.

Myelomeningocele. The sac will show clinical evidence of ulceration at the fundus as neuro-epithelium replaces true skin. Abnormal blood-vessels supply the neural tissue, so a seal of serum sets over the raw surface and granulation tissue begins to form. Fibroblastic reaction forms a scar over the fundus in 4–8 weeks, unless secondary infection is severe. The thin transparent membrane around the periphery of the ulcerated fundus is formed from arachnoid membrane, and is liable to break down where infection interferes with its nutrition, leading to slow leakage of CSF; in due course it thickens up due to inflammatory reaction. True skin around the base of the sac is present, but varies in amount dependent upon the width of the spinal defect and the amount of neural tissue present in the sac. A myelomeningocele in the sacral region is often covered by skin which is normal apart from hæmangiomatous changes or which overlies a lipoma (Figs. 5, 6), since the amount of neural tissue in the sac is small. Hæmangiomatous tissue overlying the spinal defect usually denotes abnormality of the neural element underlying it.

Clinical Evidence of Paralysis in Relation to Meningoceles and Myelomeningoceles

The pure *meningocele* seen in infancy shows no paralysis, but the older child may develop motor weakness in muscles below the level of the sac. This is due to a mild degree of dysplasia of the underlying spinal cord giving rise to clinical signs as full function develops. (It is not due to the membranes of the sac fixing the spinal cord and differential rate of growth between spinal column and cord setting up pressure on nerve roots.) The lesion lies within the spinal cord and may show itself by failure of full growth of a limb or by poor function of a small group of muscles. Pain due to pressure on nerve roots never presents as a symptom.

On the other hand, the majority of cases of *myelomeningocele* have a flaccid paralysis below the level of the lesion. When this is sacral in position the lower limbs escape involvement, because the nerves serving these muscles pass out through the intervertebral foramina above the level of the lesion.

Sharrard, Zachary, Lorber and Bruce (1963) have pointed out that the newborn baby when awake uses every muscle in its lower limbs, making it possible to assess paralysis by a system of grading the power of seven muscle groups—hip flexors, hip adductors, glutei, quadriceps, hamstrings, ankle dorsiflexors and ankle plantar flexors. They stressed the danger of drawing conclusions from the presence of reflex movements, which may be elicited in the newborn by stimulation of the skin of the limb. If reflex activity alone was present they considered the muscles to be paralysed, only true voluntary movements being significant. They noted also that in the newborn child a positive response to direct electrical stimulation of short duration, or to nerve conduction stimulation, was sometimes present in muscles showing no voluntary activity. At a later date only muscles showing voluntary activity would respond to nerve stimulation. Furthermore, muscles which had shown no voluntary activity at birth but only a response to nerve stimulation, later often exhibited voluntary activity, provided that the exposed neural tissue of the fundus of the sac had been covered over and received no further damage. The psoas muscle often escapes, due to the high level of its innervation. This causes flexion movements of the hip, the impetus in turn causing extension of the knee and making the whole limb appear to move. Misinterpretation of this false movement may lead the parents to consider that the lower limbs move voluntarily.

There is no doubt that some motor power can return to what have seemed completely flaccid muscles, the return being patchy in distribution. This is due to the fact that there is some degree of dysplasia present in the spinal cord with cystic changes, causing distortion of the tracts and leading to delay in myelinisation, which is not complete until the 18th month of life.

Where the paralysis is not severe it tends to remain localised below the knee, the child having a varying amount of power present in the flexors and extensors of the knee. Where motor power in the quadriceps muscle is sufficient to keep the knee extended the child can learn to walk, provided the feet are stabilised at a right angle by the use of boots with metal inside stiffening, and uppers to mid-calf, and by the use of calipers and T-straps, or by the operations of tendon transplant or arthrodesis of joints at a later date.

Sensory loss is difficult to detect in the infant, and the loss of trophic influence will not reveal itself until weight-bearing takes place or splints have to be applied to correct the deformities of the feet.

Some of these children suffer from paralytic dislocation of the hip-joints; after reduction of the dislocation the head can be held in the acetabulum by transferring the insertion of the psoas muscle from the lesser trochanter into the greater tochanter, the muscle passing through an opening in the iliac bone.

Paralysis of the Bladder

With a myelomeningocele of the lumbar spine associated with severe paralysis of the lower limbs, the bladder will inevitably be involved. Two types of neurogenic bladder can be recognised. 1. The flaccid bladder without contractions of the detrusor muscle and with a continuous leak of urine. There is anæsthesia of the perineum and light suprapubic pressure will cause a flow of urine. 2. The distended bladder with overflow incontinence. As the child grows up there may be short intervals of dryness, but in many cases manual expression by suprapubic pressure is of no avail in this respect.

The first type is the common one. In spite of constant dribbling of urine cystography may reveal trabeculation of the bladder. After expression of the bladder half the cases still have residual urine. This leads to stagnation of urine in the bladder and predisposes to infection. It is interesting to note that ureteric reflux is more common in the first type, where there is no obstruction to the outflow of urine, than in the second type where the distended bladder can only be emptied by heavy pressure. It is thought by some that the dilatation of the ureters is due to infection, but there is no proof of this. The point to make is that in the first type manual expression of the bladder will not get rid of such urine as has refluxed up the ureters. As infection invades the ureters they lose their peristaltic power and progressive hydronephrosis and renal damage develop.

The second type is more commonly seen where the myelomeningocele is sacral in position, and paralysis of the lower limbs is slight. As the degree of paralysis in the bladder wall is by no means complete, it is often difficult to detect the lesion in the first few months of life when the normal baby has an automatic bladder.

Infants born with the first type of lesion are easily managed during the first two to three years of life. Daily suprapubic pressure by the mother to evacuate as much urine from the bladder as possible is carried out, and as the child grows older 2-hourly manual expression may prevent urinary infection. As soon as urinary infection develops it should be treated with a sulphonamide or nitrofurantoin, for prolonged periods of time. Intravenous pyelograms to note the congenital defects and the state of dilatation present in the urinary tract must be made, and any threat to renal damage by back-pressure requires relief of urinary obstruction.

The second type does not show itself until the end of the first year of life. In spite of the distended bladder, from time to time a normal voiding stream will be seen and dry intervals develop. Manual evacuation of the bladder is again the keynote of success in conservative treatment; many of these children can have the bladder emptied with some ease and, as they grow up, have dry periods which permit them to attend school. When manual expression of the bladder fails, the question of bladder neck obstruction arises. In those patients with more than about 60 ml. of residual urine after manual expression Nash (1957) advised that resection of the bladder neck should be carried out. Other workers are not convinced that bladder neck obstruction is the cause of failure to pass urine, and in girls the operation has often led to complete incontinence.

At what stage should conservative treatment be abandoned? If a girl reaches the age of 9 and still has a continuous leak of urine associated with vulval ulceration, then diversion of the urinary stream is justified. In the boy, incontinence can be controlled by use of a portable urinal such as the Chailey apparatus. It is essential that the fitting around the penis is leakproof, for once the urine has entered the bag it cannot return due to a valve mechanism. Penile clamps are of no value as they set up ulceration of the prepuce and may lead to meatal stenosis. In rare cases in boys, where urinary control is almost complete, Nash (1956) carried out urethral plication on the bulbous portion of the penile urethra by tightening the ischio-cavernosa muscle.

The true indication for abandonment of the conservative programme is when renal function is threatened. This is shown by dilatation of the upper and lower urinary tracts, associated with infection that cannot be controlled, and a rising blood urea. One of two operations can be carried out dependent upon the size of the ureter. If the ureters are very large they can be divided at the level of the bladder and threaded retroperitoneally up to the anterior abdominal wall in the region of the right iliac fossa. An opening being made in the anterior abdominal wall, the two ends of the ureters are brought through the skin. The medial wall of each ureter is divided vertically for one inch and the edges sutured together, thus turning two ureters into one large opening. The mucosa of this opening is everted so that a cup of ureteric mucous membrane projects above the skin for 0·5 cm. An ileostomy bag is then fitted over the protruding ureteric orifice and the urine collected in the bag without leakage. This operation can only be carried out where the ureters are grossly dilated and elongated, for a great deal of their blood-supply has to be cut off in order to mobilise them. Sloughing of a ureter in the retroperitoneal tissues can cause complete disaster.

Alternatively, if the ureters are not grossly dilated, they can be divided at the level of the bladder and brought through a retro-peritoneal opening, where they are anastomosed to an isolated loop of ileum, the proximal end of the loop having been closed. The isolated loop of ileum is then threaded retro-peritoneally up to the anterior abdominal wall through an opening in the skin in the region of the right iliac fossa. The end of the loop of ileum is everted on itself to form a stump projecting above the skin, in order to fit a leak-proof ileostomy bag. In the majority of cases mucous secretion from the isolated bladder is not a problem, but occasionally heavy infection takes place and then the bladder has to be excised.

Paralysis of the Bowel

The clinical sign of this condition in the infant is a patulous anus, usually associated with marked paralysis of the lower limbs. Where the paralysis of the bowel is not severe it is difficult to detect lowered sphincter tone by rectal examination. If the infant survives into childhood full fæcal continence is never gained where the anus has been patulous, but in the cases where some sphincter tone remains the child may gain a kind of partial continence by forming a firm plug of fæces in the anal canal. Where paralysis of the bowel is present the infants are constipated, so the mother is not at first aware of the severity of paralysis present. Firm fæces can accumulate in the rectum and fill the pelvic colon and give rise to acquired megacolon. Rectal sensation is lowered in these children so that the stimulus to evacuation of the bowel is lacking. In mild cases the mother must persist in regular pottraining in an attempt to educate the child in reflex evacuation of the bowel. When the lower bowel content becomes inspissated, bowel washouts are required. (It is essential to order bowel washouts and not enemas, for an enema depends upon the presence of rectal sensation, bowel distension leading to reflex evacuation.) In cases of partial paralysis, bowel training and the use of suppositories will often lead to fæcal continence by about 7. Bisacodyl ("Dulcolax") has proved to be of great value in dealing with constipation, insertion of a suppository (5 or 10 mg) effectively breaking up the firm fæces and emptying the rectum. But if a paste-like mass of fæces already fills the whole rectum and lower pelvic colon, manual evacuation must first be carried out. The suppositories can thereafter be inserted, one each day for a week. As soon as constipation has been overcome Dulcolax can be taken by mouth, one 5 mg. tablet each night, until a formed bowel action takes place.

Where the anal sphincter tone is almost absent continence can only be obtained by maintaining a degree of constipation. Where anal tone is completely absent, detachment of the insertion of the gracilis muscle at the level of the tibia, stripping of the muscle up to the thigh with preservation of its nerve-supply, enables the muscle to be wound subcutaneously around the anal canal and fixed to the pubic bone. This does give some increase in anal tone so that a plug of fæces can remain in position and keep the child continent. Unfortunately, the lack of rectal sensation does not enable the child to use this new muscle to its full extent.

In extreme cases of paralysis of the bowel where there is ulceration of the perineum associated with fistula-in-ano I have had to perform an iliac colostomy on the left side, and if there is associated paralysis of the bladder, a uretero-ileostomy on the right side. In such a case the ulceration of the perineum rapidly clears up, there is a rapid gain in general health, and the psychological outlook of the child can be completely changed due to control of its excreta.

Sensory Loss Associated with Paralysis

In the young infant with loss of perineal sensation and incontinence of urine and fæces, ulceration is liable to develop around the perineum and in relation to the vulva. At this stage the ulceration is not severe and can usually be kept under control with adequate protection of the perineum, using a silicone barrier cream, expression of bladder and bowel, and repeated change of napkins. In the older female child, ulceration around the vulva and the perineum can become severe due to urinary incontinence. If there is no response to prolonged in-patient treatment, then diversion of the urinary stream has to be undertaken. Ulceration in relation to toes and feet does not usually occur until weight-bearing takes place, but all aparatus used in correcting deformities or preventing contractures must be well fitted and the skin at the site of the pressure points should be hardened by the use of surgical spirit. Ulceration of the feet will often respond well to operations which correct deformity and restore normal weight-bearing. Where there is loss of vasomotor control lumbar sympathectomy to the ulcerated cold limb will often permit healing to take place. Where ulceration occurs in the skin of a weight-bearing surface in relation to the os calcis, secondary infection can enter this bone and set up a low-grade osteomyelitis. This is a difficult condition to cure, but prolonged antibiotic treatment associated with curettage of all diseased bone may succeed. If this fails, amputation below the knee may have to be undertaken, provided that quadriceps power is present to extend the knee and normal sensation is present in the skin-flaps fashioned to cover the stump.

Infection and Leakage of CSF from the Sac

This complication is confined to the myelomeningocele where ulceration is present. An acute meningitis occurs in about 20% of cases. In addition, low-grade infection can enter the sub-arachnoid space and remain temporarily loculated. But if a valve is inserted to control hydrocephalus a free flow of CSF proceeds from the lateral ventricle back to the blood-stream. Organisms tend thus to be drawn up into the ventricular system setting up ventriculitis, and into the blood stream causing septicæmia. In a few cases gross infection can take place in the sac with pus formation, but the infection remains shut off from the spinal subarachnoid space.

Complete rupture of the thin-walled sac can give rise to a severe loss of CSF, but simple suture of the defect enables some 20% of such cases to survive. In other cases, the leakage is small and intermittent and as fibrosis develops perforations are sealed off.

Hydrocephalus

Hydrocephalus is not present in association with a true meningocele nor does it develop after removal of the sac.

In myelomeningocele 50% show evidence of progressive hydrocephalus by the third month, 35% already showing hydrocephalus at birth. In a small proportion the head at birth appears to be microcephalic, but wide opening of the occipito-mastoid sutures is present and ventriculography will demonstrate gross dilatation of the ventricular system.

The common cause of hydrocephalus in these cases is the presence of an *Arnold-Chiari malformation.* The Arnold portion consists of a tongue of cerebellum formed by the vermis projecting down into the cervical spinal canal, the cerebellar lobes being small or within normal limits. The Chiari portion consists of an elongated medulla with a stretched-out fourth ventricle opening into the spinal subarachnoid space below the level of the foramen magnum. The cisterna magna leading to the basal subarachnoid cisterns is usually distorted and adhesions may be present across it. There is also thickening of the arachnoid over the deformity causing further obliteration of the subarachnoid space. Stenosis of the aqueduct of Sylvius and stenosis of the foramina in the roof of the fourth ventricle are sometimes associated with this malformation. As there is usually a free flow of ventricular fluid into the spinal canal, which in many cases is in communication with a sac of a myelomeningocele, low-grade infection can pass up from the free surface of the sac setting up ventriculitis or infection in the subarachnoid space, leading to the formation of further adhesions which in turn obliterate it. In a few cases the Arnold-Chiari malformation is small in size leading to only partial obliteration of the subarachnoid space, so that the hydrocephalus can undergo arrest by recanalisation due to the pumping action of the CSF.

Treatment

The meningocele. The accurate diagnosis of pure meningocele cannot be made until exploration is carried out. At operation the neck of the sac is exposed and proved to be narrow. The skin over the sac is then removed to expose the dura and the sac is opened. A few fibrils of connective tissue are usually present, running across the sac close to its neck. If these fibrils are accompanied by fine blood-vessels then we are dealing with the neural element of a myelomeningocele. If any doubt exists about the presence of nerve fibrils, that portion of the sac to which they are adherent is left *in situ* and the redundant portion of the sac removed. If no nerve fibrils are present, transfixation and ligation of the neck of the sac is carried out. It is important to free the neck of the sac from the connective tissue forming the rim of the spinal defect. The spinal cord and its covering must lie free in the spinal canal. A fascial flap is then formed and sutured over the bony defect. As the meningocele is covered by skin there is no danger of leakage of CSF, so one can afford to wait until the end of the third month of life before undertaking operation. The reason for delay is to make certain that the sac is not that of a myelomeningocele. The majority of myelomeningoceles are associated with the presence of an Arnold-Chiari malformation which can obstruct the circulation of the CSF and give rise to slow development of hydrocephalus. Clinical evidence of progressive hydrocephalus is established by the third month of life, so operation should be postponed until that time if any doubt exists as to the true nature of the swelling.

The myelomeningocele. Treatment has undergone a revolutionary change in the past five years, with the trend towards early operation within the first 48 hours of life. Sharrard, Zachary, Lorber and Bruce (1963) have shown that immediate operation will reduce mortality, local sepsis, meningitis and ventriculitis, and also muscle paralysis. Lorber (1961) has shown that the development of antibiotics to control meningitis, and the advent of the Holter valve in the control of hydrocephalus, have so greatly altered the immediate prognosis that even a child with an extensive myelomeningocele must be considered to have a good chance of survival.

Sharrard *et al.* (1962) carried out a controlled experiment, performing the immediate operation in 20 infants and giving conservative treatment to the other 20. 14 out of 20 operated infants survived; at the end of the third week their muscular paralysis showed no deterioration and in one or two cases had improved. On the other hand, in the unoperated group where 18 infants had survived three weeks, paralysis in 9 remained unchanged, but in the other 9 had increased.

Operation is easier to carry out early, skin flaps are more easily mobilised and the size of the defect in relation to the surface area of skin present in the young infant permits approximation of the skin edges without tension. As soon as the operation has been completed the nursing problem associated with the prevention of sepsis is removed. If hydrocephalus is going to develop it will be seen by the second or third week of life and can be controlled by the insertion of a Holter valve.

Decapping of the sac in the newborn. An incision is made around the margin of true skin and arachnoid membrane, all islets of true skin being preserved and used in covering the defect. The plane of dissection is then found that leads down between the dura and the skin until the bony defect is met. All loculated areas in the sac are punctured and the neural content preserved and dropped back into the spinal canal. An attempt is then made to suture the edges of the dura over the neural content. It is most important to raise flaps of dorsi-lumbar fascia to cover the spinal defect, otherwise leakage of CSF is liable to occur. By preservation of all islets of skin in relation to the sac wall skin flaps can be mobilised to permit suture without tension. The islets of skin though often thickened and bluish in colour will survive. Major plastic operations, such as forming rotation flaps, are no longer required and skin-grafting has no place in this repair operation.

Decapping of the sac in the older child. When healing has taken place by scar formation decapping is indicated if the swelling is painful and if it prevents the child being strapped into a wheel-chair or play-chair. It is also interesting to note that where the paralysis in the lower limbs is only below the level of the knee-joint, decapping of the sac will permit movement of the spinal nerves and enable the physiotherapist to get rid of the flexion contractures present at the hip-joint. Decapping of the sac in such a case depends on defining the layer between neural element and scar tissue. Neural element is then freed from the fundus of the sac and the arachnoid traced down to the dura which leads to the neck of the sac. The dura is freed from the edge of the bony spinal defect. Cystic loculations are then evacuated and the neural element returned into the spinal canal and a dural flap sutured over it. Flaps of lumbo-dorsal fascia are finally formed to cover the spinal defect and the skin flaps sutured together after mobilisation.

Hydrocephalus. This is controlled by the insertion of a Holter or Pudenz-Heyer valve connecting the right lateral ventricle with the right atrium of the heart (Chapter 14, p. 322). In hydrocephalus associated with an Arnold-Chiari malformation there is free communication of CSF from the lateral ventricle to the spinal canal, but operations of spino-peritoneal and spino-ureteric drainage cannot be carried out owing to the position of the myelomeningocele, which in many cases has no true communication with the spinal sub-arachnoid space.

Prognosis after surgical treatment. It may be useful to summarise conclusions.

Removal of a *meningocele* does not give rise to post-operative hydrocephalus, even though pre-operative ventriculography may have shown slight dilatation of the ventricular system in relation to a cervical meningocele. These children grow up with good function, but over the years some of them may show lack of full growth in a limb or weakness in action in a muscle group.

Of cases of *myelomeningocele* 50% develop progressive hydrocephalus. The hydrocephalus can be controlled by the use of a Holter valve, but there is great danger of infection of the CSF leading to septicæmia. If the hydrocephalus can be controlled and the paralysis in the lower limbs is confined below the level of the knee, the child will walk with the use of apparatus. In some cases transplant of tendons and stabilising operations for the joints of the foot will lead to the child walking without apparatus. If the paralysis involves the quadriceps muscle, then calipers will have to be worn to keep the knee in extension.

Paralysis of the bowel usually comes under control by about 7, the child gaining a kind of continence by forming a plug of fæces in the anal canal. Pot training and avoidance of a loaded rectum, by the use of Dulcolax suppositories or a bowel washout,will prevent the onset of false diarrhœa due to impacted fæces. Where paralysis of the bladder is present the danger to life is infection of the urinary tract. This is avoided, where possible, by manual expression of the bladder, and the long-term use of antibacterial drugs, which in many cases keep infection at bay. Where there is true obstruction to the outlet from the bladder then diversion of the urinary stream has to be carried out.

In the case of the sacral myelomeningocele there is usually full motor power in the lower limbs so we have an active child. Prevention or urinary infection in such cases is essential, and early diversion of the urinary stream by the operation of uretero-ileostomy, where there is any evidence of dilatation and damage to renal function, should be carried out. As these children do not require calipers with pelvic bands to control paralysed limbs, it is a simple procedure to fit an ileostomy bag to collect the urine.

REFERENCES

AREY, L. B. (1946) *Developmental Anatomy, A Textbook and Laboratory Manual of Embryology*, 5th Ed., Saunders, Philadelphia

CAMERON, A. H. (1956) The spinal cord lesion in spina bifida cystica. *Lancet*, **2**, 171

DORAN, P. A., GUTHKELCH, A. N. (1961) Studies in spina bifida cystica. *J. Neurol. Neurosurg. Psychiat.* **24**, 331

HAMILTON, W. J., BOYD, J. D., MOSSMAN, H. W. (1952) *Human Embryology*, 2nd Ed., Heffer, Cambridge

LAURENCE, K. M. (1964) The natural history of spina bifida cystica. Detailed analysis of 407 cases. *Arch. Dis. Childh.* **39**, 41

LAURENCE, K. M., DAVID, P. A. (1963) The incidence of the major central nervous system malformations in South Wales. *Arch. Dis. Childh.* **38**, 98

LORBER, J. (1961) Systematic ventriculographic studies in infants born with meningo-myelocœle and encephalocœle. The incidence and development of hydrocephalus. *Arch. Dis. Childh.* **36**, 381

NASH, D. F. E. (1956) Ileal loop bladder in congenital spinal palsy. *Brit. J. Urol.* **28**, 387

NASH, D. F. E. (1957) The management of fæcal and urinary incontinence in spina bifida. *Proc. roy. Soc. Med.* **50**, 740

NASH, D. F. E. (1963) Meningomyelocele. *Proc. roy. Soc. Med.* **56**, 506

PATTEN, B. M. (1946) *Human Embryology*, Blakiston, Philadelphia

RECORD, R. G., McKEOWN, T. (1949) Congenital malformations of the central nervous system. A survey of 930 cases. *Brit. J. soc. Med.* **3**, 183

SHARRARD, W. J. W., ZACHARY, R. B., LORBER, J., BRUCE, A. M. (1962) A controlled, trial of immediate and delayed closure of spina bifida cystica. *Arch. Dis. Childh.* **38**, 18

Figures 1, and 3–6 are taken by permission from The Medical Press.

INDEX